Medical Tests

SOURCEBOOK

Fifth Edition

Health Reference Series

Fifth Edition

Medical Tests

SOURCEBOOK

Basic Consumer Health Information about Preventive Care Guidelines, Routine Health Screenings, Home-Use Tests, Blood, and Stool Tests, Genetic Testing, Newborn Screening, Endoscopic Exams, and Imaging Tests, Such as X-Ray, Ultrasound, Computed Tomography (CT), Mammography, Fluoroscopy, and Nuclear and Magnetic Resonance Imaging (MRI) Exams

Along with Facts about Diagnostic Tests for Allergies, Cancer, Diabetes, Heart and Lung Disease, Infectious Diseases, Sleep Problems, and Other Specific Conditions, a Glossary of Related Terms, and Directories of Additional Resources

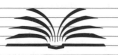

OMNIGRAPHICS

155 W. Congress, Suite 200 Detroit, MI 48226

Bibliographic Note

Because this page cannot legibly accommodate all the copyright notices, the Bibliographic Note portion of the Preface constitutes an extension of the copyright notice.

* * *

Omnigraphics, Inc.
Editorial Services provided by Omnigraphics, Inc.,
a division of Relevant Information, Inc.

Keith Jones, *Managing Editor*

* * *

Copyright © 2016 Relevant Information, Inc.
ISBN 978-0-7808-1382-3
E-ISBN 978-0-7808-1409-7

Library of Congress Cataloging-in-Publication Data

Medical tests sourcebook : basic consumer health information about preventive care guidelines, routine health screenings, home-use tests, blood, stool, and urine tests, genetic testing, biopsies, endoscopic exams, and imaging tests, such as X-ray, ultrasound, computed tomography (CT), and nuclear and magnetic resonance imaging (MRI) exams; along with facts about diagnostic tests for allergies, cancer, diabetes, heart and lung disease, infertility, osteoporosis, sleep problems, and other specific conditions, a glossary of related terms, and directories of additional resources / Keith Jones, managing editor. -- Fifth edition.
     pages cm. – (Health reference series)
   Includes bibliographical references and index.
   Summary: "Provides basic consumer health information about endoscopic, imaging, laboratory, and other types of medical testing for disease diagnosis and monitoring, along with guidelines for screening and preventive care testing in children and adults. Includes index, glossary of related terms, and other resources" – Provided by publisher.
   ISBN 978-0-7808-1382-3 (hardcover : alk. paper) – ISBN 978-0-7808-1409-7 (ebook)
   1. Diagnosis–Popular works. 2. Diagnosis, Laboratory–Popular works. 3. Medicine, Popular. I. Jones, Keith.
   RC71.3.M45 2015
   616.07'5–dc23

                                                                    2015032678

Table of Contents

Part IV: Imaging Tests and Risks

Part V: Catheterization, Endoscopic, and Electrical Tests and Assessments

Part VI: Screening and Assessments for Specific Conditions and Diseases

Preface

About This Book

Informed decisions about health and the treatment of disease are guided by the wealth of information discovered though medical screening and diagnostic tests. Screening tests identify risk factors for specific disorders, while diagnostic tests find markers of disease or dysfunction. Medical tests assist in diagnosing the causes of symptoms, making treatment decisions, and assessing treatment effectiveness. When faced with decisions about health, consumers need to understand the benefits and limitations of medical tests and how test results guide treatment and lifestyle choices.

Medical Tests Sourcebook, Fifth Edition provides updated information about exams, tests, and other screening, diagnostic, and disease monitoring procedures. It discusses preventive care guidelines and the screening tests used for such specific conditions as allergies, cancer, celiac disease, cardiovascular disorders, diabetes, kidney and thyroid dysfunction, and others. Details about laboratory blood tests, biopsies, urinalysis, and genetic tests are also presented. Imaging tests, such as X-ray, ultrasound, computed tomography, coronary calcium scan and magnetic resonance and nuclear imaging are described, and facts are offered about electrical, endoscopic, and home-use tests. The book concludes with a glossary of related terms, a list of online health screening tools, and directories of breast and cervical cancer early detection programs and other resources for more information.

How to Use This Book

This book is divided into parts and chapters. Parts focus on broad areas of interest. Chapters are devoted to single topics within a part.

Part I: Medical Tests for Healthy Living provides an introduction to medical tests and explains why regular health tests are important. It also describes the need to know family history in order to understand a particular health condition. In addition it addresses frequently asked questions on medical tests.

Part II: Screening and Preventive Care Tests are used to identify individuals with specific risk factors for which the timely provision of medical care or other interventions can help avoid or reduce health consequences. These include high blood pressure, high cholesterol, and certain genetic characteristics. Information about regular health exams, new-born screening tests, and preventive screening recommendations for children, adults, and seniors are also included.

Part III: Laboratory Tests begins with an overview of lab tests. It identifies the features that distinguish quality services and provides help for understanding lab reports. Information about commonly used diagnostic and preventive care tests is provided along with details about tests of body fluids, such as those that analyze blood, stool and urine. Specific biopsies and cultures are also explained.

Part IV: Imaging Tests and Risks describes the many types of medical imaging tests available and the accompanying risks associated with exposure to radiation emissions. Imaging tests include radiography (X-rays), contrast studies, ultrasound exams, computed tomography (CT) scans, magnetic resonance imaging (MRI), nuclear imaging, coronary calcium scan, mammograms and fluoroscopy.

Part V: Catheterization, Endoscopic, and Electrical Tests and Assessments describes tests that use scopes, cameras, and electrical data. Cardiac catheterization and endoscopy enable physicians to see the structure of the heart, esophagus, colon, and other areas inside the body. Electrical tests provide data about the functioning of the cardiovascular, brain, and nervous systems.

Part VI: Screening and Assessments for Specific Conditions and Diseases explains tests used to identify and monitor conditions such as allergy, cancer, celiac disease, cystic fibrosis, diabetes, heart disease, infectious diseases, kidney disease, lung disease, and sleep disorders. Information is also provided about hearing assessments and vision tests.

Part VII: Home and Self-Ordered Tests discusses products that offer consumers a private option for the initial screening of fecal occult blood, drug abuse, human immunodeficiency virus (HIV), and other health concerns. The pros and cons of each test are given, and consumers are cautioned to use only tests approved by the U.S. Food and Drug Administration. All questions about home or self-ordered test results should be discussed with a health care provider.

Part VIII: Additional Help and Information provides a glossary of important terms related to medical tests and a list of online health screening tools. A directory of organizations that provide health information about medical tests is also included.

Bibliographic Note

This volume contains documents and excerpts from publications issued by the following U.S. government agencies: Agency for Healthcare Research and Quality (AHRQ); Centers for Disease Control and Prevention (CDC); Genetics Home Reference (GHR); National Cancer Institute (NCI); National Eye Institute (NEI); National Heart, Lung, and Blood Institute (NHLBI); National Institute of Allergy and Infectious Diseases (NIAID); National Institute of Biomedical Imaging and Bioengineering (NIBIB); National Institute of Diabetes and Digestive and Kidney Diseases (NIDDK); National Institute on Deafness and Other Communication Disorders (NIDCD); National Institutes of Health (NIH); National Kidney Disease Education Program (NKDEP); Office of Disease Prevention and Health Promotion (ODPHP); Office of Drug & Alcohol Policy & Compliance (ODAPC); Office on Women's Health (OWH); United States Environmental Protection Agency (EPA); and U.S. Food and Drug Administration (FDA).

About the Health Reference Series

The *Health Reference Series* is designed to provide basic medical information for patients, families, caregivers, and the general public. Each volume takes a particular topic and provides comprehensive coverage. This is especially important for people who may be dealing with a newly diagnosed disease or a chronic disorder in themselves or in a family member. People looking for preventive guidance, information about disease warning signs, medical statistics, and risk factors for health problems will also find answers to their questions in the *Health Reference Series*. The *Series*, however, is not intended to serve as a tool for diagnosing illness, in prescribing treatments, or as a substitute for the physician/patient relationship. All people concerned about medical symptoms or the possibility of disease are encouraged to seek professional care from an appropriate health care provider.

A Note about Spelling and Style

Health Reference Series editors use *Stedman's Medical Dictionary* as an authority for questions related to the spelling of medical terms and the *Chicago Manual of Style* for questions related to grammatical structures, punctuation, and other editorial concerns. Consistent adherence is not always possible, however, because the individual volumes within the *Series* include many documents from a wide variety of different producers, and the editor's primary goal is to present material from each source as accurately as is possible. This sometimes means that information in different chapters or sections may follow other guidelines and alternate spelling authorities.

Medical Review

Omnigraphics contracts with a team of qualified, senior medical professionals who serve as medical consultants for the Health Reference Series. As necessary, medical consultants review reprinted and originally written material for currency and accuracy. Citations including the phrase, "Reviewed (month, year)" indicate material reviewed by this team. Medical consultation services are provided to the Health Reference Series editors by:

Dr. Vijayalakshmi, MBBS, DGO, MD
Dr. Senthil Selvan, MBBS, DCH, MD
Dr. K. Sivanandham MBBS, DCH, MS (Research), PhD

Our Advisory Board

We would like to thank the following board members for providing guidance to the development of this Series:

- Dr. Lynda Baker, Associate Professor of Library and Information Science, Wayne State University, Detroit, MI

- Nancy Bulgarelli, William Beaumont Hospital Library, Royal Oak, MI

- Karen Imarisio, Bloomfield Township Public Library, Bloomfield Township, MI

- Karen Morgan, Mardigian Library, University of Michigan-Dearborn, Dearborn, MI

- Rosemary Orlando, St. Clair Shores Public Library, St. Clair Shores, MI

Health Reference Series Update Policy

The inaugural book in the *Health Reference Series* was the first edition of Cancer Sourcebook published in 1989. Since then, the Series has been enthusiastically received by librarians and in the medical community. In order to maintain the standard of providing high-quality health information for the layperson the editorial staff at Omnigraphics felt it was necessary to implement a policy of updating volumes when warranted.

Medical researchers have been making tremendous strides, and it is the purpose of the *Health Reference Series* to stay current with the most recent advances. Each decision to update a volume is made on an individual basis. Some of the considerations include how much new information is available and the feedback we receive from people who use the books. If there is a topic you would like to see added to the update list, or an area of medical concern you feel has not been adequately addressed, please write to:

Managing Editor
Health Reference Series
Omnigraphics, Inc.
155 W. Congress, Ste. 200
Detroit, MI 48226

Part One

Medical Tests for Healthy Living

Chapter 1

Regular Health Exams Are Important

Chapter Contents

Section 1.1

Healthy Men

Text in this section is excerpted from "Healthy Men," Agency for
Healthcare Research and Quality (AHRQ), December 2012.

Learn the Facts

When you get a preventive medical test, you're not just doing it for
yourself. You're doing it for your family and loved ones:

- Men are 24 percent less likely than women to have visited a doctor within the past year and are 22 percent more likely to have neglected their cholesterol tests.

- Men are 28 percent more likely than women to be hospitalized for congestive heart failure.

- Men are 32 percent more likely than women to be hospitalized for long-term complications of diabetes and are more than twice as likely than women to have a leg or foot amputated due to complications related to diabetes.

- Men are 24 percent more likely than women to be hospitalized for pneumonia that could have been prevented by getting an immunization.

The single most important way you can take care of yourself and
those you love is to actively take part in your health care. Educate
yourself on health care and participate in decisions with your doctor.

Stay Healthy

You can make healthy choices every day.

Be physically active.

Walking briskly, mowing the lawn, playing team sports, and biking are just a few examples of how you can get moving. If you are not
already physically active, start small and work up to 30 minutes a day
of moderate physical activity for most days of the week.

Eat a healthy diet.

Fruits, vegetables, whole grains, and fat-free or low-fat dairy products are healthy choices. Lean meats, poultry, fish, beans, eggs, and nuts are good, too. Try to eat foods that are low in saturated fats, trans fats, cholesterol, salt, and added sugars.

Stay at a healthy weight.

Try to balance the calories you take in with the calories you burn with your physical activities. As you age, eat fewer calories and increase your physical activity. This will prevent gradual weight gain over time.

Drink alcohol in moderation or not at all.

Current dietary guidelines for Americans recommend that if you choose to drink alcoholic beverages, you do not exceed 2 drinks per day for men (1 drink per day for women). Some people should not drink alcoholic beverages at all, including

- Individuals who cannot restrict their drinking to moderate levels.

- Individuals who plan to drive, operate machinery, or take part in other activities that requires attention, skill, or coordination.

- Individuals taking prescription or over-the-counter medications that can interact with alcohol.

- Individuals with specific medical conditions.

- Persons recovering from alcoholism.

Don't smoke.

Take aspirin to avoid a heart attack.

If you are at risk for a heart attack (you're over 45, smoke, or have diabetes, high blood pressure, high cholesterol, or a family history of heart disease), check with your doctor and find out if taking aspirin is the right choice for you.

Get Preventive Tests

Screening tests can find diseases early, when they're easiest to treat. Talk to your doctor about which preventive medical tests you need to stay healthy.

Body Mass Index (BMI)

Your body mass index, or BMI, is a measure of your body fat based on your height and weight. It is used to screen for obesity.

Cholesterol

Once you turn 35 (or once you turn 20 if you have risk factors like diabetes, history of heart disease, tobacco use, high blood pressure, or BMI of 30 or over), have your cholesterol checked regularly. High blood cholesterol is one of the major risk factors for heart disease.

Blood Pressure

Have your blood pressure checked every 2 years. High blood pressure increases your chance of getting heart or kidney disease and for having a stroke. If you have high blood pressure, you may need medication to control it.

Cardiovascular Disease

Beginning at age 45 and through age 79, ask your doctor if you should take aspirin every day to help lower your risk of a heart attack. How much aspirin you should take depends on your age, your health, and your lifestyle.

Colorectal Cancer

Beginning at age 50 and through age 75, get tested for colorectal cancer. You and your doctor can decide which test is best. How often you'll have the test depends on which test you choose. If you have a family history of colorectal cancer, you may need to be tested before you turn 50.

Other Cancers

Ask your doctor if you should be tested for prostate, lung, oral, skin, or other cancers.

Sexually Transmitted Diseases

Talk to your doctor to see whether you should be tested for gonorrhea, syphilis, chlamydia, or other sexually transmitted diseases.

HIV

Your doctor may recommend screening for HIV if you:

- Had unprotected sex with multiple partners.
- Have used injected drugs.
- Pay for sex or have sex partners who do.
- Have past or current sex partners who are infected with HIV.
- Are being treated for sexually transmitted diseases.
- Had a blood transfusion between 1978 and 1985.

Depression

If you have felt "down" or hopeless during the past 2 weeks or you have had little interest in doing things you usually enjoy, talk to your doctor about depression. Depression is a treatable illness.

Abdominal Aortic Aneurysm

If you are between the ages of 65 and 75 and have smoked 100 or more cigarettes in your lifetime, ask your doctor to screen you for an abdominal aortic aneurysm. This is an abnormally large or swollen blood vessel in your stomach that can burst without warning.

Diabetes

If your blood pressure is higher than 135/80, ask your doctor to test you for diabetes. Diabetes, or high blood sugar, can cause problems with your heart, eyes, feet, kidneys, nerves, and other body parts.

Tobacco Use

If you smoke or use tobacco, talk to your doctor about quitting.

Know Your Prescriptions

If your doctor prescribes medicine for you, make sure you've told him or her about any other medicines you are currently taking, including over-the-counter drugs, vitamins, and supplements. You also need to talk about any allergies you have or any side effects you've had with other drugs. When you get a new prescription, make sure you understand what your doctor is prescribing, why you need to take it, and how often you should take it.

When your doctor prescribes a new medication, find out:

- The name of the medication and what it's supposed to do for you.

- If it's okay to substitute a less-expensive generic brand for the name brand drug.

- What the dose is and if you should avoid any other medicines, drinks, or food while you're taking it.

- How many refills you should get.

- What you should do it you miss a dose or if you take too much of it.

When you pick up your prescription, ask the pharmacist:

- If the drug is what your doctor ordered.

- If an information sheet is available on the medication that explains possible side effects.

- What the medicine label means. If the label says you need to take it three times a day, ask if that means you should take it every 8 hours or if you should take it at breakfast, lunch, and dinner.

- How you should measure the medication if it's a liquid.

You should schedule a followup visit with your doctor to track your progress. If you've gotten any new prescriptions from other doctors or have started taking new over-the-counter medications, be sure to let your doctor know during your office visit.

Find Advice and Support

If your doctor tells you that you have a health problem, you will need to make decisions about your treatment. For many conditions, you may have several treatment options. How do you decide what's best for you?

Find good information.

Contact a group that has information about your condition. You can also visit a local library to research your conditions. Use medical sites, like www.healthfinder.gov, to help you find information.

Make your decision with your doctor.

Once you've learned as much as you can about your condition, you and your doctor can choose what to do next. Look at the benefits and risks of each treatment for your condition and choose the treatment with which you're most comfortable. When you've made your decision, work with your doctor to create a treatment plan so you stay on track and know what to expect.

Ask questions.

If your doctor says you need surgery, ask:

- Why do I need an operation?

- Are there alternatives to surgery?

- What are the benefits of surgery? What are the risks?

- What happens if I don't have the surgery?

- Where can I get a second opinion?

- How many times have you performed this surgery?
- Where will the surgery be done?
- Will I need anesthesia? What kind?
- How long will it take for me to recover?
- How much will the operation cost?

Get support.

It's normal to be concerned about your condition. You may want to ask your family and friends for their help. If you have a tough time asking for help, think of what you need and ask one person to help you with the easiest chore on your list. You may also want to speak to a counselor or join a support group.

Section 1.2

Healthy Women

Text in this section is excerpted from "Women: Stay Healthy at Any Age," Agency for Healthcare Research and Quality (AHRQ), May 2014.

Get the Screenings You Need

Screenings are tests that look for diseases before you have symptoms. Blood pressure checks and mammograms are examples of screenings.

You can get some screenings, such as blood pressure readings, in your doctor's office. Others, such as mammograms, need special equipment, so you may need to go to a different office.

After a screening test, ask when you will see the results and who to talk to about them.

Breast Cancer. Talk with your health care team about whether you need a mammogram.

BRCA 1 and 2 Genes. If you have a family member with breast, ovarian, or peritoneal cancer, talk with your doctor or nurse about your family history. Women with a strong family history of certain cancers may benefit from genetic counseling and BRCA genetic testing.

Cervical Cancer. Starting at age 21, get a Pap smear every 3 years until you are 65 years old. Women 30 years of age or older can choose to switch to a combination Pap smear and human papillomavirus (HPV) test every 5 years until the age of 65. If you are older than 65 or have had a hysterectomy, talk with your doctor or nurse about whether you still need to be screened.

Colon Cancer. Between the ages of 50 and 75, get a screening test for colorectal cancer. Several tests—for example, a stool test or a colonoscopy—can detect this cancer. Your health care team can help you decide which is best for you. If you are between the ages of 76 and 85, talk with your doctor or nurse about whether you should continue to be screened.

Depression. Your emotional health is as important as your physical health. Talk to your health care team about being screened for depression, especially if during the last 2 weeks:

- You have felt down, sad, or hopeless.
- You have felt little interest or pleasure in doing things.

Diabetes. Get screened for diabetes (high blood sugar) if you have high blood pressure or if you take medication for high blood pressure.

Diabetes can cause problems with your heart, brain, eyes, feet, kidneys, nerves, and other body parts.

Hepatitis C Virus (HCV). Get screened one time for HCV infection if:

- You were born between 1945 and 1965.
- You have ever injected drugs.
- You received a blood transfusion before 1992.

If you currently are an injection drug user, you should be screened regularly.

> You know your body better than anyone else. Always tell your health care team about any changes in your health,

including your **vision** and **hearing**. Ask them about being checked for any condition you are concerned about, not just the ones here. If you are wondering about diseases such as **Alzheimer's disease** or **skin cancer**, for example, ask about them.

High Blood Cholesterol. Have your blood cholesterol checked regularly with a blood test if:

- You use tobacco.

- You are overweight or obese.

- You have a personal history of heart disease or blocked arteries.

- A male relative in your family had a heart attack before age 50 or a female relative, before age 60.

High Blood Pressure. Have your blood pressure checked at least every 2 years. High blood pressure can cause strokes, heart attacks, kidney and eye problems, and heart failure.

HIV. If you are 65 or younger, get screened for HIV. If you are older than 65, talk to your doctor or nurse about whether you should be screened.

Lung Cancer. Talk to your doctor or nurse about getting screened for lung cancer if you are between the ages of 55 and 80, have a 30 pack-year smoking history, and smoke now or have quit within the past 15 years. (Your pack-year history is the number of packs of cigarettes smoked per day times the number of years you have smoked.) Know that quitting smoking is the best thing you can do for your health.

Overweight and Obesity. The best way to learn if you are overweight or obese is to find your body mass index (BMI).

A BMI between 18.5 and 25 indicates a normal weight. Persons with a BMI of 30 or higher may be obese. If you are obese, talk to your doctor or nurse about getting intensive counseling and help with changing your behaviors to lose weight. Overweight and obesity can lead to diabetes and cardiovascular disease.

Osteoporosis (Bone Thinning). Have a screening test at age 65 to make sure your bones are strong. The most common test is a DEXA scan—a low-dose X-ray of the spine and hip. If you are younger than 65 and at high risk for bone fractures, you should also be screened. Talk with your health care team about your risk for bone fractures.

Sexually Transmitted Infections. Sexually transmitted infections can make it hard to get pregnant, may affect your baby, and can cause other health problems.

- Get screened for chlamydia and gonorrhea infections if you are 24 years or younger and sexually active. If you are older than 24 years, talk to your doctor or nurse about whether you should be screened.

- Ask your doctor or nurse whether you should be screened for other sexually transmitted infection.

Get Preventive Medicines If You Need Them

Aspirin. If you are 55 or older, ask your health care team if you should take aspirin to prevent strokes. Your health care team can help you decide whether taking aspirin to prevent stroke is right for you.

Breast Cancer Drugs. Talk to your doctor about your risks for breast cancer and whether you should take medicines that may reduce those risks. Medications to reduce breast cancer have some potentially serious harms, so think through both the potential benefits and harms.

Folic Acid. If you of an age at which you can get pregnant, you should take a daily supplement containing 0.4 to 0.8 mg of folic acid.

Vitamin D to Avoid Falls. If you are 65 or older and have a history of falls, mobility problems, or other risks for falling, ask your doctor about taking a vitamin D supplement to help reduce your chances of falling. Exercise and physical therapy may also help.

Immunizations:
- Get a flu shot every year.
- Get shots for tetanus, diphtheria, and whooping cough. Get tetanus booster if it has been more than 10 years since your last shot.
- If you are 60 or older, get a shot to prevent shingles.
- If you are 65 or older, get a pneumonia shot.
- Talk with your health care team about whether you need other vaccinations.

Take Steps to Good Health

- **Be physically active and make healthy food choices.**

- **Get to a healthy weight and stay there.** Balance the calories you take in from food and drink with the calories you burn off by your activities.

- **Be tobacco free.**

- **If you drink alcohol, have no more than one drink per day.** A standard drink is one 12-ounce bottle of beer or wine cooler, one 5-ounce glass of wine, or 1.5 ounces of 80-proof distilled spirits.

Section 1.3

Five Minutes (or Less) for Health

Text in this section is excerpted from "Five Minutes for Health,"
Centers for Disease Control and Prevention (CDC), April 13, 2015.

Take five for your health! Being healthy and safe takes commitment, but it doesn't have to be time-consuming. Most things are so simple and take so little time, that you'll wonder why you've been avoiding them. Taking just a few of the 1440 minutes in a day is worth having a safer and healthier life for you and your family. Below are some steps you can take to help protect your health and safety in five minutes or less.

One Minute or Less for Health

Take folic acid

The B vitamin folic acid helps prevent certain birth defects. If a woman has enough folic acid in her body before and while she is pregnant, her baby is less likely to have a major birth defect of the brain or spine. All women who could possibly get pregnant should take 400 micrograms of folic acid every day in a vitamin or in foods that have been enriched with it.

Wash hands

Wash hands to lower the risk of spreading germs and getting sick. It is best to wash hands with soap and clean running water for 20 seconds.

Check cruise ship inspection scores before you travel

If you're planning a cruise, check cruise ship inspection scores before your voyage. Cruise ships are subject to health and safety inspections twice a year to ensure that vessels are maintaining adequate levels of sanitation and to provide guidance to vessel staff when needed. CDC staff members inspect cruise ships with a foreign itinerary that call on U.S. ports and that carry 13 or more passengers.

Know local travel laws

Most people think about travel vaccines when they're planning an international trip, but few people consider the possibility that they might be involved in a car crash. Motor vehicle crashes are the leading cause of death among healthy travelers, and no vaccine can prevent a car wreck. Fortunately, a little bit of knowledge and awareness can go a long way toward keeping you safe.

Prevent poisonings

Whether they're drugs, medications, or household chemicals, follow instructions, and keep products out of the reach of children. Put the poison control number (800-222-1222) on all phones, and make sure all family members know when to call it.

Protect your skin

- Wear sunscreen, seek shade, and cover up to help lower your risk for sunburn and skin cancer.

- Wear insect repellent with DEET or Picaridin to protect yourself from mosquito and tick bites, which can cause disease.

- Set your water heater's thermostat to 120 degrees Fahrenheit or lower to help prevent burns.

Buckle up

Lower the risk for motor vehicle-related injuries. Make sure everyone is properly restrained in safety seats or safety belts. Children ages 12 and younger should always be buckled up and seated in the rear seat of vehicles. Placing children in age- and size-appropriate restraint systems lowers the risk of serious and fatal injuries by more than half.

Pledge to protect your teen driver

Parents can help protect their teen drivers from crashes—the leading killer of U.S. teens. It's proven that parents can make a positive difference when it comes to preventing the number one killer of teens in the United States—car crashes.

Gear up

When playing active sports or riding a motorcycle or bike, make sure you and your family wear protective gear, such as helmets, wrist guards, and knee and elbow pads.

Fight the urge to smoke or use tobacco

The urge will usually pass in 2-3 minutes. When you feel the urge, do something else. Take deep breaths and let them out slowly. Drink a glass of water. Carry things to put in your mouth, such as gum, hard candy, or toothpicks. Smoking even a few cigarettes a day and being around secondhand smoke (smoke from someone else smoking) can hurt you and your family's health. The only safe choice is to quit completely.

Protect your hearing

Hearing loss can result from damage to structures and/or nerve fibers in the inner ear that respond to sound. This type of hearing loss, termed "noise-induced hearing loss," is usually caused by exposure to excessively loud sounds and cannot be medically or surgically corrected. Use hearing protectors such as ear plugs and ear muffs when you can't lower noise to a safe level.

Wear a life jacket

All boat occupants should wear a life jacket to lower the risk of drowning. U.S. Coast Guard-approved life jackets are now more attractive in appearance and comfortable to wear. When properly fitted, a life jacket can help prevent a tragedy.

Read food labels

See how much fat, cholesterol, sodium, sugars, protein, and other ingredients are in the product. Note what the serving size is to make sure you don't eat more calories than you think you're getting.

Place infants back-to-sleep

To help lower the risk of sudden infant death syndrome (SIDS), always place infants on their backs (face-up) when they are resting, sleeping, or left alone.

Send a health-e-card

Health-e-cards are a quick and easy way to remind someone that you care about their health. Choose from a growing list of electronic greeting cards featuring a variety of health and safety topics.

Five Minutes or Less for Health

Test smoke alarms

Every month, check your smoke alarms to ensure they work properly. Check or replace the battery to your smoke alarm and carbon monoxide detector when you change the time on your clocks each spring and fall. If the alarm or detector sounds, leave your home immediately, and call 911.

- Fire Deaths and Injuries: Fact Sheet
- You Can Prevent Carbon Monoxide Exposure

Do a skin and body check

Check your skin and body regularly for lumps, rashes, sores, discolorations, limitations, and other changes. Do checks during and after bathing. Take note of other changes such as those related to urine or bowel habits, thirst, hunger, fatigue, discharge, vision, and weight. If you find or experience anything suspicious, see your health care provider.

Make an appointment

One of the best and easiest ways for adults to keep themselves healthy is to make sure they get recommended exams, screenings and immunizations. Screenings are designed to help detect some diseases in their early, most treatable stages. Make the appointment now.

Know your numbers

Keep track of your numbers for blood pressure, blood sugar, cholesterol, body mass index (BMI), and others. These numbers can provide a glimpse of your health status and risk for certain diseases and conditions, including heart disease, diabetes, obesity, and more. Be sure to ask your health care provider what tests you need and how often. If your numbers are too high or too low, he/she can make recommendations to help you get them to a healthier range.

Make sure you are up-to-date on your vaccinations

Keep track of your and your family's vaccinations, and make sure they stay up-to-date. Children, young adults, and older adults all need vaccinations. Vaccinations help protect people from diseases and save lives.

Eat healthy

Take the extra time to make better food choices. Eat more fruits and vegetables as a meal, less saturated fat, and healthy grab-and-go snacks. There are many quick and easy ways to add healthier choices to your day.

Wash children's hands and toys regularly

Hands and toys can become contaminated from household dust or exterior soil, both of which are sources of harmful lead.

Know important asthma triggers

An asthma attack can occur when you are exposed to things in the environment, such as house dust mites and tobacco smoke. These are called asthma triggers. Your personal triggers can be very different from those of another person. Some of the most important triggers are:

- Environmental Tobacco Smoke (Secondhand Smoke)
- Dust Mites
- Outdoor Air Pollution
- Cockroach Allergen
- Pets
- Mold
- Wood Smoke

Learn the signs for developmental problems

Check to see if your children can do the things associated with their age. From birth to 5 years, your children should reach milestones in how they play, learn, speak, and act. A delay in any of these areas could be a sign of a developmental problem.

Know the signs and symptoms for heart attack and stroke

If you or someone you know is having a heart attack or stroke, call 911 immediately. With timely treatment, a person's chance of surviving a heart attack is increased, and the risk of death and disability from stroke can be lowered.

Encourage health through play

Encourage kids to adopt safe and healthy habits with these fun pages and activity book. Children and adolescents should do 60 minutes (1 hour) or more of physical activity each day.

Take a break

If you think you're getting sick, feel yourself losing control, or are dealing with stress, take a break. Just taking a few minutes can give you the opportunity to clear your head so you can make better decisions about your and your family's health and safety.

Take care of your teeth and gums

Drink fluoridated water and use a fluoride toothpaste. Fluoride's protection against tooth decay works at all ages. Brush and floss your teeth thoroughly to reduce dental plaque and help prevent gingivitis (a form of gum disease).

Keep foods safe

Refrigerate leftovers promptly. Bacteria can grow quickly at room temperature, so refrigerate leftover foods if they are not going to be eaten within 4 hours. Wash hands, utensils, and cutting boards after they have been in contact with raw meat or poultry and before they touch another food. Wash produce. Cook meat, poultry, and eggs thoroughly. Report suspected foodborne illnesses to your local health department.

Ask questions

Before seeing your health care provider, write down all of your questions and bring the list with you to your appointment. Write down the answers during your discussion. Make sure all of your questions are answered before you leave and you know exactly what the next steps are. Don't risk injury or other problems because you are not clear on what to do.

If instructions are confusing, get help. Talk to your health care provider. Call or visit the website of the pharmacy, clinic, equipment manufacturer, or business for information. Make sure you use credible sources and websites and ask your health care provider if the information you found applies to you. With more knowledge, you can make better decisions about your health.

Listen to a health podcast

Podcasts on a variety of health and safety topics are available online. Most are one to five minutes long, and some are longer.

Disinfect surfaces to keep germs away

Cleaning removes germs from surfaces, and disinfecting destroys germs from surfaces. Disinfecting after cleaning gives an extra level of protection from germs. Areas with the largest amounts of germs and frequently used areas- such as the kitchen and bathroom- should be disinfected with a bleach solution or another disinfectant as often as possible to avoid the spread of germs.

If you have diabetes, check for sores and vision changes

If you have diabetes, check your feet every day for cuts, blisters, red spots, and swelling. Call your doctor immediately if you have sores that will not heal. Also, tell your doctor if you notice any changes in your eyesight.

Get a radon test for your home

Radon is a cancer-causing natural radioactive gas that you can't see, smell or taste. Its presence in your home can pose a danger to your family's health. Radon is the second leading cause of lung cancer in America and claims about 20,000 lives annually. Nearly 1 out of every 15 homes in the U.S. is estimated to have elevated radon levels. Testing is inexpensive and easy.

Go green

Lower greenhouse gases in the environment, reuse products, and recycle items that can no longer be used.

Learn healthy contact lens wear and care

You only have one pair of eyes, so take care of them! Healthy Habits = Healthy Eyes. Enjoy the comfort and benefits of contact lenses while lowering your chance of complications. Failure to wear, clean, and store your lenses as directed by your eye doctor raises the risk of developing serious infections. Your habits, supplies, and eye doctor are all essential to keeping your eyes healthy.

More than Five Minutes and Worth It

Be active

Be active for at least 2½ hours a week. Include activities that raise your breathing and heart rates and that strengthen your muscles. Doing 10 minutes at a time is fine. Help kids and teens be active for at least 1 hour a day. Include activities that raise their breathing and heart rates and that strengthen their muscles and bones.

Be prepared

Practice family drills at home to make sure everyone knows exactly what to do in case of an emergency. Although some people feel it is impossible to be prepared for unexpected events, the truth is that taking preparedness actions helps people deal with disasters of all sorts much more effectively when they do occur. Have an escape plan in case of fire or other emergency, and practice it as part of your family drills. Know your local weather conditions and forecast so you can prepare for any severe weather.

Know your family's health history

If you have a close relative with a chronic disease, such as heart disease, stroke, diabetes, or cancer, then you could have an increased risk for developing that disease. Keep track of your family health history by writing down the health conditions of each family member. Take a few minutes to update this information from time to time. This way, you'll have organized and accurate information ready to share with your health care provider. Family health history can help him/ her determine which tests and screenings you should have. In many cases, adopting a healthier lifestyle can lower your risk for diseases that run in your family.

Prevent falls

Check for hazards around the home to prevent falls. Each year, thousands of older Americans fall at home. Falls are often due to hazards that are easy to overlook but easy to fix.

Get involved

Get to know the people your children are around on a regular basis. Engage in conversation, participate in activities, review Internet networks to people and sites, observe, and learn more. Talk to your kids about how to protect themselves from disease and injury and to avoid risky behaviors related to tobacco, sex, and more.

Pack a traveler's health kit

Pack items that you will need to stay healthy and safe on your trip, such as sunscreen, insect repellent, prescription medicines, and basic first-aid items.

Learn tips for caregiving

Whether your family member with special needs is a child or an adult, combining personal, caregiving, and everyday needs can be challenging. Being informed, getting support, and taking care of yourself can help you and those you care for stay safe and healthy.

Section 1.4

Check-Up Checklist: Things to Do before Your Next Check-Up

Text in this section is excerpted from "Check-Up Checklist," Centers for Disease Control and Prevention (CDC), April 1, 2015.

Getting check-ups is one of many things you can do to help stay healthy and prevent disease and disability.

You've made the appointment to see your health care provider. You've reviewed the instructions on how to prepare for certain tests. You've done the usual paperwork. Done, right? Not quite.

Before your next check-up, make sure you do these four things.

Review your family health history.

Are there any new conditions or diseases that have occurred in your close relatives since your last visit? If so, let your health care provider know. Family history might influence your risk of developing heart disease, stroke, diabetes, or cancer. Your provider will assess your risk of disease based on your family history and other factors. Your provider may also recommend things you can do to help prevent disease, such as exercising more, changing your diet, or using screening tests to help detect disease early.

Find out if you are due for any general screenings or vaccinations.

Have you had the recommended screening tests based on your age, general health, family history, and lifestyle? Check with your health care provider to see if its time for any vaccinations, follow-up exams, or tests. For example, it might be time for you to get a Pap test, mammogram, prostate cancer screening, colon cancer screening, sexually transmitted disease screening, blood pressure check, tetanus shot, eye check, or other screening.

Write down a list of issues and questions to take with you.

Review any existing health problems and note any changes.

- Have you noticed any body changes, including lumps or skin changes?

- Are you having pain, dizziness, fatigue, problems with urine or stool, or menstrual cycle changes?

- Have your eating habits changed?

- Are you experiencing depression, anxiety, trauma, distress, or sleeping problems?

If so, note when the change began, how it's different from before, and any other observation that you think might be helpful.

Be honest with your provider. If you haven't been taking your medication as directed, exercising as much, or anything else, say so. You may be at risk for certain diseases and conditions because of how you live, work, and play. Your provider develops a plan based partly on what you say you do. Help ensure that you get the best guidance by providing the most up-to-date and accurate information about you.

Be sure to write your questions down beforehand. Once you're in the office or exam room, it can be hard to remember everything you want to know. Leave room between questions to write down your provider's answers.

Consider your future.

Are there specific health issues that need addressing concerning your future? Are you thinking about having infertility treatment, losing weight, taking a hazardous job, or quitting smoking? Discuss any issues with your provider so that you can make better decisions regarding your health and safety.

Section 1.5

When Getting Medical Tests

Text in this section is excerpted from "When Getting Medical
Tests," Agency for Healthcare Research and Quality (AHRQ),
September 2012.

Quick Tips

The single most important way you can stay healthy is to be an
active member of your own health care team. One way to get high-quality health care is to find and use information and take an active role
in all of the decisions made about your care.

This information will help you when making decisions about medical tests.

Doctors order blood tests, X-rays, and other tests to help diagnose medical problems. Perhaps you do not know why you need a particular test or
you don't understand how it will help you. Here are some questions to ask:

- How is the test done?

- What kind of information will the test provide?

- Is this test the only way to find out that information?

- What are the benefits and risks of having this test?

- How accurate is the test?

- What do I need to do to prepare for the test? (What you do or
  don't do may affect the accuracy of the test results.)

- Will the test be uncomfortable?

- How long will it take to get the results, and how will I get them?

- What's the next step after the test?

One study found that anywhere from 10 percent to 30 percent of
Pap smear test results that were called "normal" were not. Errors such
as this can lead to a wrong or delayed diagnosis. You want your tests
to be done the right way, and you want accurate results.

23

What can you do?

- For tests your doctor sends to a lab, ask which lab he or she uses, and why. You may want to know that the doctor chooses a certain lab because he or she has business ties to it. Or, the health plan may require that the tests go there.

- Check to see that the lab is accredited by a group such as the College of American Pathologists (800-323-4040) or the Joint Commission on Accreditation of Healthcare Organizations (telephone, 630-792-5800; Web site, http://www.jcaho.org).

- If you need a mammogram, make sure the facility is approved by the Food and Drug Administration. You can find out by checking the certificate in the facility

What about the test results?

- Do not assume that no news is good news. If you do not hear from your doctor, call to get your test results.

- If you and your doctor think the test results may not be right, have the test done again.

Remember, quality matters, especially when it comes to your health.

Chapter 2

Family History

Chapter Contents

Section 2.1

Importance of Knowing Family History

Text in this section is excerpted from "Inheriting Genetic Conditions,"
Genetic Home Reference (GHR), August 24, 2015.

Why is it important to know my family medical history?

A family medical history is a record of health information about
a person and his or her close relatives. A complete record includes
information from three generations of relatives, including children,
brothers and sisters, parents, aunts and uncles, nieces and nephews,
grandparents, and cousins.

Families have many factors in common, including their genes, environment, and lifestyle. Together, these factors can give clues to medical
conditions that may run in a family. By noticing patterns of disorders
among relatives, healthcare professionals can determine whether an
individual, other family members, or future generations may be at an
increased risk of developing a particular condition.

A family medical history can identify people with a higher-than-
usual chance of having common disorders, such as heart disease,
high blood pressure, stroke, certain cancers, and diabetes. These
complex disorders are influenced by a combination of genetic factors,
environmental conditions, and lifestyle choices. A family history also
can provide information about the risk of rarer conditions caused
by mutations in a single gene, such as cystic fibrosis and sickle cell
anemia.

While a family medical history provides information about the risk
of specific health concerns, having relatives with a medical condition
does not mean that an individual will definitely develop that condition.
On the other hand, a person with no family history of a disorder may
still be at risk of developing that disorder.

Knowing one's family medical history allows a person to take steps
to reduce his or her risk. For people at an increased risk of certain
cancers, healthcare professionals may recommend more frequent
screening (such as mammography or colonoscopy) starting at an

earlier age. Healthcare providers may also encourage regular check-ups or testing for people with a medical condition that runs in their family. Additionally, lifestyle changes such as adopting a healthier diet, getting regular exercise, and quitting smoking help many people lower their chances of developing heart disease and other common illnesses.

The easiest way to get information about family medical history is to talk to relatives about their health. Have they had any medical problems, and when did they occur? A family gathering could be a good time to discuss these issues. Additionally, obtaining medical records and other documents (such as obituaries and death certificates) can help complete a family medical history. It is important to keep this information up-to-date and to share it with a healthcare professional regularly.

Section 2.2

FAQs on Family History

Text in this section is excerpted from "Family History," Centers for Disease Control and Prevention (CDC), May 11, 2015.

What is family health history?

Family health history refers to health information about you and your close relatives. Family health history is one of the most important risk factors for health problems like heart disease, stroke, diabetes and cancer. (A risk factor is anything that increases your chance of getting a disease.)

Why is knowing my family health history important?

Family members share their genes, as well as their environment, lifestyles and habits. A family health history helps identify people at increased risk for disease because it reflects both a person's genes and these other shared risk factors.

My mother had breast cancer. Does this mean I will get cancer, too?

Having a family member with a disease suggests that you may have a higher chance of developing that disease than someone without a similar family history. It does not mean that you will definitely develop the disease. Genes are only one of many factors that contribute to disease. Other factors to consider include lifestyle habits, such as diet and physical activity.

If you are at risk for breast cancer, consider following national guidelines for a healthy diet and regular exercise. It is also important to talk with your physician about your risk and follow recommendations for screening tests (such as mammograms) that may help to detect disease early, when it is most treatable.

Because both of my parents had heart disease, I know I have "bad" genes. Is there anything I can do to protect myself?

First of all, there are no "good" or "bad" genes. Most human diseases, especially common diseases such as heart disease, result from the interaction of genes with environmental and behavioral risk factors that can be changed. The best disease prevention strategy for anyone, especially for someone with a family health history, includes reducing risky behaviors (such as smoking) and increasing healthy behaviors (such as regular exercise).

How can knowing my family health history help lower my risk of disease?

You can't change your genes, but you can change behaviors that affect your health, such as smoking, inactivity and poor eating habits. People with a family health history of chronic disease may have the most to gain from making lifestyle changes. In many cases, making these changes can reduce your risk of disease even if the disease runs in your family.

Another change you can make is to participate in screening tests, such as mammograms and colorectal cancer screening, for early detection of disease. People who have a family history of a chronic disease may benefit the most from screening tests that look for risk factors or early signs of disease. Finding disease early, before symptoms appear, can mean better health in the long run.

How can I learn about my family health history?

The best way to learn about your family health history is to ask questions, talk at family gatherings, draw a family tree and record health information. If possible, look at death certificates and family medical records.

How do I learn about my family health history if I'm adopted?

Learning about your family health history may be hard if you are adopted. Some adoption agencies collect medical information on birth relatives. This is becoming more common but is not routine. Laws concerning collection of information vary by state. Contact the health and social service agency in your state for information about how to access medical or legal records. The National Adoption Clearinghouse offers information on adoption and could be helpful if you decide to search for your birth parents.

What should I do with the information?

First, write down the information you collect about your family health history and share it with your doctor. Second, remember to keep your information updated and share it with your siblings and children. Third, pass it on to your children, so that they too will have a family health history record.

If I don't have a family health history of disease, does that mean I am not at risk?

Even if you don't have a history of a particular health problem in your family, you could still be at risk. This is because you may be unaware of disease in some family members, or you could have family members who died young, before they had a chance to develop chronic conditions. Your risk of developing a chronic disease is also influenced by many other factors, including your habits and personal health history.

Chapter 3

Questions about Medical Tests

A wide array of medical tests are available today that can detect disease or illness at an early stage, when many conditions can be treated effectively. Your physician shouldn't prescribe tests that you don't need, but you should get the tests that are right for your age, gender, and medical history.

Maybe you don't know why you need a particular test or don't understand how it will help you. Here are some that my agency, the Agency for Healthcare Research and Quality (AHRQ), developed to help you talk to your doctor.

Ask your doctor:

- How is the test done?

- What kind of information will the test provide?

- Is this test the only way to find out that information?

- What are the risks and benefits of having this test?

- How accurate is the test?

- What do I need to do to prepare for the test?

- Will the test be uncomfortable?

Text in this chapter is excerpted from "Asking Questions About Medical Tests," Agency for Healthcare Research and Quality (AHRQ), October 2014.

- How long will it take to get the results, and how will I get them?

- What's the next step after the test?

Your doctor should be able to tell you when the results of your medical test will be ready. Do not assume that everything is fine if you don't hear from your doctor. Tests results can get lost, or people can think someone else gave you the results. No news is not necessarily good news.

In fact, a study conducted at Harvard Medical School found that up to 33 percent of doctors did not always notify patients about abnormal test results. If you don't hear from your doctor, call to get your results.

It is also possible that your test results are incorrect. If you or your doctor think the test results may not be right, retake the test. A second test can confirm or rule out a diagnosis.

It's also a good idea to get information on the lab your doctor uses to analyze test results. For example, you may want to know if your doctor uses a lab because he or she has a business arrangement with them or if a health insurance company requires your doctor to use a certain lab.

You can find out if a lab is accredited by or has a seal of approval from groups such as the College of American Pathologists or the Joint Commission. Both groups require labs to meet certain standards, which are linked to better-quality services.

If you need a mammogram, which is a test to detect breast cancer, make sure the test is performed at a facility that is approved by the Food and Drug Administration.

By asking your doctor questions about medical tests and your test results, you will have the information that you need to make smart decisions about your health care.

Part Two

Screening and Preventive Care Tests

Chapter 4

Newborn Screening Tests

Chapter Contents

Section 4.1

Importance of Newborn Screening

Text in this section is excerpted from "Newborn Screening," Centers for Disease Control and Prevention (CDC), March 3, 2015.

When and How Babies are Screened

Babies that are born in a hospital should be screened before they leave the hospital. Parents should take babies that are *not* born in a hospital or those that were *not* screened before leaving the hospital to a hospital or clinic to be checked within a few days of birth. In some states all babies are screened a second time, about two weeks after birth.

Blood Test

A health professional will take a few drops of blood from the baby's heel. The blood sample is sent to a newborn screening lab for testing.

Hearing Screening

Hearing screening is a short test to tell if people might have hearing loss. Hearing screening is easy and not painful. In fact, babies are often asleep while being screened. All babies should be screened for hearing loss no later than 1 month of age. It is best if they are screened before leaving the hospital after birth.

Screening for Critical Congenital Heart Defects

Babies with a critical congenital heart defect (CCHD) are at significant risk of disability or death if their condition is not diagnosed soon after birth. Newborn screening using pulse oximetry can identify some infants with a CCHD before they show signs of the condition. Once identified, babies with a CCHD can be seen by cardiologists (doctors that know a lot about the heart) and can receive special care and treatment that can prevent disability and death early in life.

Many hospitals routinely screen all newborns for CCHDs. However, CCHD screening is not currently included in all state newborn screening panels.

Conditions Tested

Each state runs its own newborn screening program. The conditions include sickle cell disease and other hemoglobin disorders, conditions where a child is unable to process certain nutrients (such as PKU), or conditions where there is a hormonal insufficiency (such as hypothyroidism). Most states screen for a standard number of conditions, but some states may screen for more. That means that there are differences in the screening process and the number and types of conditions included in screening in each state.

Screening Results

If the results are "negative" ("pass" or in-range result) it means that the baby's test results did not show signs of any of the conditions included in the screening.

If the results are "positive" ("fail" or out-of-range result) it means that the baby's test results showed signs of one or more of the conditions included in the newborn screening. This does *not* always mean that the baby has the condition. It may just mean that more testing is needed.

The child's doctor might recommend that the child get screened again or have more specific tests to diagnose a condition. For example, all babies who do not pass a hearing screening should have a full hearing test by three months and sometimes also at six months of age to confirm if there is a hearing loss.

Get Help!

If your baby's newborn screening tests show that there could be a problem, work with your baby's doctor to get any needed follow-up tests as soon as possible – don't wait!

Finding and treating some of the conditions at an early age can prevent serious problems, such as brain damage, organ damage, and even death. Many of the conditions can be treated with medication or changes to the baby's diet.

In order to make sure your baby reaches his or her full potential, it is very important to get help for any medical condition as soon as possible.

Section 4.2

Talk with Your Doctor about Newborn Screening

Text in this section is excerpted from "Talk with Your Doctor about Newborn Screening," Office of Disease Prevention and Health Promotion (ODPHP), July 16, 2015.

The Basics

Newborn screenings are tests that check for diseases or disorders in newborn babies. Most tests are done before your baby leaves the hospital.

Newborn screenings let doctors find problems early and start treatment to keep your baby healthy. They don't cause any harm or risk to your baby.

Talk about newborn screening with your doctor or midwife **before** your baby is born. This can help you make sure your baby grows up healthy.

What tests will my baby need?

All states require newborn screening. But the number and types of tests vary from state to state. Depending on your family health history, you may want to ask for extra tests.

Most newborn screening tests use a few drops of blood taken from the heel of your baby's foot. The same sample of blood can be used to test for many different diseases, including:

- *Hypothyroid disorder* – The thyroid is a gland in the neck that makes hormones. Hypothyroid disorder can cause problems with growth and development, but it can be treated if it's found early.

- *PKU (phenylketonuria)* – PKU means babies can't process certain foods and must be fed special formula. It can cause intellectual disability (mental skills that are below average) if it's not treated early.

- *Sickle cell disease* – This is a serious blood disorder that can be watched and treated if it's found early.

Hearing loss

A hearing test uses a small microphone or earphone to check how your baby responds to sounds. Finding out early if your baby has hearing loss can help reduce or avoid speech and language delays.

If your hospital doesn't screen for hearing loss, make sure to have your baby's hearing checked within the first month.

It's also important to have your baby's hearing checked regularly, since some hearing loss starts after the time when newborn screening tests are done.

Heart defects

Heart defects (problems with the heart) can cause serious problems or death if they're not found and treated early.

Testing for heart defects uses a small sensor that is placed on your baby's hand or foot. The test is painless and only takes a few minutes.

Take Action!

If you are pregnant, talk with your doctor about newborn screening before your baby is born.

Find out which tests your hospital offers.

Ask your doctor or midwife about newborn screening. Find out which screening tests are offered at the hospital where your baby will be born.

If you aren't planning to give birth at a hospital, your baby still needs to get screened. Ask your midwife if she can screen your baby for you. Or, take your baby to a hospital or clinic to get checked a few days after birth.

Follow up.

Ask the doctor when you will get your baby's test results. Some tests may need to be repeated after 1 or 2 weeks, especially if you leave the hospital before your baby is 24 hours old. Make a plan with your doctor.

What about cost?

Some newborn screening tests are covered under the Affordable Care Act, the health care reform law passed in 2010. Depending on your insurance plan, you may be able to get your baby screened at no cost to you.

Check with your insurance provider to find out what's included in your plan.

If you don't have insurance, you can still get medical care for yourself and your baby.

Schedule well-baby checkups.

Most babies have their first checkup 2 to 3 days after coming home from the hospital. A well-baby visit is when you take your baby to the doctor for a full checkup. This is different from other visits for sickness or injury.

Start building your child's health record now.

Keep track of your baby's test results and shots. Put medical information in a safe place – you will need it for child care, school, and other activities.

Your family's health history is an important part of your baby's health record.

Section 4.3

Facts about Birth Defects

Text in this section is excerpted from "Facts about Birth Defects,"
Centers for Disease Control and Prevention (CDC), October 20, 2014.

Birth defects are serious conditions that are changes to the structure of one or more parts of the body. Birth defects affect 1 in every 33 babies born in the United States each year.

Birth Defects Are Common

Every 4 ½ minutes, a baby is born with a birth defect in the United States. That translates into nearly 120,000 babies affected by birth defects each year.

Birth defects can affect almost any part of the body (e.g., heart, brain, foot). They may affect how the body looks, works, or both. Birth defects can vary from mild to severe. The well-being of each child affected with a birth defect depends mostly on which organ or body part is involved and how much it is affected. Depending on the severity of the defect and what body part is affected, the expected lifespan of a person with a birth defect may or may not be affected.

Identifying Birth Defects

A birth defect can be found before birth, at birth, or any time after birth. Most birth defects are found within the first year of life. Some birth defects (such as cleft lip) are easy to see, but others (such as heart defects or hearing loss) are found using special tests, such as echocardiograms (an ultrasound picture of the heart), X-rays or hearing tests.

Prevention

Not all birth defects can be prevented. But, there are things that a woman can do before and during pregnancy to increase her chance of having a healthy baby. If you are pregnant or planning to get pregnant, see your healthcare provider. Seeing your healthcare provider before you get pregnant (called the preconception period) can help you have a healthy pregnancy. Prenatal care, which is health care received during pregnancy, can help find some problems early in pregnancy so that they can be monitored or treated before birth.

There are other steps a woman can take to increase her chances of having a healthy baby:

- Get 400 micrograms (mcg) of folic acid every day, starting at least one month before getting pregnant.

- Don't drink alcohol, smoke, or use "street" drugs.

- Talk to a healthcare provider about taking any medications, including prescription and over-the-counter medications and dietary or herbal supplements. Also talk to a doctor before stopping any medications that are needed to treat health conditions.

- Learn how to prevent infections during pregnancy.

- If possible, be sure any medical conditions are under control, before becoming pregnant. Some conditions that increase the risk for birth defects include diabetes and obesity.

Causes

Birth defects can occur during any stage of pregnancy. Most birth defects occur in the first 3 months of pregnancy, when the organs of the baby are forming. This is a very important stage of development. However, some birth defects occur later in pregnancy. During the last six months of pregnancy, the tissues and organs continue to grow and develop.

Most birth defects are thought to be caused by a complex mix of factors. These factors include our genes (information inherited from our parents), our behaviors, and things in the environment. For some birth defects, we know the cause. But for most, we don't.

Certain things can increase the chance that a pregnancy will be affected by a birth defect. These are called risk factors. There are some things that you can change to reduce your chances, while other things cannot be changed. Some risk factors that can increase the chances of having a baby with a birth defect: include:

- Smoking, drinking alcohol, or taking certain "street" drugs during pregnancy.

- Having certain medical conditions, such as being obese or having uncontrolled diabetes before and during pregnancy.

- Taking certain medications, such as isotretinoin (a drug used to treat severe acne).

- Having someone in your family with a birth defect. To learn more about your risk of having a baby with a birth defect, you can talk with a clinical geneticist or a genetic counselor.

- Being an older mother, typically over the age of 34 years.

Having one or more of these risks doesn't mean you'll have a pregnancy affected by a birth defect. Also, women can have a baby born with a birth defect even when they don't have any of these risks. It is important to talk to your doctor about what you can do to lower your risk.

Living with a Birth Defect

Babies who have birth defects often need special care and interventions to survive and to thrive developmentally. State birth defects tracking programs provide one way to identify and refer children as early as possible for services they need. Early intervention is vital to improving outcomes for these babies. If your child has a birth defect, you should ask his or her doctor about local resources and treatment. Geneticists, genetic counselors, and other specialists are another resource.

Section 4.4

Developmental Monitoring and Screening

Text in this section is excerpted from "Developmental Monitoring and Screening," Centers for Disease Control and Prevention (CDC), August 24, 2015.

Developmental Monitoring

Your child's growth and development are kept track of through a partnership between you and your health professional. At each well-child visit the doctor looks for developmental delays or problems and talks with you about any concerns you might have. This is called *developmental monitoring (or surveillance)*. Any problems noticed during developmental monitoring should be followed-up with *developmental screening*.

Children with special health care needs should have developmental monitoring and screening just like those without special needs. Monitoring healthy development means paying attention not only to symptoms related to the child's condition, but also to the child's physical, mental, social, and emotional well-being.

Developmental Screening

Well-child visits allow doctors and nurses to have regular contact with children to keep track of, or *monitor*, your child's health and development through periodic developmental screening. Developmental screening is a short test to tell if a child is learning basic skills when he or she should, or if there are delays. Developmental screening can also be done by other professionals in health care, community, or school settings.

The doctor might ask you some questions or talk and play with the child during an examination to see how he or she plays, learns,

43

speaks, behaves, and moves. A delay in any of these areas could be a sign of a problem.

The American Academy of Pediatrics recommends that all children be screened for developmental delays and disabilities during regular well-child doctor visits at:

- 9 months

- 18 months

- 24 or 30 months

Additional screening might be needed if a child is at high risk for developmental problems due to preterm birth, low birthweight, or other reasons.

If your child's doctor does not routinely check your child with this type of developmental screening test, you can ask that it be done.

Why It's Important

Many children with developmental delays are not being identified as early as possible. As a result, these children must wait to get the help they need to do well in social and educational settings (for example, in school).

In the United States, about 13% of children 3 to 17 years of age have a developmental or behavioral disability such as autism, intellectual disability (also known as mental retardation), and attention-deficit/hyperactivity disorder. In addition, many children have delays in language or other areas that can affect school readiness. However, many children with developmental disabilities are not identified before age 10, by which time significant delays already might have occurred and opportunities for treatment might have been missed.

Early Intervention Services

Research shows that early intervention treatment services can greatly improve a child's development. Early intervention services help children from birth through 3 years of age (36 months) learn important skills. Services include therapy to help the child talk, walk, and interact with others.

The Individuals with Disabilities Education Act (IDEA) says that children younger than 3 years of age (36 months) who are at risk of having developmental delays, might be eligible for early intervention treatment services even if the child has not received a formal diagnosis.

These services are provided through an early intervention system in each state.

In addition, treatment for particular symptoms, such as speech therapy for language delays, often does not require a formal diagnosis. Although early intervention is extremely important, intervention at any age can be helpful.

Section 4.5

Screening Test for Baby's Hearing Capabilities

Text in this section is excerpted from "It's Important to Have Your Baby's Hearing Screened," National Institute on Deafness and Other Communication Disorders (NIDCD), July 13, 2015.

It's Important to Have Your Baby's Hearing Screened

Most children hear and listen to sounds from birth. They learn to talk by imitating the sounds around them and the voices of their parents and caregivers. But that's not true for all children. In fact, about two or three out of every 1,000 children in the United States are born deaf or hard-of-hearing. More lose their hearing later during childhood. Many of these children may need to learn speech and language differently, so it's important to detect deafness or hearing loss as early as possible. For this reason, universal newborn hearing screening programs currently operate in all U.S. states and most of the territories. With help from the federal government, every state has established an Early Hearing Detection and Intervention program as part of its public health system. As a result, more than 95 percent of babies have their hearing screened soon after they are born.

When will my baby's hearing be screened?

Your baby's hearing should be screened before he or she leaves the hospital or birthing center. If you and your baby are already home and you haven't been told the results of the hearing screening, ask your doctor. If the results indicate your baby may have hearing loss, it's important to work with your doctor to make an appointment with a hearing expert, called an audiologist, to perform a more thorough hearing test before your baby is 3 months old.

How will my baby's hearing be screened?

Two different tests are used to screen for hearing loss in babies. In both tests, no activity is required from your child other than lying still.

- The **otoacoustic emissions (OAE)** test shows whether parts of the ear respond properly to sound. During this test, a soft sponge earphone is inserted into your baby's ear canal and emits a series of sounds to measure an "echo" response that occurs in normal hearing ears. If there is no echo, it could indicate hearing loss.

- The **auditory brain stem response (ABR)** test checks how the auditory brain stem (the part of the nerve that carries sound from the ear to the brain) and the brain respond to sound by measuring their electrical activity as your child listens. During this test, your baby wears small earphones in the ears and electrodes on the head. Your baby might be given a mild sedative to keep him or her calm and quiet during the test. If your child doesn't respond consistently to the sounds presented during either of these tests, your doctor will suggest a follow-up hearing screening and a referral to an audiologist for a more comprehensive hearing evaluation. If hearing loss is confirmed, it's important to consider the use of hearing devices and other communication options before your baby is 6 months old.

Why is it important to have my baby's hearing screened early?

The most important time for a child to learn language is in the first 3 years of life. In fact, children begin learning speech and language in the first 6 months of life. Research suggests that children with hearing loss who get help early develop better language skills than those who don't. The earlier you know about a child's hearing loss, the sooner you can make sure your child benefits from strategies that will help him or her learn to successfully communicate.

How can I recognize if my child develops hearing loss later in childhood?

Even though the screening tests are designed to detect hearing loss as early as possible, some children may not develop hearing loss until later in childhood. In those instances, parents, caregivers, or grandparents are often the first to notice. This means that, even if your baby has passed the hearing screening, you should still continue to look for signs that your baby is hearing well.

For example, during the first year, notice whether your baby reacts to loud noises, imitates sounds, and begins to respond to his or her name. When your child is age 2, ask yourself whether he or she makes playful sounds with his or her voice, imitates simple words, and enjoys games like peek-a-boo and pat-a-cake. Is he or she using two-word sentences to talk about and ask for things? When your child is age 3, notice whether he or she begins to understand "not now" and "no more" and follows simple directions. If for any reason you think your child is not hearing well, talk to your doctor.

If my child has hearing loss, can hearing be improved?

A variety of assistive devices and strategies are helpful for children who are hard-of-hearing. Some examples of these devices are listed here. An audiologist can help you determine whether these or other devices will help your child.

- **Hearing aids** are devices that make sounds louder. They are worn in or behind the ear and come in several different shapes and sizes. Hearing aids can be used for varying degrees of hearing loss from mild to severe. An audiologist will fit a hearing aid that will work best for your child's degree of loss. Hearing aids can be expensive, so you'll want to find out whether they have a warranty or trial period. You'll also want to talk with your insurance provider to understand what, and how much, it will pay for.

- **Cochlear implants** are small electronic devices that help provide a sense of sound to people who are profoundly deaf or hard-of-hearing. They consist of a microphone worn just behind the ear, which picks up sound from the environment; a speech processor, which selects and arranges the sounds; a transmitter and receiver/stimulator, which receive signals from the speech processor and convert them into electric impulses; and an implanted electrode array, which collects the impulses from the stimulator and sends them to the auditory nerve.

Not all children who have hearing loss should get cochlear implants. Doctors and hearing experts think they're best for children who have such severe hearing loss that they can't benefit from hearing aids. Some doctors now recommend the use of two cochlear implants, one for each ear, to help children identify the directions of sounds.

As children get older, many other devices are available to help their hearing. Some devices help children hear better in a classroom. Others make talking on the phone or watching television easier. For example, induction loop systems and FM systems can help eliminate or reduce distracting noises and make it easier to hear individual voices in a crowded room or group setting. Others, such as personal amplifiers, are better for one-on-one conversations.

How can I help my child communicate?

There are a variety of ways to help children with hearing loss express themselves and interact with others. The main options are listed below. The option you choose will depend on what you think is best for your child. Find out as much as you can about all of the choices, and ask your doctor to refer you to experts if you want to know more.

- **Auditory-oral and auditory-verbal options** combine natural hearing ability and hearing devices such as hearing aids and cochlear implants with other strategies to help children develop speech and English-language skills. Auditory-oral options use visual cues such as lipreading and sign language, while auditory-verbal options work to strengthen listening skills.

- **American Sign Language (ASL)** is a language used by some children who are deaf and their families. ASL consists of hand signs, body movements, and facial expressions. ASL has its own grammar and syntax, which are different from English, but it has no written form.

- **Cued speech** is a system that uses handshapes along with natural mouth movements to represent speech sounds. Watching the mouth movements and the handshapes can help some children learn to speech-read English; this is especially important in discriminating between sounds that look the same on the lips.

- **Signed English** is a system that uses signs to represent words or phrases in English. Signed English is designed to enhance the use of both spoken and written English.

- **Combined options** use portions of the various methods listed above. For example, some deaf children who use auditory-oral options also learn sign language. Children who use ASL also learn to read and write in English. Combined options can expose children who are deaf or hard-of-hearing to many different ways to communicate with others.

Will my child have a tough time in school?

Just like other children, children who are deaf or hard-of-hearing can develop strong academic, social, and emotional skills and succeed in school. You can do a lot to make sure this happens. Find out how your school system helps children with hearing loss.

With your input, your child's school will develop an Individualized Education Program for your child. Explore programs outside of school that may help you and your child, and talk with other parents who have already dealt with these issues. Remember, the Individuals with Disabilities Education Act ensures that children with hearing loss receive free, appropriate, early intervention services from birth throughout the school years. Consult the U.S. Department of Education, along with other resources below.

Section 4.6

Vaccine Recommendations for Infants and Children

Text in this section is excerpted from "International Travel with Infants & Children," Centers for Disease Control and Prevention (CDC), July 10, 2015.

Vaccinating children for travel requires careful evaluation. Whenever possible, children should complete the routine immunizations of childhood on a normal schedule. However, travel at an earlier age may require accelerated schedules. **Not all travel-related vaccines are effective in infants, and some are specifically contraindicated.**

Country-specific vaccination recommendations and requirements for departure and entry vary over time. For example, at the time of this publication, proof of yellow fever vaccination is required for entry into certain countries. Meningococcal vaccination is required for travelers entering Saudi Arabia for the annual Hajj. The World Health Organization issued temporary vaccination requirements for residents of and long-term visitors to countries with active wild poliovirus transmission.

Modifying the Immunization Schedule for Inadequately Immunized Infants and Younger Children before International Travel

Several factors influence recommendations for the age at which a vaccine is administered, including age-specific risks of the disease and its complications, the ability of people of a given age to develop an adequate immune response to the vaccine, and potential interference with the immune response by passively transferred maternal antibodies.

The routine immunization schedules for infants and children in the United States do not provide specific guidelines for those traveling internationally before the age when specific vaccines and toxoids are routinely recommended. Recommended age limitations are based on potential adverse events (yellow fever vaccine), lack of efficacy data or inadequate immune response (polysaccharide vaccines and influenza vaccine), maternal antibody interference (measles-mumps-rubella [MMR] vaccine), or lack of safety data. In deciding when to travel with a young infant or child, parents should be advised that the earliest opportunity to receive routinely recommended immunizations in the United States (except for the dose of hepatitis B vaccine at birth) is at age 6 weeks.

Routine Infant and Childhood Vaccinations

Children should receive routine vaccination for hepatitis A virus; hepatitis B virus; diphtheria, tetanus, pertussis; *Haemophilus influenzae* type b (Hib); human papillomavirus; influenza; MMR; *Neisseria meningitidis*; polio; rotavirus; *Streptococcus pneumoniae*; and varicella. In order to complete vaccine series before travel, vaccine doses can be administered at the minimum intervals. Parents should be informed that infants and children who have not received all recommended doses might not be fully protected. Rotavirus vaccine is unique among the routine vaccines given to U.S. infants because it has maximum ages for the first and last doses; specific consideration should be given to the timing of an infant's travel so that the infant will still be able to receive the vaccine series, if at all possible.

Travel-specific vaccine considerations include the following:

- **Hepatitis A vaccine:** Although hepatitis A is often not severe in infants and children aged <5 years, infected children may transmit the infection to older children and adults, who are at risk for severe disease. Vaccination should be ensured for all children traveling to areas where there is an intermediate or high risk of hepatitis A. Because of the potential interference by maternal antibodies, the hepatitis A vaccine is not approved for children aged <1 year. The vaccine series consists of 2 doses ≥6 months apart. One dose of monovalent hepatitis A vaccine administered at any time before departure can provide adequate protection for most healthy children. The second dose is necessary for long-term protection.

- **Immune globulin (IG) for hepatitis A protection:** Children aged <1 year or who are allergic to a vaccine component and who are traveling to high-risk areas can receive IG. One dose of 0.02 mL/kg intramuscularly provides protection for up to 3 months, and 1 dose of 0.06 mL/kg IM provides protection for 3–5 months. Children should receive a second dose after 5 months if travel continues. For optimal protection, children aged ≥1 year who are immunocompromised or have chronic medical conditions and who are planning to depart to a high-risk area in <2 weeks should receive the initial dose of vaccine along with IG at a separate anatomic injection site. IG does not interfere with the response to yellow fever vaccine but can interfere with the response to other live injected vaccines (such as MMR and varicella vaccines). Administration of MMR and varicella vaccines should be delayed for >3 months after administration of IG for hepatitis A prophylaxis. IG should not be administered <2 weeks after MMR or varicella vaccines unless the benefits exceed those of vaccination. If IG is given during this time, the child should be revaccinated with the live MMR or varicella vaccines but not sooner than 3 months after IG administration. When travel plans do not allow adequate time to administer live vaccines and IG before travel, the severity of the diseases and their epidemiology at the destination will help determine the course of preparation.

- **Hepatitis B vaccine:** Vaccine can be administered with an accelerated schedule of 4 doses of vaccine given at 0, 1, 2, and 12 months; the last dose may be given on return from travel.

- **Influenza vaccine:** Influenza viruses circulate predominantly in the winter months in temperate regions (typically November–April in the Northern Hemisphere and April–September in the Southern Hemisphere) but can occur year-round in tropical climates. Since influenza viruses may be circulating at any time of the year, travelers aged ≥6 months who were not vaccinated during the influenza season of their country of residence should be vaccinated ≥2 weeks before departure if vaccine is available. Children aged 6 months through 8 years who are receiving influenza vaccine for the first time require 2 doses administered ≥4 weeks apart. For 2014–2015, Advisory Committee on Immunization Practices (ACIP) has recommended that live, attenuated influenza vaccine is preferred for healthy children 2–8 years if it is readily available. Check the CDC website annually for updated recommendations about seasonal influenza vaccination.

- **MMR or MMRV vaccine:** Children traveling abroad may need to be vaccinated at an earlier age than is routinely recommended. Infants aged 6–11 months should receive 1 dose of MMR vaccine before departure, then be vaccinated with MMR or MMRV (measles-mumps-rubella-varicella) vaccine at 12–15 months (≥28 days after the initial dose) and again at 4–6 years, according to the routinely recommended schedule. Children aged ≥12 months need 2 doses of MMR vaccine before traveling overseas. Children who have received 1 dose should receive their second dose before departure, provided the 2 doses are separated by ≥28 days.

- **Meningococcal vaccine:** Epidemics of meningococcal disease, caused by the bacterium *Neisseria meningitidis*, occur in sub-Saharan Africa during the dry season, December through June. CDC recommends that travelers be vaccinated before traveling to this region. Meningococcal vaccination is a requirement to enter Saudi Arabia when traveling to Mecca during the annual Hajj. Health requirements and recommendations for US travelers to the Hajj are available each year on the CDC Travelers' Health website (www.cdc.gov/travel). Meningococcal vaccine is also recommended for children aged 2 months through 18 years who travel to or reside in areas where *N. meningitidis* is hyperendemic or epidemic; for these children, providers should take care to use a meningococcal vaccine that is licensed for the child's age group and contains all 4 serotypes (A, C, Y, W-135). The schedule for the primary series and booster doses varies depending on which meningococcal vaccine is administered (see CDC's Immunization Schedules webpage at www.cdc.gov/vaccines/schedules for additional information).

- **Polio vaccine:** Polio vaccine is recommended for travelers to countries with evidence of wild poliovirus (WPV) circulation (during the last 12 months) and for travelers with a high risk of exposure to someone with imported WPV infection when traveling to some countries that border areas with WPV circulation. Refer to the CDC Travelers' Health website destination pages for the most up-to-date polio vaccine recommendations (wwwnc. cdc.gov/travel/destinations/list). Clinicians should ensure that travelers have completed the recommended age-appropriate polio vaccine series and have received a single lifetime booster dose, if necessary. See Chapter 3, Poliomyelitis and CDC's Immunization Schedules webpage (www.cdc.gov/vaccines/schedules) for information about accelerated schedules for completing the routine series. Young adults (≥18 years of age) who are traveling to areas where polio vaccine is recommended and who have received a routine series with either inactivated polio vaccine (IPV) or live oral polio vaccine in childhood should receive a single lifetime booster dose of IPV before departure. Available data do not indicate the need for more than a single lifetime booster dose with IPV. However, requirements for long-term travelers may apply when departing certain countries.

- In May 2014, the World Health Organization (WHO) declared the international spread of polio to be a Public Health Emergency of International Concern (PHEIC) under the authority of the International Health Regulations (2005). To prevent further spread of disease, WHO issued temporary polio vaccine recommendations for long-term travelers (staying >4 weeks) and residents departing from countries with WPV transmission ("exporting WPV" or "infected with WPV"). Clinicians should be aware that long-term travelers and residents may be required to show proof of polio vaccination when departing from these countries. All polio vaccination administration should be documented on an International Certificate of Vaccination or Prophylaxis

(ICVP). The polio vaccine must be received between 4 weeks and 12 months before the date of departure from the polio-infected country. Country requirements may change, so clinicians should check for updates on the CDC Travelers' Health website.

Other Vaccines

Japanese Encephalitis Vaccine

Japanese encephalitis (JE) virus is transmitted by mosquitoes and is endemic throughout Asia. The risk can be seasonal in temperate climates and year-round in more tropical climates. The risk to short-term travelers and those who confine their travel to urban centers is low. JE vaccine is recommended for travelers who plan to spend a month or longer in endemic areas during the JE virus transmission season. JE vaccine should be considered for short-term (<1 month) travelers whose itinerary or activities might increase their risk for exposure to JE virus.

An inactivated Vero cell culture– derived JE vaccine (Ixiaro [Valneva]) was licensed by the Food and Drug Administration in 2009 for use in the United States for travelers aged ≥17 years. In 2013, the recommendations were expanded and the vaccine was licensed for use in children starting at age 2 months.

The primary series is 2 intramuscular doses administered 28 days apart. For people aged ≥17 years, ACIP recommends that if the primary series was administered >1 year previously, a booster dose may be given before potential JE virus exposures. Although studies are being conducted on the need for a booster dose following a primary series of Ixiaro in children, data are not yet available.

Rabies Vaccine

Rabies virus causes an acute viral encephalitis that is virtually 100% fatal. Traveling children may be at increased risk of rabies exposure, mainly from dogs who roam the streets in developing countries. Bat bites carry a potential risk of rabies throughout the world. There are 2 strategies to prevent rabies in humans:

- Avoiding animal bites or scratches.

- A 3-shot preexposure immunization series on days 0, 7, and 21 or 28. In the event of a subsequent possible rabies virus exposure, the child will require 2 more doses of rabies vaccine on days 0 and 3.

For children who have not received preexposure immunization and may have been exposed to rabies, a weight-based dose of human rabies immune globulin and a series of 4 rabies vaccine injections are required on days 0, 3, 7, and 14.

Typhoid Vaccine

Typhoid fever is caused by the bacterium Salmonella enterica serotype Typhi. Vaccination is recommended for travelers to areas where there is a recognized risk of exposure to Salmonella Typhi.

Two typhoid vaccines are available: Vi capsular polysaccharide vaccine (ViCPS) administered intramuscularly and oral live attenuated vaccine (Ty21a). Both vaccines induce a protective response in 50%–80% of recipients. The ViCPS vaccine can be administered to children who are aged ≥2 years, with a booster dose 2 years later if continued protection is needed. The Ty21a vaccine, which consists of a series of 4 capsules (1 taken every other day) can be administered to children aged ≥6 years. A booster series for Ty21a should be taken every 5 years, if indicated. The capsule cannot be opened for administration but must be swallowed whole. All 4 doses should be taken ≥1 week before potential exposure.

Yellow Fever Vaccine

Yellow fever, a disease transmitted by mosquitoes, is endemic in certain areas of Africa and South America. Infants and children aged ≥9 months can be vaccinated if they travel to countries within the yellow fever–endemic zone.

Infants aged <9 months are at higher risk for developing encephalitis from yellow fever vaccine, which is a live virus vaccine. Studies conducted during the early 1950s identified 4 cases of encephalitis out of 1,000 children aged <6 months vaccinated with yellow fever vaccine. An additional 10 cases of encephalitis associated with yellow fever vaccine administered to infants aged <4 months were reported worldwide during the 1950s.

Travelers with infants aged <9 months should be advised against traveling to areas within the yellow fever–endemic zone. ACIP recommends that yellow fever vaccine never be given to infants aged <6 months. Infants aged 6–8 months should be vaccinated only if they must travel to areas of ongoing epidemic yellow fever and if a high level of protection against mosquito bites is not possible.

Chapter 5

Preventive Care for Children and Adolescents

Chapter Contents

Section 5.1

Recommended Screening Tests for Children and Adolescents

Text in this section is excerpted from "Guide to Clinical Preventive
Services, 2014," Agency for Healthcare Research and Quality
(AHRQ), June 2014.

The U.S. Preventive Services Task Force (USPSTF) recommends
that clinicians discuss these preventive services with eligible patients
and offer them as a priority. All these services have received an "A"
or a "B" (recommended) grade from the Task Force. Refer to the
endnotes for each recommendation for population-specific clinical
considerations.

Table 5.1. Blood Lead Levels in Children and Pregnant Women

Title	Screening for Elevated Blood Lead Levels in Children and Pregnant Women		
Population	Asymptomatic children ages 1 to 5 years who are at increased risk	Asymptomatic children ages 1 to 5 years who are at average risk	Asymptomatic pregnant women
Recommendation	No recommendation. Grade: I (Insufficient Evidence)	Do not screen for elevated blood lead levels. Grade: D	Do not screen for elevated blood lead levels. Grade: D
Risk Assessment	Children younger than age 5 years are at greater risk for elevated blood lead levels and lead toxicity because of increased hand-to-mouth activity, increased lead absorption from the gastrointestinal tract, and the greater vulnerability of the developing central nervous system.		

Table 5.1. Continued

Title	Screening for Elevated Blood Lead Levels in Children and Pregnant Women		
	Risk factors for increased blood lead levels in children and adults include: minority race/ethnicity; urban residence; low income; low educational attainment; older (pre-1950) housing; recent or ongoing home renovation or remodeling; pica; use of ethnic remedies, certain cosmetics, and exposure to lead-glazed pottery; occupational exposure; and recent immigration. Additional risk factors for pregnant women include alcohol use and smoking.		
Screening Tests	Venous sampling accurately detects elevated blood lead levels. Screening questionnaires may be of value in identifying children at risk for elevated blood lead levels, but should be tailored for and validated in specific communities for clinical use.		
Interventions	Treatment options for elevated blood lead levels include residential lead hazard-control efforts (i.e., counseling and education, dust or paint removal, and soil abatement), chelation, and nutritional interventions. Community-based interventions for the prevention of lead exposure are likely to be more effective, and may be more cost-effective, than office-based screening, treatment, and counseling. Relocating children who do not yet have elevated blood lead levels but who live in settings with high lead exposure may be especially helpful.		
Balance of Benefits and Harms	There is not enough evidence to assess the balance between the potential benefits and harms of routine screening for elevated blood lead levels in children at increased risk.	Given the significant potential harms of treatment and residential lead hazard abatement, and no evidence of treatment benefit, the harms of screening for elevated blood lead levels in children at average risk outweigh the benefits.	Given the significant potential harms of treatment and residential lead hazard abatement, and no evidence of treatment benefit, the harms of screening for elevated blood lead levels in asymptomatic pregnant women outweigh the benefits.

Table 5.2. Child Maltreatment

Title	Primary Care Interventions to Prevent Child Maltreatment
Population	**Children and adolescents aged 0 to 18 years without signs or symptoms of maltreatment**
Recommendation	**No recommendation.** **Grade: I (Insufficient Evidence)**
Risk Assessment	There are numerous risk factors associated with child maltreatment, including but not limited to: Young, single, or nonbiological parents. • Parental lack of understanding of children's needs, child development, or parenting skills. • Poor parent child relationships/negative interactions. • Parental thoughts or emotions that support maltreatment behaviors. • Family dysfunction or violence. • Parental history of abuse or neglect in family of origin. • Substance abuse within the family. • Social isolation, poverty, or other socioeconomic disadvantages. • Parental stress and distress.
Interventions	Although the evidence is insufficient to recommend specific preventive interventions, most child maltreatment prevention programs focus on home visitation. Home visitation programs usually comprise a combination of services provided by a nurse or paraprofessional in the family's home on a regularly scheduled basis; most programs are targeted to families with young children and often begin in the prenatal or postnatal period.
Balance of Benefits and Harms	The evidence on interventions in primary care to prevent child maltreatment among children without signs or symptoms of maltreatment is insufficient, and the balance of benefits and harms cannot be determined.
Other Relevant USPSTF Recommendations	The USPSTF has made recommendations on screening for intimate partner violence and abuse of elderly and vulnerable adults. These recommendations are available at http://www.uspreventiveservicestaskforce.org

Table 5.3. Congenital Hypothyroidism

Title	Screening for Congenital Hypothyroidism
Population	All newborn infants
Recommendation	Screening for congenital hypothyroidism (CH). Grade: A
Screening Tests	Two methods of screening are used most frequently in the United States: • Primary TSH with backup T4. • Primary T4 with backup TSH. Screening for congenital hypothyroidism (CH) is mandated in all 50 states and the District of Columbia. Clinicians should become familiar with the tests used in their area and the limitations of the screening strategies employed.
Timing of Screening	Infants should be tested between 2 and 4 days of age. Infants discharged from hospitals before 48 hours of life should be tested immediately before discharge. Specimens obtained in the first 24-48 hours of age may be falsely elevated for TSH regardless of the screening method used.
Suggestions for Practice	Infants with abnormal screens should receive confirmatory testing and begin appropriate treatment with thyroid hormone replacement within 2 weeks after birth. Children with positive confirmatory testing in whom no permanent cause of CH is found should undergo a 30-day trial of reduced or discontinued thyroid hormone replacement therapy to determine if the hypothyroidism is permanent or transient. This trial of reduced or discontinued therapy should take place at some time after the child reaches 3 years of age.
Other Relevant Recommendations from the USPSTF	Additional USPSTF recommendations regarding screening tests for newborns can be accessed at: http://www.uspreventiveservicestaskforce.org/tfchildcat.htm

Table 5.4. Developmental Dysplasia of the Hip

Title	Screening for Developmental Dysplasia of the Hip
Population	**Infants who do not have obvious hip dislocations or other abnormalities evident without screening**
Recommendation	**No recommendation.** **Grade: I (Insufficient Evidence)**
Risk Assessment	Risk factors for developmental dysplasia of the hip include female sex, family history, breech positioning, and in utero postural deformities. However, the majority of cases of developmental dysplasia of the hip have no identifiable risk factors.
Screening Tests	Screening tests for developmental dysplasia of the hip have limited accuracy. The most common methods of screening are serial physical examinations of the hip and lower extremities, using the Barlow and Ortolani procedures, and ultrasonography.
Interventions	Treatments for developmental dysplasia of the hip include both nonsurgical and surgical options. Nonsurgical treatment with abduction devices is used as early treatment and includes the commonly prescribed Pavlik method. Surgical intervention is used when the dysplasia is severe or diagnosed late, or after an unsuccessful trial of nonsurgical treatment. Avascular necrosis of the hip is the most common and most severe potential harm of both surgical and nonsurgical interventions, and can result in growth arrest of the hip and eventual joint destruction, with significant disability.
Balance of Benefits and Harms	The USPSTF was unable to assess the balance of benefits and harms of screening for developmental dysplasia of the hip due to insufficient evidence. There are concerns about the potential harms associated with treatment of infants identified by routine screening.
Other Relevant USPSTF Recommendations	The USPSTF has made recommendations on screening for hyperbilirubinemia, phenylketonuria, sickle cell disease, congenital hypothyroidism, and hearing loss in newborns. These recommendations are available at http://www.uspreventiveservicestaskforce.org

Table 5.5. Gonococcal Ophthalmia Neonatorum

Title	Ocular Prophylaxis for Gonococcal Ophthalmia Neonatorum
Population	All newborn infants
Recommendation	Provide prophylactic ocular topical medication for the prevention of gonococcal ophthalmia neonatorum. Grade: A
Risk Assessment	All newborns should receive prophylaxis. However, some newborns are at increased risk, including those with a maternal history of no prenatal care, sexually transmitted infections, or substance abuse.
Preventive Interventions	Preventive medications include 0.5% erythromycin ophthalmic ointment, 1.0% solution of silver nitrate, and 1.0% tetracycline ointment. All are considered equally effective; however, the latter two are no longer available in the United States.
Timing of Intervention	Within 24 hours after birth.
Other Relevant USPSTF Recommendations	Several recommendations on screening and counseling for infectious diseases and perinatal care can be found at: http://www.uspreventiveservicestaskforce.org

Table 5.6. Hearing Loss in Newborns

Title	Universal Screening for Hearing Loss in Newborns
Population	All newborns
Recommendation	Screen for hearing loss in all newborn infants. Grade: B
Risk Assessment	The prevalence of hearing loss in newborn infants with specific risk indicators is 10 to 20 times higher than in the general population of newborns. Risk indicators associated with permanent bilateral congenital hearing loss include: • Neonatal intensive care unit admission for 2 or more days. • Family history of hereditary childhood sensorineural hearing loss. • Craniofacial abnormalities. • Certain congenital syndromes and infections.

Table 5.6. Continued

Title	Universal Screening for Hearing Loss in Newborns
	Approximately 50% of newborns with permanent bilateral congenital hearing loss do not have any known risk indicators.
Screening Tests	Screening programs should be conducted using a one-step or two-step validated protocol. A frequently-used 2-step screening process involves otoacoustic emissions followed by auditory brain stem response in newborns who fail the first test. Infants with positive screening tests should receive appropriate audiologic evaluation and follow-up after discharge. Procedures for screening and follow-up should be in place for newborns delivered at home, birthing centers, or hospitals without hearing screening facilities.
Timing of Screening	All infants should have hearing screening before one month of age. Infants who do not pass the newborn screening should undergo audiologic and medical evaluation before 3 months of age.
Treatment	Early intervention services for hearing-impaired infants should meet the individualized needs of the infant and family, including acquisition of communication competence, social skills, emotional well-being, and positive self-esteem. Early intervention comprises evaluation for amplification or sensory devices, surgical and medical evaluation, and communication assessment and therapy. Cochlear implants are usually considered for children with severe-to-profound hearing loss only after inadequate response to hearing aids.
Other Relevant USPSTF Recommendations	Additional USPSTF recommendations regarding screening tests for newborns can be accessed at http://www.uspreventiveservicestaskforce.org/recommendations.htm#pediatric

Table 5.7. High Blood Pressure in Children

Title	**Screening for Primary Hypertension in Children and Adolescents**
Population	**Children and adolescents without symptoms of hypertension**
Recommendation	**No recommendation.** **Grade: I (Insufficient Evidence)**
Risk Assessment	The strongest risk factor for primary hypertension in children is elevated body mass index. Other risk factors include low birthweight, male sex, ethnicity, and a family history of hypertension.
Screening Tests	Blood pressure screening with sphygmomanometry in the clinical setting may identify children and adolescents with hypertension with reasonable sensitivity; however, false-positive results may occur with normalization of subsequent blood pressure measurements.
Treatment	Stage 1 hypertension in children is treated with lifestyle and pharmacological interventions; medications are not recommended as first-line therapy.
Balance of Benefits and Harms	The USPSTF found inadequate evidence on the diagnostic accuracy of screening for primary hypertension. The USPSTF also found inadequate evidence on the effectiveness of treatment and the harms of screening or treatment. Therefore, the USPSTF cannot determine the balance of benefits and harms of screening for hypertension in children and adolescents.
Other Relevant USPSTF Recommendations	The USPSTF has made recommendations on screening for lipid disorders in children and adolescents. These recommendations are available athttp://www.uspreventiveservicestaskforce.org

Table 5.8. Hyperbilirubinemia in Infants

Title	**Screening of Infants for Hyperbilirubinemia To Prevent Chronic Bilirubin Encephalopathy**
Population	**Healthy newborn infants ≥35 weeks' gestational age**
Recommendation	**No recommendation** **Grade: I (Insufficient Evidence)**

Table 5.8. Continued

Title	Screening of Infants for Hyperbilirubinemia To Prevent Chronic Bilirubin Encephalopathy
Risk Assessment	Risk factors for hyperbilirubinemia include family history of neonatal jaundice, exclusive breastfeeding, bruising, cephalohematoma, ethnicity (Asian, black), maternal age >25 years, male gender, G6PD deficiency, and gestational age <36 weeks. The specific contribution of these risk factors to chronic bilirubin encephalopathy in healthy children is not well understood.
Importance	Chronic bilirubin encephalopathy is a rare but devastating condition. Not all children with chronic bilirubin encepahalopathy have a history of hyperbilirubinemia.
Balance of Benefits and Harms	Evidence about the benefits and harms of screening is lacking. Therefore, the USPSTF could not determine the balance of benefits and harms of screening newborns for hyperbilirubinemia to prevent chronic bilirubin encephalopathy.
Considerations for Practice	In deciding whether to screen, clinicians should consider the following: • **Potential preventable burden.** Bilirubin encephalopathy is a relatively rare disorder. Hyperbilirubinemia alone does not account for the neurologic condition of chronic bilirubin encephalopathy. There is no known screening test that will reliably identify all infants at risk of developing chronic bilirubin encephalopathy. • **Potential harms.** Potential harms of screening are unmeasured but may be important. Evidence about the potential harms of phototherapy is lacking. Harms of treatment by exchange transfusion may include apnea, bradycardia, cyanosis, vasospasm, thrombosis, necrotizing enterocolitis, and, rarely, death. • **Current practice.** Universal screening is widespread in the United States.
Screening Tests	Screening may consist of risk-factor assessment, measurement of bilirubin level either in serum or by transcutaneous estimation, or a combination of methods.

Table 5.8. Continued

Title	Screening of Infants for Hyperbilirubinemia To Prevent Chronic Bilirubin Encephalopathy
Interventions	Phototherapy is commonly used to treat hyperbilirubinemia. Exchange transfusion is used to treat extreme hyperbilirubinemia.
Relevant USPSTF Recommendations	USPSTF recommendations on screening newborns for hearing loss, congenital hypothyroidism, hemoglobinopathies, and phenylketonuria (PKU) can be found at http://www.uspreventiveservicestaskforce.org

Table 5.9. Illicit and Prescription Drug Use in Children and Adolescents

Title	Primary Care Behavioral Interventions to Reduce Illicit Drug and Nonmedical Pharmaceutical Use in Children and Adolescents
Population	Children and adolescents younger than age 18 years who have not already been diagnosed with a substance use disorder
Recommendation	No recommendation. Grade: I statement
Risk Assessment	While the evidence is insufficient to recommend specific interventions in the primary care setting, those that have been studied include face-to-face counseling, videos, print materials, and interactive computer-based tools. Studies on these interventions were limited and findings on whether interventions significantly improved health outcomes were inconsistent.
Balance of Benefits and Harms	The evidence regarding primary care-based behavioral interventions to prevent or reduce illicit drug and nonmedical pharmaceutical use in children and adolescents is insufficient, and the balance of benefits and harms cannot be determined.

Table 5.9. Continued

Title	Primary Care Behavioral Interventions to Reduce Illicit Drug and Nonmedical Pharmaceutical Use in Children and Adolescents
Other Relevant USPSTF Recommendations	The USPSTF has made recommendations on screening for and interventions to decrease the unhealthy use of other substances, including alcohol and tobacco. These recommendations are available at http://www.uspreventiveservicestaskforce.org

Table 5.10. Iron Deficiency Anemia (Screening)

Title	Part I: Screening for Iron Deficiency Anemia in Children and Pregnant Women	
Population	Asymptomatic children ages 6 to 12 months	Asymptomatic pregnant women
Recommendation	No recommendation Grade: I (Insufficient Evidence)	Screen for iron deficiency anemia. Grade: B
Risk Assessment	Serum hemoglobin or hematocrit is the primary screening test for identifying anemia. Hemoglobin is sensitive for iron deficiency anemia; however, it is not sensitive for iron deficiency because mild deficiency states may not affect hemoglobin levels. Potential harms of screening include false-positive results, anxiety, and cost.	
Screening Tests	Serum hemoglobin or hematocrit is the primary screening test for identifying anemia. Hemoglobin is sensitive for iron deficiency anemia; however, it is not sensitive for iron deficiency because mild deficiency states may not affect hemoglobin levels. Potential harms of screening include false-positive results, anxiety, and cost.	
Interventions	Iron deficiency anemia is usually treated with oral iron preparations. The likelihood that iron deficiency anemia identified by screening will respond to treatment is unclear, because many families do not adhere to treatment and because the rate of spontaneous resolution is high.	

Table 5.10. Continued

Title	Part I: Screening for Iron Deficiency Anemia in Children and Pregnant Women	
Balance of Benefits and Harms	The USPSTF was unable to determine the balance between the benefits and harms of routine screening for iron deficiency anemia in asymptomatic children ages 6 to 12 months.	The benefits of routine screening for iron deficiency anemia in asymptomatic pregnant women outweigh the potential harms.
Other Relevant USPSTF Recommendations	The USPSTF has also made recommendations on screening for blood lead levels in children and pregnant women. These recommendations are available at http://www.uspreventiveservicestaskforce.org	

Table 5.11. Iron Deficiency Anemia (Supplementation)

Title	Part II: Iron Supplementation for Children and Pregnant Women		
Population	Asymptomatic children ages 6 to 12 months who are at increased risk for iron deficiency anemia	Asymptomatic children ages 6 to 12 months who are at average risk for iron deficiency anemia	Pregnant women who are not anemic
Recommendation	Provide routine iron supplementation Grade: B	No recommendation Grade: I (Insufficient Evidence)	No recommendation Grade: I (Insufficient Evidence)
Risk Assessment	A validated risk assessment tool to guide primary care physicians in identifying individuals who would benefit from iron supplementation has not been developed.		

Table 5.11. Continued

Title	Part II: Iron Supplementation for Children and Pregnant Women		
Preventive Medication	Iron supplementation, such as iron-fortified formula or iron supplements, may improve neurodevelopmental outcomes in children at increased risk for iron deficiency anemia. There is poor evidence that it improves neurodevelopmental or health outcomes in other populations. Oral iron supplementation increases the risk for unintentional overdose and gastrointestinal symptoms. Given appropriate protection against overdose, these harms are small.		
Balance of Benefits and Harms	The moderate benefits of iron supplementation in asymptomatic children ages 6 to 12 months who are at increased risk for iron deficiency anemia outweigh the potential harms.	The USPSTF was unable to determine the balance between the benefits and harms of iron supplementation in children ages 6 to 12 months who are at average risk for iron deficiency anemia.	The USPSTF was unable to determine the balance between the benefits and harms of iron supplementation in non-anemic pregnant women.
Other Relevant USPSTF Recommendations	The USPSTF has also made recommendations on folic acid supplementation in women planning or capable of pregnancy and vitamin D supplementation to prevent cancer and fractures. These recommendations are available at http://www.uspreventiveservicestaskforce.org		

Table 5.12. Lipid Disorders in Children

Title	Screening for Lipid Disorders in Children
Population	**Asymptomatic infants, children, adolescents, and young adults (age 20 years or younger)**
Recommendation	**No recommendation** **Grade: I (Insufficient Evidence)**
Risk Assessment	Risk factors for dyslipidemia include overweight, diabetes, and a family history of common familial dyslipidemias (e.g., familial hypercholesterolemia).

Table 5.12. Continued

Title	Screening for Lipid Disorders in Children
Screening Tests	Serum lipid (total cholesterol, high-density and low-density lipoprotein cholesterol) levels are accurate screening tests for childhood dyslipidemia, although many children with multifactorial types of dyslipidemia will have normal lipid levels in adulthood. The use of family history as a screening tool for dyslipidemia has variable accuracy, largely because definitions of a positive family history and lipid threshold values vary substantially.
Interventions	The effectiveness of treatment interventions (diet, exercise, lipid-lowering agents) in improving health outcomes in children with dyslipidemia (including multifactorial dyslipidemia) remains a critical research gap. Potential harms of screening may include labeling of children whose dyslipidemia would not persist into adulthood or cause health problems. Adverse effects from lipid-lowering medications and low-fat diets, including potential long-term harms, have been inadequately evaluated in children.
Balance of Benefits and Harms	The USPSTF was unable to determine the balance between the potential benefits and harms of routinely screening children and adolescents for dyslipidemia.
Other Relevant USPSTF Recommendations	The USPSTF has made recommendations on screening for lipid disorders in adults and screening for carotid artery stenosis, coronary heart disease, high blood pressure, and peripheral arterial disease. These recommendations are available at http://www.uspreventiveservicestaskforce.org

Table 5.13. Major Depressive Disorder in Children and Adolescents

Title	Screening and Treatment for Major Depressive Disorder in Children and Adolescents	
Adolescents (12-18 years)	Children (7-11 years)	
Recommendation	Screen when systems for diagnosis, treatment, and follow-up are in place. Grade: B	No Recommendation Grade: I (Insufficient Evidence)
Risk Assessment	Risk factors for major depressive disorder (MDD) include parental depression, having comorbid mental health or chronic medical conditions, and having experienced a major negative life event.	
Screening Tests	The following screening tests have been shown to do well in teens in primary care settings: • Patient Health Questionnaire for Adolescents (PHQ-A). • Beck Depression Inventory-Primary Care Version (BDI-PC).	Screening instruments perform less well in younger children.
Treatments	Among pharmacotherapies fluoxetine, a selective serotonin reuptake inhibitor (SSRI), has been found efficacious. However, because of risk of suicidality, SSRIs should be considered only if clinical monitoring is possible. Various modes of psychotherapy, and pharmacotherapy combined with psychotherapy, have been found efficacious.	Evidence on the balance of benefits and harms of treatment of younger children is insufficient for a recommendation.

Table 5.14. Obesity in Children and Adolescents

Title	Screening for Obesity in Children and Adolescents
Population	Children and adolescents 6 to 18 years of age
Recommendation	Screen children aged 6 years and older for obesity. Offer or refer for intensive counseling and behavioral interventions. Grade: B
Screening Tests	Body mass index (BMI) is calculated from the weight in kilograms divided by the square of the height in meters. Height and weight, from which BMI is calculated, are routinely measured during health maintenance visits. BMI percentile can be plotted on a chart or obtained from online calculators. Overweight = age- and gender-specific BMI at ≥85th to 94th percentile Obesity = age- and gender-specific BMI at ≥95th percentile
Timing of Screening	No evidence was found on appropriate screening intervals.
Interventions	Refer patients to comprehensive moderate- to high-intensity programs that include dietary, physical activity, and behavioral counseling components.
Balance of Benefits and Harms	Moderate- to high-intensity programs were found to yield modest weight changes. Limited evidence suggests that these improvements can be sustained over the year after treatment. Harms of screening were judged to be minimal.
Other Relevant USPSTF Recommendations	Recommendations on other pediatric and behavioral counseling topics can be found at http://www.uspreventiveservicestaskforce.org

Table 5.15. Phenylketonuria (PKU)

Title	Screening for Phenylketonuria
Population	**All newborn infants**
Recommendation	**Screen for Phenykeltonuria (PKU).** **Grade: A**
Screening Tests	Screening for PKU is mandated in all 50 states. Methods of screening vary. Three main methods are used to screen for PKU in the United States: 1. Guthrie Bacterial Inhibition Assay (BIA) 2. Automated fluorometric assay 3. Tandem mass spectrometry
Timing of Screening	Infants who are tested within the first 24 hours after birth should receive a repeat screening test by 2 weeks of age. Optimal timing of screening for premature infants and infants with illnesses is at or near 7 days of age, but in all cases before discharge from the newborn nursery.
Treatment	It is essential that phenylalanine restrictions be instituted shortly after birth to prevent the neurodevelopmental effects of PKU.
Other Relevant USPSTF Recommendations	Additional USPSTF recommendations regarding screening tests for newborns can be accessed at: http://www.uspreventiveservicestaskforce.org/recommendations.htm#pediatric

Table 5.16. Sickle Cell Disease in Newborns

Title	Screening for Sickle Cell Disease in Newborns
Population	**All newborn infants**
Recommendation	**Screen for sickle cell disease.** **Grade: A**
Screening Tests	Screening for sickle cell disease in newborns is mandated in all 50 states and the District of Columbia. In most states, one of these tests is used for the initial screening: Thin-layer isoelectric focusing (IEF). High performance liquid chromatography (HPLC). Both IEF and HPLC have extremely high sensitivity and specificity for sickle cell anemia.

Table 5.16. Continued

Title	Screening for Sickle Cell Disease in Newborns
Timing of Screening	All newborns should undergo screening regardless of birth setting. Birth attendants should make arrangements for samples to be obtained. The first clinician to see the infant at an office visit should verify screening results. Confirmatory testing should occur no later than 2 months of age.
Treatment	Infants with sickle cell anemia should receive: Prophylactic penicillin starting by age 2 months. Pneumococcal immunizations at recommended intervals.
Other Relevant USPSTF Recommendations	Additional USPSTF recommendations regarding screening tests for newborns can be accessed at http://www.uspreventiveservicestaskforce.org/recommendations.htm#vision.

Table 5.17. Speech and Language Delay

Title	Screening for Speech and Language Delay in Preschool Children
Population	Children ages 5 years and younger who have not already been identified as at increased risk for speech and language delays
Recommendation	No Recommendation Grade: I (Insufficient Evidence)
Risk Assessment	The most consistently reported risk factors include a family history of speech and language delay, male sex, and perinatal factors, such as prematurity and low birth-weight. Other risk factors reported less consistently include levels of parental education, specific childhood illnesses, birth order, and larger family size.

Table 5.17. Continued

Title	Screening for Speech and Language Delay in Preschool Children
Screening Tests	There is insufficient evidence that brief, formal screening instruments that are suitable for use in primary care for assessing speech and language development can accurately identify children who would benefit from further evaluation and intervention.
Balance of Benefits and Harms	The USPSTF could not determine the balance of benefits and harms of using brief, formal screening instruments to screen for speech and language delay in the primary care setting.
Other Relevant USPSTF Recommendations	The USPSTF has also made recommendations on screening for hearing loss in newborns and vision impairment in children ages 1 to 5 years. These recommendations are available at http://www.uspreventiveservicestaskforce.org

Table 5.18. Tobacco Use in Children and Adolescents

Title	Primary Care Interventions to Prevent Tobacco Use in Children and Adolescents
Population	School-aged children and adolescents
Recommendation	Provide interventions to prevent initiation of tobacco use. Grade: B
Risk Assessment	The strongest factors associated with smoking initiation in children and adolescents are parental smoking and parental nicotine dependence. Other factors include low levels of parental monitoring, easy access to cigarettes, perception that peers smoke, and exposure to tobacco promotions.
Behavioral Counseling Interventions	Behavioral counseling interventions, such as face-to-face or phone interaction with a health care provider, print materials, and computer applications, can reduce the risk for smoking initiation in school-aged children and adolescents. The type and intensity of effective behavioral interventions substantially varies.

Table 5.18. Continued

Title	Primary Care Interventions to Prevent Tobacco Use in Children and Adolescents
Balance of Benefits and Harms	There is a moderate net benefit to providing primary care interventions to prevent tobacco use in school-aged children and adolescents.

Table 5.19. Visual Impairment in Children Ages 1–5

Title	Screening for Visual Impairment in Children Ages 1-5	
Population	Children ages 3 to 5 years	Children younger than 3 years of age
Recommendation	Provide vision screening Grade: B	No recommendation Grade: I (Insufficient Evidence)
Screening Tests	Various screening tests are used in primary care to identify visual impairment in children, including: Visual acuity test Stereoacuity test Cover-uncover test Hirschberg light reflex test Autorefraction Photoscreening	
Timing of Screening	No evidence was found regarding appropriate screening intervals.	
Interventions	Primary treatment for amblyopia includes the use of corrective lenses, patching, or atropine therapy of the non-affected eye. Treatment may also consist of a combination of interventions.	
Balance of Benefits and Harms	There is adequate evidence that early treatment of amblyopia in children ages 3 to 5 years leads to improved visual outcomes. There is limited evidence on harms of screening, including psychosocial effects, in children ages 3 years and older. There is inadequate evidence that early treatment of amblyopia in children younger than 3 years of age leads to improved visual outcomes.	

Table 5.19. Continued

Title	Screening for Visual Impairment in Children Ages 1-5
Suggestions for Practice Regarding the I Statement	In deciding whether to refer children younger than 3 years of age for screening, clinicians should consider: *Potential preventable burden*: screening later in the preschool years seems to be as effective as screening earlier *Costs*: initial high costs associated with autorefractors and photoscreeners *Current practice*: typical vision screening includes assessment of visual acuity, strabismus, and stereoacuity; children with positive findings should be referred for a comprehensive ophthalmologist exam

Section 5.2

Child and Teen BMI

Text in this section is excerpted from "About Child & Teen BMI,"
Centers for Disease Control and Prevention (CDC), May 15, 2015.

What is body mass index (BMI)?

Body mass index (BMI) is a person's weight in kilograms divided by the square of height in meters. For children and teens, BMI is age- and sex-specific and is often referred to as BMI-for-age. In children, a high amount of body fat can lead to weight-related diseases and other health issues and being underweight can also put one at risk for health issues.

A high BMI can be an indicator of high body fatness. BMI does not measure body fat directly, but research has shown that BMI is cor-related with more direct measures of body fat, such as skinfold thick-ness measurements, bioelectrical impedance, densitometry (under-water weighing), dual energy X-ray absorptiometry (DXA) and other methods. BMI can be considered an alternative to direct measures of body fat. In general, BMI is an inexpensive and easy-to-perform method of screening for weight categories that may lead to health problems.

How is BMI calculated for children and teens?

Calculating BMI using the BMI Percentile Calculator involves the following steps:

1. Measure height and weight.

2. Use the Child and Teen BMI Calculator (http://nccd.cdc.gov/ dnpabmi/Calculator.aspx) to calculate BMI. The BMI number is calculated using standard formulas.

What is a BMI percentile and how is it interpreted?

After BMI is calculated for children and teens, it is expressed as a percentile which can be obtained from either a graph or a percentile calculator. These percentiles express a child's BMI relative to children in the U.S. who participated in national surveys that were conducted from 1963-65 to 1988-94. Because weight and height change during growth and development, as does their relation to body fatness, a child's BMI must be interpreted relative to other children of the same sex and age.

The BMI-for-age percentile growth charts are the most commonly used indicator to measure the size and growth patterns of children and teens in the United States. BMI-for-age weight status categories and the corresponding percentiles were based on expert committee recommendations and are shown in the following table.

Table 5.20. Weight Status Category versus Percentile Range

Weight Status Category	Percentile Range
Underweight	Less than the 5th percentile
Normal or Healthy Weight	5th percentile to less than the 85th percentile
Overweight	85th to less than the 95th percentile
Obese	Equal to or greater than the 95th percentile

How is BMI used with children and teens?

For children and teens, BMI is not a diagnostic tool and is used to screen for potential weight and health-related issues. For example, a child may have a high BMI for their age and sex, but to determine if excess fat is a problem, a health care provider would need to perform further assessments. These assessments might include skinfold thickness measurements, evaluations of diet, physical activity, family history, and other appropriate health screenings. The American Academy of Pediatrics recommends the use of BMI to screen for overweight and obesity in children beginning at 2 years old. For children under the age of 2 years old, consult the WHO standards.

Is BMI interpreted the same way for children and teens as it is for adults?

BMI is interpreted differently for children and teens even though it is calculated as weight ÷ height. Because there are changes in weight and height with age, as well as their relation to body fatness, BMI levels among children and teens need to be expressed relative to other children of the same sex and age. These percentiles are calculated from the CDC growth charts, which were based on national survey data collected from 1963-65 to 1988-94.

Obesity is defined as a BMI at or above the 95th percentile for children and teens of the same age and sex. For example, a 10-year-old boy of average height (56 inches) who weighs 102 pounds would have a BMI of 22.9 kg/m^2. This would place the boy in the 95th percentile for BMI, and he would be considered to have obesity. This means that the child's BMI is greater than the BMI of 95% of 10-year-old boys in the reference population.

For adults, BMI is interpreted as weight status categories that are not dependent on sex or age.

Why can't healthy weight ranges be provided for children and teens?

Normal or healthy weight weight status is based on BMI between the 5th and 85th percentile on the CDC growth chart. It is difficult to provide healthy weight ranges for children and teens because the interpretation of BMI depends on weight, height, age, and sex.

What are the BMI trends for children and teens in the United States?

The prevalence of children and teens who measure in the 95th percentile or greater on the CDC growth charts has greatly increased over the past 40 years. Recently, however, this trend has leveled off and has even declined in certain age groups.

How can I tell if my child is overweight or obese?

CDC and the American Academy of Pediatrics (AAP) recommend the use of BMI to screen for overweight and obesity in children and teens age 2 through 19 years. For children under the age of 2 years old, consult the WHO standards. Although BMI is used to screen for overweight and obesity in children and teens, BMI is not a diagnostic tool. To determine whether the child has excess fat, further assessment by a trained health professional would be needed.

Can I determine if my child or teen is obese by using an adult BMI calculator?

In general, it's not possible to do this.

The adult calculator provides only the BMI value (weight/height^2) and not the BMI percentile that is needed to interpret BMI among children and teens. It is not appropriate to use the BMI categories for adults to interpret the BMI of children and teens.

However, if a child or teen has a BMI of ≥ 30 kg/m^2, the child is almost certainly obese. A BMI of 30 kg/m^2 is approximately the 95th percentile among 17-year-old girls and 18-year-old boys.

My two children have the same BMI values, but one is considered obese and the other is not. Why is that?

The interpretation of BMI varies by age and sex. So if the children are not the same age and the same sex, the interpretation of BMI has different meanings. For children of different age and sex, the same BMI could represent different BMI percentiles and possibly different weight status categories.

See the following graphic for an example for a 10-year-old boy and a 15-year-old boy who both have a BMI-for-age of 23. (Note that two children of different ages are plotted on the same growth chart to illustrate a point. Normally the measurement for only one child is plotted on a growth chart.)

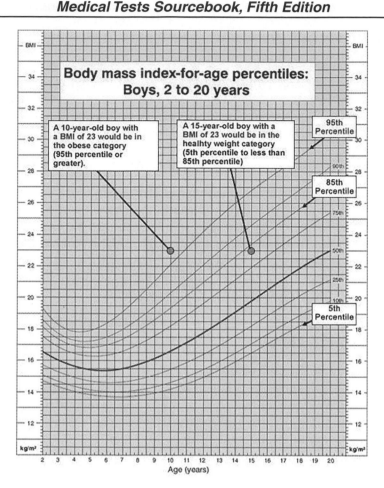

Figure 5.1. Sample BMI numbers would be interpreted for a 10-year-old boy

What are the health consequences of obesity during childhood?

Health risks now

- Childhood obesity can have a harmful effect on the body in a variety of ways.

- High blood pressure and high cholesterol, which are risk factors for cardiovascular disease (CVD). In one study, 70% of obese children had at least one CVD risk factor, and 39% had two or more.

- Increased risk of impaired glucose tolerance, insulin resistance and type 2 diabetes.

- Breathing problems, such as sleep apnea, and asthma.

- Joint problems and musculoskeletal discomfort.

- Fatty liver disease, gallstones, and gastro-esophageal reflux (i.e., heartburn).

- Psychological stress such as depression, behavioral problems, and issues in school.

- Low self-esteem and low self-reported quality of life.

- Impaired social, physical, and emotional functioning.

Health risks later

- Obese children are more likely to become obese adults. Adult obesity is associated with a number of serious health conditions including heart disease, diabetes, and some cancers.

- If children are overweight, obesity in adulthood is likely to be more severe.

Section 5.3

Tips for Parents – Ideas to Help Children Maintain a Healthy Weight

Text in this section is excerpted from "Tips for Parents—Ideas to Help Children Maintain a Healthy Weight," Centers for Disease Control and Prevention (CDC), June 5, 2015.

You've probably read about it in newspapers and seen it on the news: in the United States, the number of obese children and teens has continued to rise over the past two decades. You may wonder: Why are doctors and scientists troubled by this trend? And as parents or other concerned adults, you may also ask: What steps can we take to help prevent obesity in our children? This part provides answers to some of the questions you may have and provides you with resources to help you keep your family healthy.

Why is childhood obesity considered a health problem?

Doctors and scientists are concerned about the rise of obesity in children and youth because obesity may lead to the following health problems:

Heart disease, caused by:

- high cholesterol and/or
- high blood pressure
- Type 2 diabetes
- Asthma
- Sleep apnea
- Social discrimination

Childhood obesity is associated with various health-related consequences. Obese children and adolescents may experience immediate health consequences and may be at risk for weight-related health problems in adulthood.

Psychosocial Risks

Some consequences of childhood and adolescent overweight are psychosocial. Obese children and adolescents are targets of early and systematic social discrimination. The psychological stress of social stigmatization can cause low self-esteem which, in turn, can hinder academic and social functioning, and persist into adulthood.

Cardiovascular Disease Risks

Obese children and teens have been found to have risk factors for cardiovascular disease (CVD), including high cholesterol levels, high blood pressure, and abnormal glucose tolerance. In a population-based sample of 5- to 17-year-olds, almost 60% of overweight children had at least one CVD risk factor while 25 percent of overweight children had two or more CVD risk factors.

Additional Health Risks

Less common health conditions associated with increased weight include asthma, hepatic steatosis, sleep apnea and Type 2 diabetes.

- Asthma is a disease of the lungs in which the airways become blocked or narrowed causing breathing difficulty. Studies have identified an association between childhood overweight and asthma.

- Hepatic steatosis is the fatty degeneration of the liver caused by a high concentration of liver enzymes. Weight reduction causes liver enzymes to normalize.

- Sleep apnea is a less common complication of overweight for children and adolescents. Sleep apnea is a sleep-associated breathing disorder defined as the cessation of breathing during sleep that lasts for at least 10 seconds. Sleep apnea is characterized by loud snoring and labored breathing. During sleep apnea, oxygen levels in the blood can fall dramatically. One study estimated that sleep apnea occurs in about 7% of overweight children.

- Type 2 diabetes is increasingly being reported among children and adolescents who are overweight. While diabetes and glucose intolerance, a precursor of diabetes, are common health effects of adult obesity, only in recent years has Type 2 diabetes begun to emerge as a health-related problem among children and adolescents. Onset of diabetes in children and adolescents can result in advanced complications such as CVD and kidney failure.

In addition, studies have shown that obese children and teens are more likely to become obese as adults.

What can I do as a parent or guardian to help prevent childhood overweight and obesity?

To help your child maintain a healthy weight, balance the calories your child consumes from foods and beverages with the calories your child uses through physical activity and normal growth.

Remember that the goal for overweight and obese children and teens is to reduce the rate of weight gain while allowing normal growth and development. Children and teens should NOT be placed on a weight reduction diet without the consultation of a health care provider.

Balancing Calories: Help Kids Develop Healthy Eating Habits

One part of balancing calories is to eat foods that provide adequate nutrition and an appropriate number of calories. You can help children learn to be aware of what they eat by developing healthy eating habits, looking for ways to make favorite dishes healthier, and reducing calorie-rich temptations.

Encourage healthy eating habits.

There's no great secret to healthy eating. To help your children and family develop healthy eating habits:

- Provide plenty of vegetables, fruits, and whole-grain products.
- Include low-fat or non-fat milk or dairy products.
- Choose lean meats, poultry, fish, lentils, and beans for protein.
- Serve reasonably-sized portions.
- Encourage your family to drink lots of water.
- Limit sugar-sweetened beverages.
- Limit consumption of sugar and saturated fat.

Remember that small changes every day can lead to a recipe for success

Look for ways to make favorite dishes healthier.

The recipes that you may prepare regularly, and that your family enjoys, with just a few changes can be healthier and just as satisfying.

Remove calorie-rich temptations!

Although everything can be enjoyed in moderation, reducing the calorie-rich temptations of high-fat and high-sugar, or salty snacks can also help your children develop healthy eating habits. Instead only allow your children to eat them sometimes, so that they truly will be treats! Here are examples of easy-to-prepare, low-fat and low-sugar treats that are 100 calories or less:

- A medium-size apple
- A medium-size banana
- 1 cup blueberries
- 1 cup grapes
- 1 cup carrots, broccoli, or bell peppers with 2 tbsp. hummus

Balancing Calories: Help Kids Stay Active

Another part of balancing calories is to engage in an appropriate amount of physical activity and avoid too much sedentary time. In addition to being fun for children and teens, regular physical activity has many health benefits, including:

- Strengthening bones
- Decreasing blood pressure
- Reducing stress and anxiety
- Increasing self-esteem
- Helping with weight management

Help kids stay active.

Children and teens should participate in at least 60 minutes of moderate intensity physical activity most days of the week, preferably daily. Remember that children imitate adults. Start adding physical activity to your own daily routine and encourage your child to join you.

Some examples of moderate intensity physical activity include:

- Brisk walking
- Playing tag
- Jumping rope
- Playing soccer
- Swimming
- Dancing

Reduce sedentary time.

In addition to encouraging physical activity, help children avoid too much sedentary time. Although quiet time for reading and homework is fine, limit the time your children watch television, play video games, or surf the web to no more than 2 hours per day. Additionally, the American Academy of Pediatrics (AAP) does not recommend television viewing for children age 2 or younger. Instead, encourage your children to find fun activities to do with family members or on their own that simply involve more activity.

Section 5.4

Screening Test for Child's Vision

Text in this section is excerpted from "Get Your Child's Vision
Checked," Office of Disease Prevention and Health Promotion
(ODPHP), July 10, 2015.

The Basics

It's important for children to have their vision checked at least once
before age 6, even if there aren't any signs of eye problems. Finding
and treating eye problems early on can save a child's sight.

Healthy eyes and vision are very important to a child's development. Growing children constantly use their eyes, both at play and
in the classroom.

What are common eye problems in children?

These common eye problems can be treated if they are found early
enough:

- Lazy eye (amblyopia)

- Crossed eyes (strabismus)

Other conditions – like being nearsighted or farsighted – can be
corrected with glasses or contact lenses. Conditions like these are
called refractive errors.

Is my child at risk for vision problems?

If your family has a history of childhood vision problems, your child
may be more likely to have eye problems. Talk to the doctor about eye
problems in your family.

Eye exams are part of regular checkups.

The doctor will check your child's eyes during each checkup, beginning with your child's first well-baby visit.

Around age 3 or 4, the doctor will give your child a more complete eye exam to make sure her vision is developing normally. If there are any problems, the doctor may send your child to an eye doctor.

Take Action!

Follow these steps to protect your child's vision.

Talk to your child's doctor.

Ask the doctor or nurse if there are any problems with your child's vision.

If the doctor recommends a visit to an eye specialist:

- Ask your child's doctor for the name of an eye doctor who is good with kids.
- Write down any information about your child's vision problem.
- Plan your child's visit to the eye doctor.

What about cost?

Vision screening for kids is covered under the Affordable Care Act, the health care reform law passed in 2010.

- If you have private insurance, your child may be able to get screened at no cost to you. Check with your insurance provider.
- Medicaid and CHIP also cover vision care for kids.

Look out for problems.

Schedule an eye exam for your child if you see signs of an eye problem, like if your child's eyes:

- Are crossed all the time
- Turn out
- Don't focus together
- Are red, crusted, or swollen around the eyelids

Protect your child's eyes.

- Don't let your child play with toys that have sharp edges or points.

- Keep sharp or pointed objects, like knives and scissors, away from your child.

- Protect your child's eyes from the sun. Look for kids' sunglasses that block 100% of UVA and UVB rays.

- Keep chemicals and sprays (like cleaners and bug spray) where kids can't reach them.

- Make sure your child wears the right eye protection for sports.

Help develop your child's vision.

It takes skill to match what we see with what we want to do – like when we want to bounce a ball or read a book.

Here are ways to help your child develop vision skills:

- Read to your child. As you read, let your child see what you are reading.

- Play with your child using a chalkboard, finger paints, or different shaped blocks.

- Take your child to the playground to climb the jungle gym and walk on the balance beam.

- Play catch with your child.

Section 5.5

Get Your Teen Screened for Depression

Text in this section is excerpted from "Get Your Teen Screened for Depression," Office of Disease Prevention and Health Promotion (ODPHP), July 15, 2015.

The Basics

If your child is between ages 12 and 18, ask the doctor about screening (checking) for depression even if you don't see signs of a problem.

Why do I need to get my teen screened for depression?

More than 1 in 10 teens show some signs of depression. Depression can be serious, and most teens with depression don't get the help they need.

The good news is that depression can be treated with counseling or medicine. When you ask the doctor about screening for depression, find out what services are available (like therapy or counseling) in case your teen needs follow-up care.

What is depression?

Teen depression can be a serious mental health problem. If your child is depressed, she may:

- Feel sad or irritable (easily upset) most of the time

- Lose interest in favorite activities

- Have aches and pains for no reason

- Sleep too much or be unable to sleep

- Eat too much or have trouble eating

- Use drugs or alcohol

- Think about death or suicide

It's normal for teens to have mood swings, and it can be hard to tell if your child is just feeling down or if she's depressed. That's why it's so important for all teens to be screened for depression.

What causes depression?

Depression can happen to anyone. It's not your fault or your teen's fault. Some experiences may make it more likely that a teen will develop depression, like:

- Dealing with a big loss, like a death or divorce in the family

- Living with someone who is depressed

- Having another mental health problem, like anxiety or an eating disorder

- Feeling stressed at school or at home

- Having a family history of depression

Teen girls are more likely to get depressed than teen boys.

What happens during a depression screening?

The doctor will ask your teen questions about his feelings and behaviors. This may include asking how often your teen:

- Feels hopeless or sad
- Has low energy or feels tired during the day
- Has trouble paying attention at school
- Eats too much or has trouble eating

Screening for depression usually takes about 5 minutes. It can be done as part of your teen's yearly checkup.

What if the doctor finds signs of depression?

If your child is showing signs of depression, the doctor will:

- Refer your teen to a therapist or doctor with special training in helping young people with emotional or behavioral problems
- Talk about medicines or other treatments that could help your teen with depression
- Order tests to check for other health problems

Make sure to include your teen when you make any decisions about treatment.

Take Action!

Take steps to protect your teen's mental health.

Talk to your teen's doctor about depression screening.

Ask the doctor to screen your child for depression. If you are worried about your teen, be sure to let the doctor know. Find out what services are available in case your teen needs treatment.

What about cost?

Screening for depression is covered under the Affordable Care Act, the health care reform law passed in 2010. Depending on your insurance plan, your teen may be able to get screened at no cost to you. Check with your insurance provider.

If you don't have health insurance, Some programs offer free or low-cost treatment for depression.

Write down any concerns you have.

Keep track of your teen's actions and words that make you think she might be depressed. If you see a change in your child's behavior, make a note about the change and when it happened. Include details like:

- How long the behavior has been going on
- How often the behavior happens
- How serious you think it is

Share these notes with your teen's doctor. You can also use them to start a conversation with your teen.

Watch for signs that your teen may be thinking about suicide.

Most people who are depressed don't attempt suicide, but depression can increase the risk of suicide and suicide attempts. Suicide is the second leading cause of death for people ages 15 to 24.

These behaviors may be signs your teen is thinking about suicide:

- Talking about wanting to kill or hurt himself
- Taking dangerous risks, like driving recklessly
- Spending less and less time with friends and family
- Talking about not being around in the future or "going away"
- Giving away prized possessions
- Increasing the use of alcohol or drugs
- Talking about feeling hopeless, or very angry

If your child is showing some or all of these warning signs, get help right away. Visit the National Suicide Prevention Lifeline or call 1-800-273-TALK (1-800-273-8255) to learn how to help.

If you think your child may be in immediate danger, call 911 or take him to the emergency room.

Find resources for your teen.

If your child isn't ready to talk to you about her feelings, there are still things you can do. Help your teen find resources online and in the community.

Make a list with your teen of other people she can go to with problems or questions – like a teacher, guidance counselor, or adult friend. Tell her about ways she can get information anonymously (without giving her name).

Remind your teen that you are always there if she wants to talk.

Chapter 6

Preventive Care and Screening Test Guidelines for Adults

Chapter Contents

Section 6.1

Recommended Screening Tests for Adults

Text in this section is excerpted from "Guide to Clinical Preventive Services, 2014," Agency for Healthcare Research and Quality (AHRQ), June 2014.

The following tables illustrate various important screening tests recommended for the adults.

Table 6.1. Carotid Artery Stenosis

Title	Screening for Carotid Artery Stenosis
Population	Adult general population [1]
Recommendation	Do not screen with ultrasound or other screening tests. Grade: D
Risk Assessment	The major risk factors for carotid artery stenosis (CAS) include: older age, male gender, hypertension, smoking, hypercholesterolemia, and heart disease. However, accurate, reliable risk assessment tools are not available.
Balance of Benefits and Harms	Harms outweigh benefits. In the general population, screening with carotid duplex ultrasound would result in more false-positive results than true positive results. This would lead either to surgeries that are not indicated or to confirmatory angiography. As the result of these procedures, some people would suffer serious harms (death, stroke, and myocardial infarction) that outweigh the potential benefit surgical treatment may have in preventing stroke.
Other Relevant Recommendations from the USPSTF	Adults should be screened for hypertension, hyperlipidemia, and smoking. Clinicians should discuss aspirin chemoprevention with patients at increased risk for cardiovascular disease. These recommendations and related evidence are available at http://www.uspreventiveservicestaskforce.org

[1] *This recommendation applies to adults without neurological symptoms and without a history of transient ischemic attacks (TIA) or stroke. If otherwise eligible, an individual who has a carotid area TIA should be evaluated promptly for consideration of carotid endarterectomy.*

Table 6.2. Cervical Cancer

Title	Screening for Cervical Cancer					
Population	Women ages 21 to 65	Women ages 30 to 65	Women younger than age 21	Women older than age 65 who have had adequate prior screening and are not high risk	Women after hysterectomy with removal of the cervix and with no history of high-grade precancer or cervical cancer	Women younger than age 30
Recommendation	Screen with cytology (Pap smear) every 3 years. Grade: A	Screen with cytology every 3 years or co-testing (cytology/HPV testing) every 5 years. Grade: A	Do not screen. Grade: D	Do not screen. Grade: D	Do not screen. Grade: D	Do not screen with HPV testing (alone or with cytology) Grade: D
Risk Assessment	Human papillomavirus (HPV) infection is associated with nearly all cases of cervical cancer. Other factors that put a woman at increased risk of cervical cancer include HIV infection, a compromised immune system, in utero exposure to diethylstilbestrol, and previous treatment of a high-grade precancerous lesion or cervical cancer.					

Table 6.2. Continued

Title	Screening for Cervical Cancer				
Screening Tests and Interval	Screening women ages 21 to 65 years every 3 years with cytology provides a reasonable balance between benefits and harms. Screening with cytology more often than every 3 years confers little additional benefit, with large increases in harms. HPV testing combined with cytology (co-testing) every 5 years in women ages 30 to 65 years offers a comparable balance of benefits and harms, and is therefore a reasonable alternative for women in this age group who would prefer to extend the screening interval.				
Timing of Screening	Screening earlier than age 21 years, regardless of sexual history, leads to more harms than benefits. Clinicians and patients should base the decision to end screening on whether the patient meets the criteria for adequate prior testing and appropriate follow-up, per established guidelines.				

Table 6.2. Continued

Title	Screening for Cervical Cancer					
Interventions	Screening aims to identify high-grade precancerous cervical lesions to prevent development of cervical cancer and early-stage asymptomatic invasive cervical cancer. High-grade lesions may be treated with ablative and excisional therapies, including cryotherapy, laser ablation, loop excision, and cold knife conization. Early-stage cervical cancer may be treated with surgery (hysterectomy) or chemoradiation.					
Balance of Benefits and Harms	The benefits of screening with cytology every 3 years substantially outweigh the harms.	The benefits of screening with co-testing (cytology/HPV testing) every 5 years outweigh the harms.	The harms of screening earlier than age 21 years outweigh the benefits.	The benefits of screening after age 65 years do not outweigh the potential harms.	The harms of screening after hysterectomy outweigh the benefits.	The potential harms of screening with HPV testing (alone or with cytology) outweigh the potential benefits.
Other Relevant USPSTF Recommendations	The USPSTF has made recommendations on screening for breast cancer and ovarian cancer, as well as genetic risk assessment and BRCA mutation testing for breast and ovarian cancer susceptibility. These recommendations are available at http://www.uspreventiveservicestaskforce.org/.					

Table 6.3. Chlamydial Infection

Title	Screening for Chlamydial Infection						
opulation	**Non-pregnant women**			**Pregnant women**			**Men**
	24 years and younger	**25 years and older**		**24 years and younger**	**25 years and older**		
	Includes adolescents	Not at increased risk	At increased risk	Includes adolescents	Not at increased risk	At increased risk	
Recommendation	Screen if sexually active Grade A	Do not automatically screen. Grade: C	Screen. Grade: A	Screen. Grade: B	Do not automatically screen. Grade: C	Screen. Grade: B	No recommendation. Grade: I (Insufficient Evidence [1])
Risk Assessment	**Age:** Women and men aged 24 years and younger are at greatest risk. **History of:** Previous Chlamydial infection or other sexually transmitted infections, new or multiple sexual partners, inconsistent condom use, sex work. **Demographics:** African-Americans and Hispanic women and men have higher prevalence rates than the general population in many communities.						

Table 6.3. Continued

Title	Screening for Chlamydial Infection	
Screening Tests	Nucleic acid amplification tests (NAATs) can identify chlamydial infection in asymptomatic women (non-pregnant and pregnant) and asymptomatic men. NAATs have high specificity and sensitivity and can be used with urine and vaginal swabs.	
Screening Intervals	**Non-Pregnant Women** The optimal interval for screening is not known. The CDC recommends that women at increased risk be screened at least annually.[2]	**Pregnant Women** For women 24 years and younger and older women at increased risk: Screen at the first prenatal visit. For patients at continuing risk, or who are newly at risk: Screen in the 3rd trimester.	Not applicable

Table 6.3. Continued

Title	Screening for Chlamydial Infection		
Treatment	The Centers for Disease Control and Prevention has outlined appropriate treatment at: http://www.cdc. gov/STD/treatment. Test and/ or treat partners of patients treated for Chlamydial infection.		

[1] Chlamydial infection results in few sequelae in men. Therefore, the major benefit of screening men would be to reduce the likelihood that infected and untreated men would pass the infection to sexual partners. There is no evidence that screening men reduces the long-term consequences of chlamydial infection in women. Because of this lack of evidence, the USPSTF was not able to assess the balance of benefits and harms, and concluded that the evidence is insufficient to recommend for or against routinely screening men.

[2] Centers for Disease Control and Prevention, Sexually transmitted diseases treatment guidelines, 2006. MMWR 2006. 55(No. RR-11).

Table 6.4. Chronic Kidney Disease

Title	Screening for Chronic Kidney Disease
Population	**Asymptomatic adults without diagnosed chronic kidney disease (CKD)**
Recommendation	**No recommendation** **Grade: I (Insufficient Evidence)**
Risk Assessment	There is no generally accepted risk assessment tool for CKD or risk for complications of CKD. Diabetes and hypertension are well-established risk factors with strong links to CKD. Other risk factors for CKD include older age, cardiovascular disease, obesity, and family history.
Screening Tests	While there is insufficient evidence to recommend routine screening, the tests often suggested for screening that are feasible in primary care include testing the urine for protein (microalbuminuria or macroalbuminuria) and testing the blood for serum creatinine to estimate glomerular filtration rate.
Balance of Harms and Benefits	The USPSTF could not determine the balance between the benefits and harms of screening for CKD in asymptomatic adults.
Relevant USPSTF Recommendations	The USPSTF has made recommendations on screening for diabetes, hypertension, and obesity, as well as aspirin use for the prevention of cardiovascular disease. These recommendations are available at http://www.uspreventiveservicestaskforce.org/

Table 6.5. Chronic Obstructive Pulmonary Disease

Title	Screening for Chronic Obstructive Pulmonary Disease Using Spirometry
Population	**Adult general population**
Recommendation	**Do not screen for chronic obstructive pulmonary disease using spirometry** **Grade: D**
Additional Population Information	This screening recommendation applies to healthy adults who do not recognize or report respiratory symptoms to a clinician. It does not apply to individuals with a family history of alpha-1 antitrypsin deficiency.

Table 6.5. Continued

Title	Screening for Chronic Obstructive Pulmonary Disease Using Spirometry
Risk Assessment	Risk factors for COPD include: Current or past tobacco use. Exposure to occupational and environmental pollutants. Age 40 or older.
Screening Tests [1]	Spirometry can be performed in a primary care physician's office or a pulmonary testing laboratory. The USPSTF did not review evidence comparing the accuracy of spirometry performed in primary care versus referral settings. For individuals who present to clinicians complaining of chronic cough, increased sputum production, wheezing, or dyspnea, spirometry would be indicated as a diagnostic test for COPD, asthma, and other pulmonary diseases.
Other Approaches to the Prevention of Pulmonary Illnesses	These services should be offered to patients regardless of COPD status: All current smokers should receive smoking cessation counseling and be offered pharmacologic therapies demonstrated to increase cessation rates. All patients 50 years of age or older should be offered **influenza immunization** annually. All patients 65 years of age or older should be offered one-time **pneumococcal immunization**.
Other Relevant USPSTF Recommendations	Clinicians should screen all adults for tobacco use and provide tobacco cessation interventions for those who use tobacco products. The USPSTF tobacco cessation counseling recommendation and supporting evidence are available at http://www.uspreventiveservicestaskforce.org/uspstf/uspstbac.htm

[1] *The potential benefit of spirometry-based screening for COPD is prevention of one or more exacerbations by treating patients found to have an airflow obstruction previously undetected. However, even in groups with the greatest prevalence of airflow obstruction, hundreds of patients would need to be screened with spirometry to defer one exacerbation.*

Table 6.6. Cognitive Impairment

Title	Screening for Cognitive Impairment in Older Adults
Population	**Community-dwelling adults who are older than age 65 years and have no signs or symptoms of cognitive impairment**
Recommendation	**No recommendation.** **Grade: I statement**
Risk Assessment	Increasing age is the strongest known risk factor for cognitive impairment. Other reported risk factors for cognitive impairment include cardiovascular risk factors (such as diabetes, tobacco use, hypercholesterolemia, and hypertension), head trauma, learning disabilities (such as Down syndrome), depression, alcohol abuse, physical frailty, low education level, low social support, and having never been married.
Screening Tests	Screening tests for cognitive impairment in the clinical setting generally include asking patients to perform a series of tasks that assess 1 or more cognitive domains (memory, attention, language, and visuospatial or executive functioning). The most widely studied instrument is the Mini-Mental State Examination. Other instruments with more limited evidence include the Clock Draw Test, Mini-Cog, Memory Impairment Screen, Abbreviated Mental Test, Short Portable Mental Status Questionnaire, Free and Cued Selective Reminding Test, 7-Minute Screen, Telephone Interview for Cognitive Status, and Informant Questionnaire on Cognitive Decline in the Elderly.
Treatment	Pharmacologic treatments approved by the U.S. Food and Drug Administration include acetylcholinesterase inhibitors and memantine. Nonpharmacologic interventions include cognitive training, lifestyle behavioral interventions, exercise, educational interventions, and multidisciplinary care interventions. Some interventions focus on the caregiver and aim to improve caregiver morbidity and delay institutionalization of persons with dementia.
Balance of Benefits and Harms	The evidence on screening for cognitive impairment is lacking, and the balance of benefits and harms cannot be determined.
Other Relevant USPSTF Recommendations	The USPSTF has made recommendations related to several of the risk factors for cognitive impairment, including counseling on tobacco cessation, alcohol use, healthful diet, physical activity, and falls prevention and screening for high cholesterol, hypertension, and depression. This recommendation is available at http://www.uspreventiveservicestaskforce.org

Table 6.7. Colorectal Cancer

Title	Screening for Colorectal Cancer		
Population[1]	Adults age 50 to 75	Adults age 76 to 85 years	Adults older than 85
Recommendation	Screen with high sensitivity fecal occult blood testing (FOBT), sigmoidoscopy, or colonoscopy. Grade: A	Do not screen routinely Grade: C	Do not screen Grade: D
	For all populations, evidence is insufficient to assess the benefits and harms of screening with computerized tomography colonography (CTC) and fecal DNA testing. **Grade: I (insufficient evidence)**		
Screening Tests	High sensitivity FOBT, sigmoidoscopy with FOBT, and colonoscopy are effective in decreasing colorectal cancer mortality. The risks and benefits of these screening methods vary. Colonoscopy and flexible sigmoidoscopy (to a lesser degree) entail possible serious complications.		
Screening Test Intervals	Intervals for recommended screening strategies: • Annual screening with high-sensitivity fecal occult blood testing • Sigmoidoscopy every 5 years, with high-sensitivity fecal occult blood testing every 3 years • Screening colonoscopy every 10 years		
Balance of Benefits and Harms	The benefits of screening outweigh the potential harms for 50- to 75-year-olds.	The likelihood that detection and early intervention will yield a mortality benefit declines after age 75 because of the long average time between adenoma development and cancer diagnosis.	
Implementation	Focus on strategies that maximize the number of individuals who get screened. Practice shared decisionmaking; discussions with patients should incorporate information on test quality and availability. Individuals with a personal history of cancer or adenomatous polyps are followed by a surveillance regimen, and screening guidelines are not applicable.		

Table 6.7. Continued

Title	Screening for Colorectal Cancer		
Other Relevant USPSTF Recommendations	The USPSTF recommends against the use of aspirin or nonsteroidal anti-inflammatory drugs for the primary prevention of colorectal cancer. This recommendation is available at http://www.uspreventiveservicestaskforce.org		

[1] *These recommendations do not apply to individuals with specific inherited syndromes (Lynch Syndrome or Familial Adenomatous Polyposis) or those with inflammatory bowel disease.*

Table 6.8. Coronary Heart Disease (Risk Assessment, Nontraditional Risk Factors)

Title	Using Nontraditional Risk Factors In Coronary Heart Disease Risk Assessment
Population	Asymptomatic men and women with no history of coronary heart disease (CHD), diabetes, or any CHD risk equivalent
Recommendation	No recommendation. Grade: I (Insufficient Evidence)
Risk Assessment	This recommendation applies to adult men and women classified at intermediate 10-year risk for CHD (10% to 20%) by traditional risk factors.
Importance	Coronary heart disease (CHD) is the most common cause of death in adults in the United States. Treatment to prevent CHD events by modifying risk factors is currently based on the Framingham risk model. If the classification of individuals at intermediate risk could be improved by using additional risk factors, treatment to prevent CHD might be targeted more effectively. Risk factors not currently part of the Framingham model (nontraditional risk factors) include high sensitivity C-reactive protein (hs-CRP), ankle-brachial index (ABI), leukocyte count. fasting blood glucose level, periodontal disease, carotid intima-media thickness,; electron beam computed tomography,; homocysteine level, and lipoprotein(a) level.

Table 6.8. Continued

Title	Using Nontraditional Risk Factors In Coronary Heart Disease Risk Assessment
Balance of Benefits and Harms	There is insufficient evidence to determine the percentage of intermediate-risk individuals who would be reclassified by screening with nontraditional risk factors, other than hs-CRP and ABI. For individuals reclassified as high-risk on the basis of hs-CRP or ABI scores, data are not available to determine whether they benefit from additional treatments. Little evidence is available to determine the harms of using nontraditional risk factors in screening. Potential harms include lifelong use of medications without proven benefit and psychological and other harms from being misclassified in a higher risk category.
Suggestions for Practice	Clinicians should continue to use the Framingham model to assess CHD risk and guide risk-based preventive therapy. Adding nontraditional risk factors to CHD assessment would require additional patient and clinical staff time and effort. Routinely screening with nontraditional risk factors could result in lost opportunities to provide other important health services of proven benefit.
Other Relevant USPSTF Recommendations	USPSTF recommendations on risk assessment for CHD, the use of aspirin to prevent cardiovascular disease, and screening for high blood pressure can be accessed at http://www.uspreventiveservicestaskforce.org

Table 6.9. Coronary Heart Disease (Electrocardiography)

Title	Screening for Coronary Heart Disease with Electrocardiography	
Population	Asymptomatic adults at low risk for coronary heart disease (CHD) events	Asymptomatic adults at intermediate or high risk for CHD events
Recommendation	Do not screen with resting or exercise electrocardiography (ECG). Grade: D	No recommendation. Grade: I (Insufficient Evidence)

Table 6.9. Continued

Title	Screening for Coronary Heart Disease with Electrocardiography	
Risk Assessment	Several factors are associated with a higher risk for CHD events, including older age, male sex, high blood pressure, smoking, abnormal lipid levels, diabetes, obesity, and sedentary lifestyle. Calculators are available to ascertain a person's 10-year risk for a CHD event. Persons with a 10-year risk >20% are considered to be high-risk, those with a 10-year risk <10% are considered to be low-risk, and those in the 10%–20% range are considered to be intermediate-risk.	
Screening Tests	Several abnormalities on resting and exercise ECG are associated with an increased risk for a serious CHD event. However, the incremental information offered by screening asymptomatic adults at low risk for a CHD event with resting or exercise ECG (beyond that obtained with conventional CHD risk factors) is highly unlikely to result in changes in risk stratification that would prompt interventions and ultimately reduce CHD-related events.	
Balance of Harms and Benefits	The potential harms of screening for CHD with exercise or resting ECG equal or exceed the potential benefits in this population.	The USPSTF could not determine the balance between the benefits and harms of screening for CHD with resting or exercise ECG in this population.
Other Relevant USPSTF Recommendations	The USPSTF has made recommendations on screening for carotid artery stenosis, high blood pressure, lipid disorders, peripheral arterial disease, and obesity. These recommendations are available at http://www.uspreventiveservicestaskforce.org	

109

Table 6.10. Depression in Adults

Title	Screening for Depression in Adults	
Population	Nonpregnant adults 18 years or older	
Recommendation	Screen when staff-assisted depression care supports are in place to assure accurate diagnosis, effective treatment, and follow-up. **Grade: B**	Do not routinely screen when staff-assisted depression care supports are not in place. **Grade: C**
Risk Assessment	Persons at increased risk for depression are considered at risk throughout their lifetime. Groups at increased risk include persons with other psychiatric disorders, including substance misuse; persons with a family history of depression; persons with chronic medical diseases; and persons who are unemployed or of lower socioeconomic status. Also, women are at increased risk compared with men. However, the presence of risk factors alone cannot distinguish depressed patients from nondepressed patients.	
Screening Tests	Simple screening questions may perform as well as more complex instruments. Any positive screening test result should trigger a full diagnostic interview using standard diagnostic criteria.	
Timing of Screening	The optimal interval for screening is unknown. In older adults, significant depressive symptoms are associated with common life events, including medical illness, cognitive decline, bereavement, and institutional placement in residential or inpatient settings.	
Balance of Benefits and Harms		Limited evidence suggests that screening for depression in the absence of staff-assisted depression care does not improve depression outcomes.

Table 6.10. Continued

Title	Screening for Depression in Adults
Suggestions for Practice	"Staff-assisted depression care supports" refers to clinical staff that assists the primary care clinician by providing some direct depression care and/or coordination, case management, or mental health treatment.
Relevant USPSTF Recommendations	Related USPSTF recommendations on screening for suicidality and screening children and adolescents for depression are available at http://www.uspreventiveservicestaskforce.org.

Table 6.11. Diabetes Mellitus

Title	Screening for Type 2 Diabetes Mellitus in Adults	
Population	**Asymptomatic adults with sustained blood pressure greater than 135/80 mm Hg**	**Asymptomatic adults with sustained blood pressure 135/80 mm Hg or lower**
Recommendation	**Screen for type 2 diabetes mellitus Grade: B**	**No recommendation Grade: I (Insufficient Evidence)**
Risk Assessment	These recommendations apply to adults with no symptoms of type 2 diabetes mellitus or evidence of possible complications of diabetes. Blood pressure measurement is an important predictor of cardiovascular complications in people with type 2 diabetes mellitus. The first step in applying this recommendation should be measurement of blood pressure (BP). Adults with treated or untreated BP >135/80 mm Hg should be screened for diabetes.	
Screening Tests	Three tests have been used to screen for diabetes: • Fasting plasma glucose (FPG). • 2-hour postload plasma. • Hemoglobin A1c. The American Diabetes Association (ADA) recommends screening with FPG, defines diabetes as FPG $\geq$ 126 mg/dL, and recommends confirmation with a repeated screening test on a separate day.	

Table 6.11. Continued

Title	Screening for Type 2 Diabetes Mellitus in Adults
Screening Intervals	The optimal screening interval is not known. The ADA, on the basis of expert opinion, recommends an interval of every 3 years.
Suggestions for practice regarding insufficient evidence	When BP is ≤ 135/80 mm Hg, screening may be considered on an individual basis when knowledge of diabetes status would help inform decisions about coronary heart disease (CHD) preventive strategies, including consideration of lipid-lowering agents or aspirin. To determine whether screening would be helpful on an individual basis, information about 10-year CHD risk must be considered. For example, if CHD risk without diabetes was 17% and risk with diabetes was >20%, screening for diabetes would be helpful because diabetes status would determine lipid treatment. In contrast, if risk without diabetes was 10% and risk with diabetes was 15%, screening would not affect the decision to use lipid-lowering treatment.
Other relevant information from the USPSTF and the Community Preventive Services Task Force	Evidence and USPSTF recommendations regarding blood pressure, diet, physical activity, and obesity are available at http://www.uspreventiveservicestaskforce.org. The reviews and recommendations of the Task Force on Community Preventive Services may be found at http://www.thecommunityguide.org

Table 6.12. Falls in Older Adults

Title	Prevention of Falls in Community-Dwelling Older Adults	
Population	Community-dwelling adults aged 65 years and older who are at increased risk for falls	Community-dwelling adults aged 65 years and older
Recommendation	Provide intervention consisting of exercise or physical therapy and/or vitamin D supplementation to prevent falls. Grade: B	Do not automatically perform an in-depth multifactorial risk assessment with comprehensive management of identified risks to prevent falls. Grade: C

Table 6.12. Continued

Title	Prevention of Falls in Community-Dwelling Older Adults	
Risk Assessment	Primary care clinicians can consider the following factors to identify older adults at increased risk for falls: a history of falls, a history of mobility problems, and poor performance on the timed Get-Up-and-Go test.	
Interventions	Effective exercise and physical therapy interventions include group classes and at-home physiotherapy strategies and range in intensity from very low ($\leq$9 hours) to high (>75 hours). Benefit from vitamin D supplementation occurs by 12 months; the efficacy of treatment of shorter duration is unknown. The recommended daily allowance for vitamin D is 600 IU for adults aged 51 to 70 years and 800 IU for adults older than 70 years. Comprehensive multifactorial assessment and management interventions include assessment of multiple risk factors for falls and providing medical and social care to address factors identified during the assessment. In determining whether this service is appropriate in individual cases, patients and clinicians should consider the balance of benefits and harms on the basis of the circumstances of prior falls, medical comorbid conditions, and patient values.	
Balance of Harms and Benefits	Exercise or physical therapy and vitamin D supplementation have a moderate benefit in preventing falls in older adults.	Multifactorial risk assessment with comprehensive management of identified risks has at least a small benefit in preventing falls in older adults.
Other Relevant USPSTF Recommendations	Recommendations on screening for other types of cancer can be found at http://www.uspreventiveservicestaskforce.org	

Table 6.13. Folic Acid Supplementation

Title	**Folic Acid for the Prevention of Neural Tube Defects**
Population	**Women planning a pregnancy or capable of becoming pregnant**
Recommendation	**Take a daily vitamin supplement containing 0.4 to 0.8 mg (400 to 800 µg) of folic acid.** **Grade: A**

Table 6.13. Continued

Title	Folic Acid for the Prevention of Neural Tube Defects
Risk Assessment	Risk factors include: • A personal or family history of a pregnancy affected by a neural tube defect • The use of certain antiseizure medications • Mutations in folate-related enzymes • Maternal diabetes • Maternal obesity **Note:** This recommendation does not apply to women who have had a previous pregnancy affected by neural tube defects or women taking certain antiseizure medicines. These women may be advised to take higher doses of folic acid.
Timing of Medication	Start supplementation at least 1 month before conception. Continue through first 2 to 3 months of pregnancy.
Recommendations of Others	ACOG, AAFP, and most other organizations recommend 4 mg/d for women with a history of a pregnancy affected by a neural tube defect.
Abbreviations: *AAFP = American Academy of Family Physicians; ACOG = American College of Obstetricians and Gynecologists.*	

Section 6.2

Facts on Adult BMI

Text in this section is excerpted from "About Adult BMI," Centers for Disease Control and Prevention (CDC), May 15, 2015.

What is BMI?

BMI is a person's weight in kilograms divided by the square of height in meters. BMI does not measure body fat directly, but research has shown that BMI is moderately correlated with more direct measures of body fat obtained from skinfold thickness measurements, bioelectrical impedance, densitometry (underwater weighing), dual energy X-ray absorptiometry (DXA) and other methods. Furthermore,

BMI appears to be as strongly correlated with various metabolic and disease outcome as are these more direct measures of body fatness. In general, BMI is an inexpensive and easy-to-perform method of screening for weight category, for example underweight, normal or healthy weight, overweight, and obesity.

How is BMI used?

A high BMI can be an indicator of high body fatness. BMI can be used as a screening tool but is not diagnostic of the body fatness or health of an individual.

To determine if a high BMI is a health risk, a healthcare provider would need to perform further assessments. These assessments might include skinfold thickness measurements, evaluations of diet, physical activity, family history, and other appropriate health screenings.

What are the BMI trends for adults in the United States?

The prevalence of adult BMI greater than or equal to 30 kg/m^2 (obese status) has greatly increased since the 1970s. Recently, however, this trend has leveled off, except for older women. Obesity has continued to increase in adult women who are age 60 years and older.

Why is BMI used to measure overweight and obesity?

BMI can be used for population assessment of overweight and obesity. Because calculation requires only height and weight, it is inexpensive and easy to use for clinicians and for the general public. BMI can be used as a screening tool for body fatness but is not diagnostic.

What are some of the other ways to assess excess body fatness besides BMI?

Other methods to measure body fatness include skinfold thickness measurements (with calipers), underwater weighing, bioelectrical impedance, dual-energy X-ray absorptiometry (DXA), and isotope dilution. However, these methods are not always readily available, and they are either expensive or need to be conducted by highly trained personnel. Furthermore, many of these methods can be difficult to standardize across observers or machines, complicating comparisons across studies and time periods.

How is BMI calculated?

BMI is calculated the same way for both adults and children. The calculation is based on the following formulas:

Table 6.14. BMI Formula and Calculation

Measurement Units	Formula and Calculation
Kilograms and meters (or centimeters)	Formula: weight (kg) / [height (m)]2 With the metric system, the formula for BMI is weight in kilograms divided by height in meters squared. Because height is commonly measured in centimeters, divide height in centimeters by 100 to obtain height in meters. Example: Weight = 68 kg, Height = 165 cm (1.65 m) Calculation: 68 ÷ (1.65)2 = 24.98
Pounds and inches	Formula: weight (lb) / [height (in)]2 x 703 Calculate BMI by dividing weight in pounds (lbs) by height in inches (in) squared and multiplying by a conversion factor of 703. Example: Weight = 150 lbs, Height = 5'5" (65") Calculation: [150 ÷ (65)2] x 703 = 24.96

How is BMI interpreted for adults?

For adults 20 years old and older, BMI is interpreted using standard weight status categories. These categories are the same for men and women of all body types and ages.

The standard weight status categories associated with BMI ranges for adults are shown in the following table.

Table 6.15. BMI and Weight Status

BMI	Weight Status
Below 18.5	Underweight
18.5 – 24.9	Normal or Healthy Weight
25.0 – 29.9	Overweight
30.0 and Above	Obese

For example, here are the weight ranges, the corresponding BMI ranges, and the weight status categories for a person who is 5' 9".

Table 6.16. Weight ranges, BMI ranges and weight status for a 5' 9" person

Height	Weight Range	BMI	Weight Status
5' 9"	124 lbs or less	Below 18.5	Underweight
	125 lbs to 168 lbs	18.5 to 24.9	Normal or Healthy Weight
	169 lbs to 202 lbs	25.0 to 29.9	Overweight
	203 lbs or more	30 or higher	Obese

For children and teens, the interpretation of BMI depends upon age and sex.

Is BMI interpreted the same way for children and teens as it is for adults?

BMI is interpreted differently for children and teens, even though it is calculated using the same formula as adult BMI. Children and teen's BMI need to be age and sex-specific because the amount of body fat changes with age and the amount of body fat differs between girls and boys. The CDC BMI-for-age growth charts take into account these differences and visually show BMI as a percentile ranking. These percentiles were determined using representative data of the U.S. population of 2- to 19-year-olds that was collected in various surveys from 1963-65 to 1988-94.

Obesity among 2- to 19-year-olds is defined as a BMI at or above the 95th percentile of children of the same age and sex in this 1963 to 1994 reference population. For example, a 10-year-old boy of average height (56 inches) who weighs 102 pounds would have a BMI of 22.9 kg/m². This would place the boy in the 95th percentile for BMI – meaning that his BMI is greater than that of 95% of similarly aged boys in this reference population – and he would be considered to have obesity.

How good is BMI as an indicator of body fatness?

The correlation between the BMI and body fatness is fairly strong, but even if 2 people have the same BMI, their level of body fatness may differ. In general,

- At the same BMI, women tend to have more body fat than men.

- At the same BMI, Blacks have less body fat than do Whites, and Asians have more body fat than do Whites

- At the same BMI, older people, on average, tend to have more body fat than younger adults.

- At the same BMI, athletes have less body fat than do non-athletes.

The accuracy of BMI as an indicator of body fatness also appears to be higher in persons with higher levels of BMI and body fatness. While, a person with a very high BMI (e.g., 35 kg/m^2) is very likely to have high body fat, a relatively high BMI can be the results of either high body fat or high lean body mass (muscle and bone). A trained healthcare provider should perform appropriate health assessments in order to evaluate an individual's health status and risks.

If an athlete or other person with a lot of muscle has a BMI over 25, is that person still considered to be overweight?

According to the BMI weight status categories, anyone with a BMI between 25 and 29.9 would be classified as overweight and anyone with a BMI over 30 would be classified as obese.

However, athletes may have a high BMI because of increased muscularity rather than increased body fatness. In general, a person who has a high BMI is likely to have body fatness and would be considered to be overweight or obese, but this may not apply to athletes. A trained healthcare provider should perform appropriate health assessments in order to evaluate an individual's health status and risks.

What are the health consequences of obesity for adults?

People who are obese are at increased risk for many diseases and health conditions, including the following:

- All-causes of death (mortality)

- High blood pressure (Hypertension)

- High LDL cholesterol, low HDL cholesterol, or high levels of triglycerides (Dyslipidemia)

- Type 2 diabetes

- Coronary heart disease

- Stroke

- Gallbladder disease

- Osteoarthritis (a breakdown of cartilage and bone within a joint)

- Sleep apnea and breathing problems

- Chronic inflammation and increased oxidative stress

- Some cancers (endometrial, breast, colon, kidney, gallbladder, and liver)

- Low quality of life

- Mental illness such as clinical depression, anxiety, and other mental disorders

- Body pain and difficulty with physical functioning

Section 6.3

Tips for Adults – Preventing Weight Gain and Importance of Physical Activity

Text in this section begins with excerpts from "Preventing Weight Gain," Centers for Disease Control and Prevention (CDC), May 15, 2015.

Text in this section beginning with "Why is physical activity important?" is excerpted from "Physical Activity for a Healthy Weight," Centers for Disease Control and Prevention (CDC), May 15, 2015.

Preventing Weight Gain

If you're currently at a healthy weight, you're already one step ahead of the game. To stay at a healthy weight, it's worth doing a little planning now.

Or maybe you are overweight but aren't ready to lose weight yet. If this is the case, preventing further weight gain is a worthy goal.

As people age, their body composition gradually shifts—the proportion of muscle decreases and the proportion of fat increases. This shift slows their metabolism, making it easier to gain weight. In addition, some people become less physically active as they get older, increasing the risk of weight gain.

The good news is that weight gain can be prevented by choosing a lifestyle that includes good eating habits and daily physical activity. By avoiding weight gain, you avoid higher risks of many chronic diseases, such as heart disease, stroke, type 2 diabetes, high blood pressure, osteoarthritis, and some forms of cancer.

Choosing an Eating Plan to Prevent Weight Gain

So, how do you choose a healthful eating plan that will enable you to maintain your current weight? The goal is to make a habit out of choosing foods that are nutritious and healthful.

If your goal is to prevent weight gain, then you'll want to choose foods that supply you with the appropriate number of calories to maintain your weight. This number varies from person to person. It depends on many factors, including your height, weight, age, sex, and activity level.

Get Moving!

In addition to a healthy eating plan, an active lifestyle will help you maintain your weight. By choosing to add more physical activity to your day, you'll increase the amount of calories your body burns. This makes it more likely you'll maintain your weight.

Although physical activity is an integral part of weight management, it's also a vital part of health in general. Regular physical activity can reduce your risk for many chronic diseases and it can help keep your body healthy and strong.

Self-monitoring

You may also find it helpful to weigh yourself on a regular basis. If you see a few pounds creeping on, take the time to examine your lifestyle. With these strategies, you make it more likely that you'll catch small weight gains more quickly.

Ask yourself—

• Has my activity level changed?

• Am I eating more than usual? You may find it helpful to keep a food diary for a few days to make you more aware of your eating choices.

If you ask yourself these questions and find that you've decreased your activity level or made some poor food choices, make a commitment to yourself to get back on track. Set some reasonable goals to help you get more physical activity and make better food choices.

Why is physical activity important?

Regular physical activity is important for good health, and it's especially important if you're trying to lose weight or to maintain a healthy weight.

- When losing weight, more physical activity increases the number of calories your body uses for energy or "burns off." The burning of calories through physical activity, combined with reducing the number of calories you eat, creates a "calorie deficit" that results in weight loss.

- Most weight loss occurs because of decreased caloric intake. However, evidence shows the only way to *maintain* weight loss is to be engaged in regular physical activity.

- Most importantly, physical activity reduces risks of cardiovascular disease and diabetes beyond that produced by weight reduction alone.

Physical activity also helps to—

- Maintain weight.
- Reduce high blood pressure.
- Reduce risk for type 2 diabetes, heart attack, stroke, and several forms of cancer.
- Reduce arthritis pain and associated disability.
- Reduce risk for osteoporosis and falls.
- Reduce symptoms of depression and anxiety.

How much physical activity do I need?

When it comes to weight management, people vary greatly in how much physical activity they need. Here are some guidelines to follow:

To maintain your weight: Work your way up to 150 minutes of moderate-intensity aerobic activity, 75 minutes of vigorous-intensity aerobic activity, or an equivalent mix of the two each week. Strong scientific evidence shows that physical activity can help you maintain your weight over time. However, the exact amount of physical activity needed to do this is not clear since it varies greatly from person to person. It's possible that you may need to do more than the equivalent of 150 minutes of moderate-intensity activity a week to maintain your weight.

To lose weight and keep it off: You will need a high amount of physical activity unless you also adjust your diet and reduce the amount of calories you're eating and drinking. Getting to and staying at a healthy weight requires both regular physical activity and a healthy eating plan.

What do moderate- and vigorous-intensity mean?

Moderate: While performing the physical activity, if your breathing and heart rate is noticeably faster but you can still carry on a conversation—it's probably moderately intense. Examples include
Walking briskly (a 15-minute mile).

- Light yard work (raking/bagging leaves or using a lawn mower).
- Light snow shoveling.
- Actively playing with children.
- Biking at a casual pace.

Vigorous: Your heart rate is increased substantially and you are breathing too hard and fast to have a conversation, it's probably vigorously intense. Examples include

- Jogging/running.
- Swimming laps.
- Rollerblading/inline skating at a brisk pace.
- Cross-country skiing.
- Most competitive sports (football, basketball, or soccer).
- Jumping rope.

How many calories are used in typical activities?

The following table shows calories used in common physical activities at both moderate and vigorous levels.

Table 6.17. Physical Activity and Calorie Used

Calories Used per Hour in Common Physical Activities		
Moderate Physical Activity	**Approximate Calories/30 Minutes for a 154 lb Person**[1]	**Approximate Calories/ Hr for a 154 lb Person**[1]
Hiking	185	370
Light gardening/yard work	165	330
Dancing	165	330
Golf (walking and carrying clubs)	165	330
Bicycling (<10 mph)	145	290
Walking (3.5 mph)	140	280
Weight lifting (general light workout)	110	220
Stretching	90	180
Vigorous Physical Activity	**Approximate Calories/30 Minutes for a 154 lb Person**[1]	**Approximate Calories/ Hr for a 154 lb Person**[1]
Running/jogging (5 mph)	295	590
Bicycling (>10 mph)	295	590
Swimming (slow freestyle laps)	255	510
Aerobics	240	480
Walking (4.5 mph)	230	460
Heavy yard work (chopping wood)	220	440
Weight lifting (vigorous effort)	220	440
Basketball (vigorous)	220	440

[1] *Calories burned per hour will be higher for persons who weigh more than 154 lbs (70 kg) and lower for persons who weigh less.*

Section 6.4

Get Your Blood Pressure Checked

Text in this section is excerpted from "Get Your Blood Pressure
Checked," Office of Disease Prevention and Health Promotion
(ODPHP), July 15, 2015.

The Basics

Check your blood pressure at least every 2 years starting at age
18. It's important to check your blood pressure often, especially if you
are over age 40.

What is blood pressure?

Blood pressure is how hard your blood pushes against the walls of
your arteries when your heart pumps blood.

Arteries are the tubes that carry blood away from your heart. Every
time your heart beats, it pumps blood through your arteries to the rest
of your body.

What is hypertension?

Hypertension is the medical term for high blood pressure. High
blood pressure has no signs or symptoms. The only way to know if you
have high blood pressure is to get tested.

By taking steps to lower your blood pressure, you can reduce your
risk of heart disease, stroke, and kidney failure. Lowering your blood
pressure can help you live a longer, healthier life.

How can I get my blood pressure checked?

To test your blood pressure, a nurse or doctor will put a cuff around
your upper arm and pump up the cuff with air until it feels tight. Then
the nurse or doctor will slowly let the air out.

This usually takes less than a minute. The nurse or doctor can
tell you what your blood pressure numbers are right after the test
is over.

You can also check your own blood pressure with a blood pressure machine. You can find blood pressure machines in shopping malls, pharmacies, and grocery stores.

What do blood pressure numbers mean?

A blood pressure test measures how hard your heart is working to pump blood through your body.

Blood pressure is measured with two numbers. The first number is the pressure in your arteries when your heart beats. The second number is the pressure in your arteries between each beat, when your heart relaxes.

Compare your blood pressure to these numbers:

- Normal blood pressure is lower than 120/80 (said "120 over 80").

- High blood pressure is 140/90 or higher.

- Blood pressure that's between normal and high (for example, 130/85) is called prehypertension, or high normal blood pressure.

Am I at risk for high blood pressure?

One in 3 Americans has high blood pressure. As you get older, your risk of high blood pressure increases. You are also at higher risk for high blood pressure if you:

- Are overweight or obese
- Are African American
- Have a family history of high blood pressure
- Eat foods high in sodium (salt)
- Get less than 30 minutes of physical activity on most days

These things may also increase your risk of high blood pressure:

- Drinking too much alcohol
- Having chronic (ongoing) stress
- Smoking

How can high blood pressure affect pregnancy?

High blood pressure can be dangerous for a pregnant woman and her unborn baby. If you have high blood pressure and you want to get pregnant, it's important to take steps to lower your blood pressure first.

Sometimes, women get high blood pressure for the first time during pregnancy. This is called gestational hypertension. Usually, this type of high blood pressure goes away after the baby is born.

If you have high blood pressure while you are pregnant, be sure to visit your doctor regularly.

What if I have high blood pressure?

If you have high blood pressure, talk to a doctor. You may need medicine to control your blood pressure.

Take these steps to lower your blood pressure:

- **Eat healthy foods** that are low in saturated fat and sodium (salt).

- **Get active**. Aim for 2 hours and 30 minutes a week of moderate aerobic activity.

- **Watch your weight** by eating healthy and getting active.

- **Remember to take medicines** as prescribed (ordered) by your doctor.

Small changes can add up. For example, losing just 10 pounds can help lower your blood pressure.

Take Action!

Take steps to prevent or lower high blood pressure. To start, get your blood pressure checked as soon as possible.

Check your blood pressure regularly.

Ask a doctor or nurse to check your blood pressure at your next visit.

You can also find blood pressure machines at many shopping malls, pharmacies, and grocery stores. Most of these machines are free to use.

What about the cost of testing?

Blood pressure testing is covered under the Affordable Care Act, the health care reform law passed in 2010. Depending on your insurance, you may be able to get your blood pressure checked by a doctor or nurse at no cost to you.

Check with your insurance provider to find out what's included in your plan.

Eat less sodium.

Eating less sodium (salt) can lower your blood pressure. Look for foods that say "low sodium," "reduced sodium," or "no salt added."

Choose foods with 5% or less of the Daily Value of sodium. Foods with a DV of 20% or more are high in sodium.

Eating more potassium can also help lower your blood pressure. Good sources of potassium include potatoes, cantaloupe, bananas, beans, and yogurt.

Get active.

Getting regular physical activity can reduce your risk of high blood pressure. Aim for 2 hours and 30 minutes a week of moderate activity, like:

- Walking fast
- Dancing
- Riding bikes
- Swimming
- Aerobics

Drink alcohol only in moderation.

If you choose to drink alcohol, limit your drinking to no more than 1 drink a day for women and no more than 2 drinks a day for men.

Manage your stress.

Managing stress can help prevent and control high blood pressure. Deep breathing and meditation are good ways to relax and manage stress.

Quit smoking.

Smoking damages your heart and blood vessels. Quit smoking to help lower your risk of high blood pressure and heart disease.

Section 6.5

Talk with Your Doctor about Depression

Text in this section is excerpted from "Talk with Your Doctor about
Depression," Office of Disease Prevention and Health Promotion
(ODPHP), July 16, 2015.

The Basics

If you think you might be depressed, talk with a doctor about how
you are feeling.

What is depression?

Depression is an illness that involves the brain. It can affect your
thoughts, mood, and daily activities. Depression is more than feeling
sad for a few days.

Depression can be mild or severe. Mild depression can become more
serious if it's not treated.

If you are diagnosed with depression, you aren't alone. Depression
is a common illness that affects millions of adults in the United States
every year.

The good news is that depression can be treated. Getting help is
the best thing you can do for yourself and your loved ones. You can
feel better.

What are the signs of depression?

It's normal to feel sad sometimes, but if you feel sad or "down" on
most days for more than 2 weeks at a time, you may be depressed.

Depression affects people differently. Some signs of depression
are:

- Losing interest in activities you used to enjoy

- Feeling hopeless or empty

- Forgetting things or having trouble making decisions

- Sleeping too much or too little

- Gaining or losing weight without meaning to
- Thinking about suicide or death

How is depression treated?

Depression can be treated with talk therapy, medicines (called anti-depressants), or both. Your doctor may refer you to a mental health professional for talk therapy or medicine.

Take Action!

Depression is a real illness. If you think you might be depressed, see your doctor.

Talk to a doctor about how you are feeling.

Get a medical checkup. Ask to see a doctor or nurse who can screen you for depression.

The doctor or nurse may also check to see if you have another health condition (like thyroid disease) that can cause depression or make it worse. If you have one of these health conditions, it's important to get treatment right away.

What about cost?

Thanks to the Affordable Care Act, the health care reform law passed in 2010, insurance plans must cover screening for depression. This means you may be able to get screened at no cost to you.

Get help and support.

When you have depression, seeking help is the best thing you can do.

Here are some places you can go to for help with depression:

- Doctor's office or health clinic
- Family service or social service agency
- Church or clergy person
- Psychologist
- Counselor or social worker
- Psychotherapist

Remember, even if asking for help seems scary, it's an important step toward feeling better.

Get help right away if you or someone you know is thinking about suicide.

To get help for yourself or someone else, visit National Suicide Prevention Lifeline (http://www.suicidepreventionlifeline.org/) or call 1-800-273-TALK (1-800-273-8255).

If someone is in immediate danger, call 911.

Get active.

Getting active can lower your stress level and help your treatment work better. It can also help keep you from getting depressed again. But it's important to know that physical activity isn't a treatment for depression.

Section 6.6

Get Your Cholesterol Checked

Text in this section is excerpted from "Get Your Cholesterol Checked," Office of Disease Prevention and Health Promotion (ODPHP), August 27, 2015.

The Basics

Too much cholesterol in your blood can cause a heart attack or a stroke. You could have high cholesterol and not know it.

The good news is that it's easy to get your cholesterol checked and if your cholesterol is high, you can take steps to control it.

Who needs to get their cholesterol checked?

- All men age 35 and older
- Men ages 20 to 35 who have heart disease or risk factors for heart disease

- Women age 20 and older who have heart disease or risk factors for heart disease

Talk to your doctor or nurse about your risk factors for heart disease. Ask if you need to get your cholesterol checked.

What are the risk factors for heart disease?

Risk factors for heart disease include:

- High blood pressure
- A family history of heart disease
- Hardening of the arteries (called atherosclerosis)
- Smoking
- Diabetes
- Being overweight or obese
- Not getting enough physical activity

What is cholesterol?

Cholesterol is a waxy substance (material) that's found naturally in your blood. Your body makes cholesterol and uses it to do important things, like making hormones and digesting fatty foods.

You also get cholesterol by eating foods like egg yolks, fatty meats, and regular cheese.

If you have too much cholesterol in your body, it can build up inside your blood vessels and make it hard for blood to flow through them. Over time, this can lead to a heart attack or a stroke.

What are the symptoms of high cholesterol?

There are no signs or symptoms of high cholesterol. That's why it's so important to get your cholesterol checked.

How often do I need to get my cholesterol checked?

The general recommendation is to get your cholesterol checked every 5 years. Some people need to get their cholesterol checked more or less often. Talk to your doctor about what's best for you.

How can I get my cholesterol checked?

Cholesterol is checked with a blood test called a lipid profile. During the test, a nurse will take a small sample of blood from your finger or arm.

Be sure to find out how to get ready for the test. For example, you may need to fast (not eat or drink anything except water) for 9 to 12 hours before the test.

There are other blood tests that can check cholesterol, but a lipid profile gives the most information.

What do the test results mean?

If you get a lipid profile test, the results will show 4 numbers. A lipid profile measures:

- Total cholesterol
- HDL (good) cholesterol
- LDL (bad) cholesterol
- Triglycerides

Total cholesterol is a measure of all the cholesterol in your blood. It's based on the HDL, LDL, and triglycerides numbers.

HDL cholesterol is the good type of cholesterol – so a higher level is better for you. Having a low HDL cholesterol level can increase your risk for heart disease.

LDL cholesterol is the bad type of cholesterol that can block your arteries – so a lower level is better for you.

Triglycerides are a type of fat in your blood that can increase your risk for heart attack and stroke.

What can cause unhealthy cholesterol levels?

- Genetic (inherited) factors
- Type 2 diabetes
- Smoking
- Being overweight
- Not getting enough physical activity
- Taking certain medicines

Causes of unhealthy HDL cholesterol levels include:

- Having a family history of high LDL cholesterol
- Eating too much saturated fat, trans fat, and cholesterol

What if my cholesterol levels aren't healthy?

As your LDL cholesterol gets higher, so does your risk of heart disease. Take these steps to lower your cholesterol and reduce your risk of heart disease:

- Eat heart-healthy foods.
- Get active.
- If you smoke, quit.

Ask your doctor if you also need to take medicine to help lower your cholesterol.

Take Action!

Find out what your cholesterol levels are. If your cholesterol is high, take steps to control it.

Make an appointment to get your cholesterol checked.

Call your doctor's office or health center to schedule the test. Be sure to ask for a complete lipid profile – and find out what instructions you'll need to follow before the test. For example, you may need to fast (not eat or drink anything except water) for 9 to 12 hours before the test.

What about cost?

Cholesterol testing is covered under the Affordable Care Act, the health care reform law passed in 2010. Depending on your insurance plan, you may be able to get your cholesterol checked at no cost to you.

- Check with your insurance provider to find out what's included in your plan. Ask about the Affordable Care Act.
- You can still get your cholesterol checked even if you don't have insurance.

Keep track of your cholesterol levels.

Remember to ask the doctor or nurse for your cholesterol levels each time you get your cholesterol checked. Write the levels down to keep track of your progress.

Eat heart-healthy foods.

Making healthy changes to your diet can help lower your cholesterol. Try to:

- Eat less saturated fat, which comes from animal products (like regular cheese, fatty meats, and dairy desserts) and tropical oils (like palm, palm kernel, and coconut oil).

- Stay away from trans fats, which may be in baked goods (like cookies and cake), snack foods (like microwave popcorn), fried foods, and margarines.

- Limit foods that are high in cholesterol, including fatty meats and organ meat (like liver and kidney).

- Limit foods that are high in salt or added sugar.

- Choose low-fat or fat-free milk, cheese, and yogurt.

- Eat more foods that are high in fiber, like oatmeal, oat bran, beans, and lentils.

- Eat more vegetables and fruits.

Get active.

Getting active can help you lose weight, lower your LDL (bad) cholesterol, and raise your HDL (good) cholesterol. Aim for 2 hours and 30 minutes a week of moderate activity, such as:

- Walking fast

- Swimming

- Aerobics

Quit smoking.

Quitting smoking will help lower your cholesterol. If you smoke, make a plan to quit today.

And if you don't smoke, don't start!

Section 6.7

Get Tested for Chlamydia and Gonorrhea

Text in this section is excerpted from "Get Tested for Chlamydia
and Gonorrhea," Office of Disease Prevention and Health Promotion
(ODPHP), July 15, 2015.

The Basics

Chlamydia and gonorrhoea are STDs (sexually transmitted diseases) that can be passed on during vaginal, anal, or oral sex. A pregnant woman can also pass these STDs to her baby before or during the baby's birth.

STDs are also sometimes called STIs (sexually transmitted infections).

How can I know if I have an STD?

Getting tested is the only way to know for sure if you have an STD. Most people who have an STD don't feel sick or have any symptoms.

It's also important to talk with a doctor or nurse if someone you recently had sex with has an STD.

Can chlamydia and gonorrhea be cured?

Yes. Chlamydia and gonorrhea can both be cured with medicine if they are treated early. If these STDs aren't treated, they can cause serious health problems, like making it dangerous or impossible for a woman to get pregnant.

If you have an STD, it's important to get treatment right away. It's also important to tell anyone you have sex with so he or she can get treatment, too. This will help prevent you from getting infected again.

Who needs to get tested for chlamydia and gonorrhea?

The recommendations for getting tested for chlamydia and for gonorrhea are the same.

For women:

- If you are age 24 or younger and having sex, get tested once every year.

- If you are age 25 or older, get tested if you have more than one sex partner or a new sex partner.

For men:

- Talk with a doctor about getting tested if you are worried about chlamydia, gonorrhea, or other STDs.

What are the signs of chlamydia or gonorrhea?

Many people who have chlamydia or gonorrhea don't have any signs or symptoms. When there are symptoms, chlamydia and gonorrhea cause very similar things.

- Women with symptoms may have abnormal discharge (fluid) from the vagina, burning when they urinate (pee), or pain during sex.

- Men with symptoms may have abnormal discharge from the penis or burning when they urinate

How do doctors test for chlamydia and gonorrhea?

A doctor or nurse can test your urine (pee) for both chlamydia and gonorrhea. Sometimes, the doctor might take a sample from the vagina or penis to test. The test is easy and painless.

Take Action!

Get tested for chlamydia and gonorrhea if you are at risk. Talk with your partner about getting tested, too.

Make an appointment at a health center or clinic.

If you think you may be at risk, talk with your doctor about getting tested for chlamydia and gonorrhea. Be sure to ask about getting tested for HIV, too.

What about cost?

Some STD testing and prevention counseling is covered under the Affordable Care Act, the health care reform law passed in 2010.

Depending on your insurance plan, you may be able to get these services at no cost to you.

Talk to your insurance company to find out what this means for you.

Stay safe.

The best way to protect yourself from STDs is to not have vaginal, anal, or oral sex. Wait to have sex until you and your partner have tested negative for STDs.

Here are some other ways to protect yourself from STDs:

- Use a latex condom the right way every time you have vaginal, anal, or oral sex.

- Make sure you and your partner have been tested for STDs.

- If you know that you or your partner has an STD, get it treated before having sex.

If you are pregnant, talk with your doctor about STD testing.

Having chlamydia, gonorrhea, or another STD while you are pregnant can be very serious for you and your baby.

Section 6.8

Get Tested for HIV

Text in this section is excerpted from "Get Tested for HIV," Office of Disease Prevention and Health Promotion (ODPHP), July 15, 2015.

The Basics

The only way to know if you have HIV is to get tested. You could have HIV and still feel healthy.

How often do I need to get tested for HIV?

Everyone ages 15 to 65 needs to get tested for HIV at least once. All pregnant women also need to get tested.

How often you need to get tested depends on your risk for HIV infection. Talk to your doctor or nurse about your risk for HIV. Ask how often you need to get tested.

Get tested for HIV at least once a year if you:

- Have sex without a condom with someone who may have HIV
- Have sex with men who have sex with other men
- Use drugs with needles
- Have a sex partner who has HIV
- Have had a sexually transmitted disease (STD)
- Have sex with more than one partner
- Have sex with people you don't know
- Have sex for drugs or money

If you are a man who has sex with men, you may need to get tested more often like every 3 to 6 months.

Why do I need to get tested for HIV?

The only way to know if you have HIV is to get tested. Many people with HIV don't have any symptoms.

Even if you don't feel sick, getting early treatment for HIV is important.

- If you don't have HIV (you are HIV-negative), you can take steps to make sure you stay HIV-free.
- If you have HIV (you are HIV-positive), you can take steps to have a healthier future. You can also take steps to protect other people.

Live longer with HIV.

If you have HIV, early treatment can help you live a longer, healthier life. The sooner you get care for HIV, the better.

Protect yourself and others.

If you have HIV, you can take steps to protect your partner from the virus. If you are pregnant or thinking about getting pregnant, you can get treatment to prevent passing HIV to your baby.

How can I get tested for HIV?

There are different types of HIV tests. The most common are:

- Lab tests – It can take from a few days to 2 weeks to get the results.

- Rapid tests – Results are ready in 10 to 20 minutes.

When you get tested, the nurse will take a sample of your blood or collect fluid from your mouth with a swab (a stick with a soft tip).

If you test positive, the doctor or nurse will give you a second HIV test to be sure.

What's the difference between confidential and anonymous testing?

When you get tested at a doctor's office or clinic, your test results are **confidential**. This means they can only be shared with people allowed to see your medical records.

If you are worried about giving your name, you can get an **anonymous** HIV test at some clinics. This means that you don't have to give your name.

What is HIV?

HIV stands for human immunodeficiency virus. This is the virus that causes AIDS. There is no cure yet for HIV/AIDS, but there are treatments that can help people live longer, healthier lives.

How do people get HIV?

HIV is spread through some of the body's fluids, like blood, semen (cum), vaginal fluids, and breast milk. HIV is passed from one person to another by:

- Having sex (vaginal, anal, or oral) without a condom or dental dam with a person who has HIV

- Sharing needles with someone who has HIV

- Breastfeeding, pregnancy, or childbirth if the mother has HIV

- Getting a transfusion of blood that's infected with HIV (very rare in the United States)

Take Action!

Take these steps to protect yourself and others from HIV.

Find a place to get tested.

Ask your doctor or nurse for an HIV test. Or visit an HIV testing center or health clinic. You also can get tested at a hospital or health department.

What about cost?

Free HIV testing is available at some testing centers and health clinics.

Thanks to the Affordable Care Act, the health care reform law passed in 2010, insurance plans must cover HIV testing. HIV counseling is covered for women who are sexually active. Talk to your insurance company to find out more.

Protect yourself from HIV.

The best way to protect yourself from HIV is to not have sex until you are in a relationship with only one person **and** you have both tested negative.

Here are other steps you can take to help prevent HIV:

- Use a latex condom with water-based lubricant every time you have vaginal or anal sex.

- When you have oral sex, use a condom or dental dam (rectangular sheet of latex placed over the vagina).

- Limit your number of sexual partners.

- Don't inject drugs or share needles.

- If you have more than one sexual partner, get tested for HIV regularly.

Talk with your partner about getting tested.

It's important to make time to talk before having sex. Ask your partner to get tested for HIV and other STDs. Offer to get tested together.

Get counseling about HIV prevention.

If you want more information about preventing HIV, ask your local testing center if they offer prevention counseling. You may want counseling if:

- You are worried about getting HIV
- You have HIV and are worried about giving it to someone else

Chapter 7

Screening Tests for Women

Chapter Contents

Section 7.1

Recommended Screening Tests for Women

Text in this section is excerpted from "Screening Tests and Vaccines,"
Office of Womenshealth (OWH), June 7, 2013.

Check the guidelines listed here to find out about important screening tests for women. These guidelines are recommended by the U.S. Preventive Services Task Force. Keep in mind that these are guidelines only. Your doctor or nurse will personalize the timing of the screening tests you need based on many factors. Ask your doctor or nurse if you don't understand why a certain test is recommended for you. Check with your insurance plan to find out which tests are covered. Insurance companies are required to cover many preventive services for women at not cost to you because of the Affordable Care Act.

Where do these guidelines come from?

The screening guidelines listed here are recommended by the U.S. Preventive Services Task Force (USPSTF). The USPSTF is a group of non-Federal experts in prevention (stopping disease before it starts). USPSTF recommendations are evidence-based. This means that science supports USPSTF screening guidelines. The USPSTF is made up of primary care providers (such as internists, pediatricians, family physicians, gynecologists/obstetricians, nurses, and health behavior specialists).

Get regular checkups

Your doctor or nurse can help you stay healthy. Ask your doctor or nurse how often you need to be seen for a routine checkup. Use this time to bring up any health concerns or questions you have. Make sure to ask about:

- Alcohol use
- Depression
- Weight

Table 7.1. Screening tests

Screening tests	Ages 18–39	Ages 40–49	Ages 50–64	Ages 65 and older
Blood pressure test	Get tested at least every 2 years if you have normal blood pressure (lower than 120/80). Get tested once a year if you have blood pressure between 120/80 and 139/89. Discuss treatment with your doctor or nurse if you have blood pressure 140/90 or higher.	Get tested at least every 2 years if you have normal blood pressure (lower than 120/80). Get tested once a year if you have blood pressure between 120/80 and 139/89. Discuss treatment with your doctor or nurse if you have blood pressure 140/90 or higher.	Get tested at least every 2 years if you have normal blood pressure (lower than 120/80). Get tested once a year if you have blood pressure between 120/80 and 139/89. Discuss treatment with your doctor or nurse if you have blood pressure 140/90 or higher.	Get tested at least every 2 years if you have normal blood pressure (lower than 120/80). Get tested once a year if you have blood pressure between 120/80 and 139/89. Discuss treatment with your doctor or nurse if you have blood pressure 140/90 or higher.
Bone mineral density test (osteoporosis screening)			Discuss with your doctor or nurse if you are at risk of osteoporosis.	Get this test at least once at age 65 or older. Talk to your doctor or nurse about repeat testing.
Breast cancer screening (mammogram)		Discuss with your doctor or nurse.	Starting at age 50, get screened every 2 years.	Get screened every 2 years through age 74. Age 75 and older, ask your doctor or nurse if you need to be screened.

145

Table 7.1. Continued

Screening tests	Ages 18–39	Ages 40–49	Ages 50–64	Ages 65 and older
Cervical cancer screening (Pap test)	Get a Pap test every 3 years if you are 21 or older and have a cervix. If you are 30 or older, you can get a Pap test and HPV test together every 5 years.	Get a Pap test and HPV test together every 5 years if you have a cervix.	Get a Pap test and HPV test together every 5 years if you have a cervix.	Ask your doctor or nurse if you need to get a Pap test.
Chlamydia test	Get tested for chlamydia yearly through age 24 if you are sexually active or pregnant. Age 25 and older, get tested for chlamydia if you are at increased risk, pregnant or not pregnant.	Get tested for chlamydia if you are sexually active and at increased risk, pregnant or not pregnant.	Get tested for chlamydia if you are sexually active and at increased risk.	Get tested for chlamydia if you are sexually active and at increased risk.
Cholesterol test	Starting at age 20, get a cholesterol test regularly if you are at increased risk for heart disease. Ask your doctor or nurse how often you need your cholesterol tested.	Get a cholesterol test regularly if you are at increased risk for heart disease. Ask your doctor or nurse how often you need your cholesterol tested.	Get a cholesterol test regularly if you are at increased risk for heart disease. Ask your doctor or nurse how often you need your cholesterol tested.	Get a cholesterol test regularly if you are at increased risk for heart disease. Ask your doctor or nurse how often you need your cholesterol tested.

Table 7.1. Continued

Screening tests	Ages 18–39	Ages 40–49	Ages 50–64	Ages 65 and older
Colorectal cancer screening (using fecal occult blood testing, sigmoidoscopy, or colonoscopy)			Starting at age 50, get screened for colorectal cancer. Talk to your doctor or nurse about which screening test is best for you and how often you need it.	Get screened for colorectal cancer through age 75. Talk to your doctor or nurse about which screening test is best for you and how often you need it.
Diabetes screening	Get screened for diabetes if your blood pressure is higher than 135/80 or if you take medicine for high blood pressure.	Get screened for diabetes if your blood pressure is higher than 135/80 or if you take medicine for high blood pressure.	Get screened for diabetes if your blood pressure is higher than 135/80 or if you take medicine for high blood pressure.	Get screened for diabetes if your blood pressure is higher than 135/80 or if you take medicine for high blood pressure.
Gonorrhea test	Get tested for gonorrhea if you are sexually active and at increased risk, pregnant or not pregnant.	Get tested for gonorrhea if you are sexually active and at increased risk, pregnant or not pregnant.	Get tested for gonorrhea if you are sexually active and at increased risk.	Get tested for gonorrhea if you are sexually active and at increased risk.

147

Table 7.1. Continued

Screening tests	Ages 18–39	Ages 40–49	Ages 50–64	Ages 65 and older
HIV test	Get tested for HIV at least once. Discuss your risk with your doctor or nurse because you may need more frequent tests. All pregnant women need to be tested for HIV.	Get tested for HIV at least once. Discuss your risk with your doctor or nurse because you may need more frequent tests. All pregnant women need to be tested for HIV.	Get tested for HIV at least once. Discuss your risk with your doctor or nurse because you may need more frequent tests.	Get tested for HIV at least once if you are age 65 and have never been tested. Get tested if you are at increased risk for HIV. Discuss your risk with your doctor or nurse.
Syphilis test	Get tested for syphilis if you are at increased risk or pregnant.	Get tested for syphilis if you are at increased risk or pregnant.	Get tested for syphilis if you are at increased risk.	Get tested for syphilis if you are at increased risk

Section 7.2

Get Tested for Breast Cancer

Text in this section is excerpted from "Get Tested for Breast Cancer,"
Office of Disease Prevention and Health promotion (ODPHP),
August 31, 2015.

The Basics

Mammograms can help find breast cancer early. Most women can survive breast cancer if it's found and treated early.

Women ages 40 to 49:

- Talk with your doctor about when to start getting mammograms and how often you need them.

Women ages 50 to 74:

- Get mammograms every 2 years. Talk with your doctor to decide if you need them more often.

What is a mammogram?

A mammogram is an X-ray of the breast. Mammograms use a very low level of X-rays, which are a type of radiation. A mammogram is very safe.

When you get mammograms, the nurse will place your breasts, one at a time, between 2 plastic plates and take pictures of them. Mammograms can be uncomfortable for some women, but they don't hurt.

It takes about 20 minutes to get mammograms.

What if the doctor finds something wrong with my breast?

Mammograms let the doctor or nurse look for small lumps inside your breast. If a lump is found, you will need other tests to find out if it's cancer.

The doctor or nurse may take a small bit of tissue from the lump for testing. This is called a biopsy ("BY-op-see")

What is breast cancer?

Abnormal (unusual) cells in the breast can turn into cancer. Breast cancer can spread to other parts of the body.

About 1 in 8 women born today in the United States will get breast cancer. After skin cancer, breast cancer is the most common kind of cancer in women. The good news is that most women survive breast cancer when it's found and treated early.

Talk with your doctor or nurse if you notice any of these changes:

- A lump in the breast

- A change in size, shape, or feel of the breast

- Fluid (called discharge) coming out of a nipple

Take Action!

Talk with your doctor about when and how often to get mammograms.

Ask the doctor about your breast cancer risk.

- Use these questions to start a conversation with your doctor about mammograms.

- Tell your doctor if anyone in your family has had breast or ovarian cancer.

- If you have a family history of breast or ovarian cancer, use these questions to talk with your doctor about genetic testing.

- Ask about ways you may be able to lower your breast cancer risk.

Together, you and your doctor can decide what's best for you.

What about cost?

The Affordable Care Act, the health care reform law passed in 2010, covers mammograms for women over age 40. Depending on your insurance plan, you may be able to get mammograms at no cost to you.

Check with your insurance company to find out what's included in your plan.

If you don't have private insurance, you can still get mammograms.

- Find a program near you that offers free or low-cost mammograms.

- Find out how often Medicare pays for mammograms.

Get support.

Use these tips to get support when you get mammograms.

- Ask other women who have had mammograms about what to expect.

- When you go to get mammograms, ask a family member or friend to go with you.

Get active.

Getting active increases your chances of living longer. Physical activity may help prevent breast cancer, colorectal cancer, and heart disease.

Get your well-woman visit.

Get a well-woman visit every year. Use this visit to talk with your doctor or nurse about important screenings and services to help you stay healthy.

Section 7.3

Get Tested for Cervical Cancer

Text in this section is excerpted from "Get Tested for Cervical Cancer," Office of Disease Prevention and Health promotion (ODPHP), July 10, 2015.

The Basics

Getting regular screening tests (called Pap tests) and follow-up care can help prevent cervical cancer. You can get a Pap test (sometimes called a Pap smear) at your doctor's office or clinic.

Most deaths from cervical cancer can be prevented if women get regular Pap tests. A Pap test can find abnormal (changed) cells **before** they turn into cancer. Pap tests can also find cervical cancer early, when it usually can be cured.

How often should I get screened (tested)?

How often you should get screened for cervical cancer depends on how old you are and which tests you get.

- If you are age 21 to 29, get a Pap test every 3 years.
- If you are age 30 to 65:
- Get screened every 3 years if you only have a Pap test.
- Get screened every 5 years if you have both a Pap test and an HPV (human papillomavirus) test.

If you are age 66 or older, ask your doctor if cervical cancer screening is recommended for you.

What is cervical cancer?

Cervical cancer is cancer of the cervix, which is the lower, narrow part of the uterus (or womb). The cervix connects the uterus to the vagina.

Abnormal cells in the cervix can turn into cancer if they aren't found early and treated. Cervical cancer is more common in women over age 30.

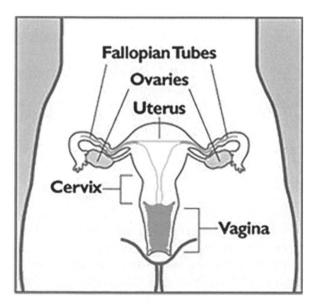

Figure 7.1. *Female reproductive system*

What happens during a Pap test?

A Pap test takes about 2 to 5 minutes. It may feel uncomfortable, but a Pap test usually doesn't hurt.

While you lie on the exam table, the doctor or nurse will put a medical tool (called a speculum) into your vagina and open it to see your cervix. The doctor or nurse will use a special brush to collect a few cells from your cervix. These cells are sent to a lab to be checked by an expert.

The doctor or nurse will also do a pelvic exam to check your uterus, ovaries, and other organs.

Take Action!

Take these steps to help prevent cervical cancer.

Schedule your Pap test.

Call a doctor's office or local health clinic to schedule your Pap test and pelvic exam.

Get ready for your Pap test.

Try to schedule your Pap test for a time when you won't have your period.

For 2 days before your test, doctors recommend that you don't:

- Use tampons
- Have sex
- Use birth control creams, foams, or jellies
- Douche (rinse the vagina with water or other liquid)

Find out your Pap test results.

When you get a Pap test, ask the doctor how you will find out the results. Pap test results can be "normal," "unclear," or "abnormal." Get help understanding your Pap test result.

What about cost?

Testing for cervical cancer is covered under the Affordable Care Act, the health care reform law passed in 2010. Depending on your insurance plan, you may be able to get tested at no cost to you.

- If you have private insurance, check with your insurance provider to find out what's included in your plan.

- If you don't have insurance, find a program near you that offers free or low-cost Pap tests.

- If you have Medicare, find out how often Medicare covers Pap tests and pelvic exams.

Lower your risk of cervical cancer.

Long-term HPV (human papillomavirus) infections are a major cause of cervical cancer. HPV is a very common infection that can spread during sex.

Some types of HPV can cause genital and anal warts. Other types of HPV can cause cervical cancer and other cancers.

You are at higher risk of getting HPV if you:

- Started having sex before age 18

- Have unprotected sex

- Have many different sex partners

- Have a sex partner who has other sex partners

Get the HPV vaccine.

Doctors recommend that women age 26 and younger get the HPV vaccine. The HPV vaccine is given in 3 shots over 6 months. The shots protect against the types of HPV that cause most cases of cervical cancer. Find out more about the HPV vaccine.

Girls and boys need the HPV vaccine, too. If you have kids, ask their doctor about the HPV vaccine.

Get your well-woman visit every year.

During your visit, talk to the doctor or nurse about other important screenings and services to help you stay healthy. Find out more about getting your well-woman visit every year.

Section 7.4

Get Tested for Colorectal Cancer

Text in this section is excerpted from "Get Tested for Colorectal Cancer," Office of Disease Prevention and Health promotion (ODPHP), July 15, 2015.

The Basics

If you are age 50 to 75, get tested regularly for colorectal cancer. All it takes is a visit to the doctor to have a special exam (called a screening).

You may need to get tested before age 50 if colorectal cancer runs in your family. Talk with your doctor and ask about your risk for colorectal cancer.

How often should I get screened?

How often you get screened will depend on your risk for colorectal cancer. It will also depend on which screening test is used.

There are different ways to test for colorectal cancer. Some tests are done every 1 to 2 years. Other tests are done every 5 to 10 years. Your doctor can help you decide which test is right for you and how often to get screened.

Most people can stop getting screened after age 75. Talk with your doctor about what's right for you.

What happens during the test?

There are different kinds of tests used to screen for colorectal cancer. Some tests you can do at home, such as a fecal occult blood test. Other tests, such as a colonoscopy, must be done in a clinic or hospital.

You may need to drink only clear liquids (like water or plain tea) the day before your test and use laxatives to clean out your colon. Your doctor will tell you how to get ready for your test.

Does it hurt to get tested?

Some people find the tests for colorectal cancer to be uncomfortable. Most people agree that the benefits to their health outweigh the discomfort.

What is colorectal cancer?

Cancer of the colon or rectum is called colorectal cancer. Like other types of cancer, colorectal cancer can spread to other parts of your body. The colon is the longest part of the large intestine. The rectum is the bottom part of the large intestine.

Am I at risk for colorectal cancer?

People over age 50 are at higher risk of developing colorectal cancer. Other risk factors are:

- Polyps (growths) inside the colon

- Family history of colorectal cancer

- Smoking

- Obesity

- Not getting enough physical activity

- Drinking too much alcohol

- Health conditions, such as Crohn's disease, which cause chronic inflammation (ongoing irritation) of the intestines

Take control – act early.

If you act early, you have a good chance of preventing colorectal cancer or finding it when it can be treated more easily.

- If your doctor finds polyps inside your colon during testing, these growths can be removed before they become cancer.

- If you find out you have cancer after you get tested, you can take steps to treat it right away.

Take Action!

The best way to prevent colorectal cancer is to get tested starting at age 50.

What about cost?

Thanks to the Affordable Care Act, the health care reform law passed in 2010, most insurance plans must cover screening for colorectal cancer. Depending on your insurance plan, you may be able to get screened at no cost to you.

- If you have Medicare, find out about Medicare coverage for different colorectal cancer tests.

- If you have private insurance, talk to your insurance company to find out what's included in your plan. Ask about the Affordable Care Act.

- If you don't have insurance, you can still get important screening tests. To learn more, find a health center near you.

Get support.

If you are nervous about getting a colorectal cancer test, get support.

- Ask a family member or friend to go with you.

- Talk with people you know who have been screened to learn what to expect.

Get active.

Regular exercise may help reduce your risk of colorectal cancer.

Drink alcohol only in moderation.

Drinking too much alcohol may increase your risk of colorectal cancer. If you choose to drink, have only a moderate (limited) amount. This means:

- No more than 1 drink a day for women

- No more than 2 drinks a day for men

Eat healthy.

Eating healthy foods that are low in fat and high in calcium and fiber may help prevent colorectal cancer.

- You can get calcium from foods like yogurt, cheese, and spinach.

- Fiber is in foods like beans, barley, and nuts.

Chapter 8

Preventive Care and Screening for Seniors

Chapter Contents

Section 8.1

FAQs on Preventive Care and Screening for Seniors

Text in this section is excerpted from "Health Screenings and Immunizations," National Institutes of Health (NIH), December 2014.

What are health screenings?

Health screenings are tests that look for diseases before you have symptoms. Screening tests can find diseases early, when they're easier to treat.

What questions should you ask your doctor before having a screening?

Before you have a health screening test, ask your doctor these questions.

- Why do I need the test? What will it show about my health?
- What will it cost and will my insurance cover it?
- What do I need to do to prepare for the test? (For example, do I need to have an empty stomach, or will I need to provide a urine sample.)
- What steps does the medical test involve?
- Are there any harms or side effects?
- How will I find out the results of my test?
- How long will it take to get the results?
- What will we know after the test?

What types of diseases are screened for?

Some conditions that doctors commonly screen for include

- breast cancer and cervical cancer in women

- colorectal cancer
- diabetes
- high blood pressure
- high cholesterol
- osteoporosis
- overweight and obesity

How often should you have a comprehensive dilated eye exam?

If you are age 60 or older, you should have a comprehensive dilated eye exam at least once a year. If you are at increased risk for or have any age-related eye disease, you may need to see your eye care professional more often.

Who should be tested for hepatitis C virus?

Get screened one time for HCV infection if

- you were born between 1945 and 1965
- you have ever injected drugs
- you received a blood transfusion before 1992.

If you currently are an injection drug user, you should be screened regularly.

When should you have a test for colon cancer?

Between the ages of 50 and 75, get a screening test for colorectal cancer. If you are between the ages of 76 and 85, talk with your doctor or nurse about whether you should continue to be screened.

Several tests – for example, a stool test or a colonoscopy – can detect colon cancer.

How can you find out if you are overweight or obese?

The best way to learn if you are overweight or obese is to find your body mass index (BMI). You can find your BMI by entering your height and weight into a BMI calculator, such as the one available at: http://www.nhlbi.nih.gov/guidelines/obesity/BMI/bmicalc.htm. A BMI between 18.5 and 25 indicates a normal weight. Persons with a BMI of 30 or higher may be obese.

How does a vaccine prevent disease?

Vaccines contain the same germs that cause disease. (For example, measles vaccine contains measles virus.) But the viruses have been either killed or weakened to the point that they don't make you sick. Some vaccines contain only a part of the disease germ.

A vaccine stimulates your immune system to produce antibodies, exactly like it would if you were exposed to the disease. After getting vaccinated, you develop immunity to that disease without having to get the disease first.

What vaccines are recommended for adults 50+?

- Get a flu shot every year.

- Get a shot for tetanus, diphtheria, and whooping cough. Get a tetanus booster if it has been more than 10 years since your last shot.

- If you are 60 or older, get a shot to prevent shingles. Even if you have had shingles, you can still get the shingles vaccine to help prevent future occurrences of the disease.

- If you are 65 or older, get a pneumonia shot (also known as a pneumococcal vaccine).

Should older adults get tested for HIV?

If you are 65 or younger, get screened for HIV. If you are older than 65, ask your doctor or nurse if you should be screened.

When should a woman get tested for osteoporosis, a bone thinning disease?

Have a screening test at age 65 to make sure your bones are strong. The most common test is a DEXA scan – a low-dose X-ray of the spine and hip. If you are younger than 65 and at high risk for bone fractures, you should also be screened. Talk with your health care team about your risk for bone fractures.

Who should be screened for abdominal aortic aneurysm?

If you are a man between the ages of 65 and 75 and have ever been a smoker (smoked 100 or more cigarettes in your lifetime), talk to your health care team about being screened for abdominal aortic aneurysm

(AAA). AAA is a bulging in your abdominal aorta, your largest artery. An AAA may burst, which can cause dangerous bleeding and death.

An ultrasound, a painless procedure in which you lie on a table while a technician slides a medical device over your abdomen, will show whether an aneurysm is present.

When should I talk to my health care team about getting screened for depression?

Talk to your health care team about being screened for depression especially if during the last 2 weeks

- you have felt down, sad, or hopeless

- you have felt little interest or pleasure in doing things.

How often should you have your blood pressure checked?

Have your blood pressure checked at least every 2 years.

Who should get checked for high blood cholesterol?

Have your blood cholesterol checked regularly with a blood test if

- you use tobacco

- you are overweight or obese

- you have a personal history of heart disease or blocked arteries

- a male relative in your family had a heart attack before age 50 or a female relative, before age 60

- you have diabetes

- you have high blood pressure.

High blood cholesterol increases your chance of heart disease, stroke, and poor circulation.

How often do older women need to be screened for cervical cancer?

Get screened for cervical cancer (a Pap smear) every 3 years or get a combination Pap smear and human papillomavirus (HPV) test every 5 years until age 65. If you are older than 65 or have had a hysterectomy, talk with your doctor or nurse about whether you still need to be screened.

Should you be screened for lung cancer?

Talk to your doctor or nurse about getting screened for lung cancer if you are between the ages of 55 and 80, have a 30 pack-year smoking history, and smoke now or have quit within the past 15 years. (Your pack-year history is the number of packs of cigarettes smoked per day times the number of years you have smoked.)

What immunizations are recommended for adults 50 and older?

Here is a list of immunizations adults 50 and older should consider. (Source: Centers for Disease Control and Prevention)

- Get a flu shot every year. Over 60 percent of seasonal flu-related hospitalizations occur in people 65 years and older.

- Get a shot for tetanus, diphtheria, and whooping cough. Get a tetanus booster if it has been more than 10 years since your last shot.

- If you are 60 or older, get a shot to prevent shingles. Even if you have had shingles, you can still get the shingles vaccine to help prevent future occurrences of the disease.

- People 65 years or older need a series of two different vaccines for pneumococcal disease. Talk with your health care team about how to schedule them. Be sure to let the team know if you have ever had a pneumococcal vaccine before.

Talk with your health care team about whether you need other vaccinations.

Section 8.2

Recommended Screenings for Seniors – Men

Text in this section is excerpted from "Health Screenings and Immunizations," National Institutes of Health (NIH), December 2014.

Abdominal Aortic Aneurysm

If you are between the ages of 65 and 75 and have ever been a smoker (smoked 100 or more cigarettes in your lifetime), talk to your health care team about being screened for abdominal aortic aneurysm (AAA). AAA is a bulging in your abdominal aorta, your largest artery. An AAA may burst, which can cause dangerous bleeding and death.

An ultrasound, a painless procedure in which you lie on a table while a technician slides a medical device over your abdomen, will show whether an aneurysm is present.

Colon Cancer

If you are 75 or younger, get a screening test for colorectal cancer. Several different tests – for example, a stool test or a colonoscopy – can detect this cancer. Your doctor or nurse can help you decide which is best for you. If you are between the ages of 76 and 85, talk to your doctor or nurse about whether you should continue to be screened.

Depression

Your emotional health is as important as your physical health. Talk to your health care team about being screened for depression, especially if during the last 2 weeks:

- You have felt down, sad, or hopeless.

- You have felt little interest or pleasure in doing things.

Diabetes

Ask your doctor if you should be screened for diabetes (high blood sugar). Diabetes can cause problems with your heart, brain, eyes, feet, kidneys, nerves, and other body parts.

Hepatitis C Virus (HCV)

Get screened one time for HCV infection if

- you were born between 1945 and 1965.
- you have ever injected drugs.
- you received a blood transfusion before 1992.

If you currently are an injection drug user, you should be screened regularly.

High Blood Cholesterol

Have your blood cholesterol checked regularly with a blood test. High blood cholesterol increases your chance of heart disease, stroke, and poor circulation.

High Blood Pressure

Have your blood pressure checked at least every 2 years. High blood pressure can cause strokes, heart attacks, kidney and eye problems, and heart failure.

HIV

If you are 65 or younger, get screened for HIV. If you are older than 65, ask your doctor or nurse if you should be screened.

Lung Cancer

Talk to your doctor or nurse about getting screened for lung cancer if you are between the ages of 55 and 80, have a 30 pack-year smoking history, and smoke now or have quit within the past 15 years. (Your pack-year history is the number of packs of cigarettes smoked per day times the number of years you have smoked.) Know that quitting smoking is the best thing you can do for your health.

Lung cancer can be detected with low-dose computed tomography (LCT). For LCT, you lie on a table while a large machine passes over you to scan your lungs.

Overweight and Obesity

The best way to learn if you are overweight or obese is to find your body mass index (BMI).

A BMI between 18.5 and 25 indicates a normal weight. Persons with a BMI of 30 or higher may be obese. If you are obese, talk to your doctor or nurse about getting intensive counseling and help with changing your behaviors to lose weight. Overweight and obesity can lead to diabetes and cardiovascular disease.

Vision Disorders

If you are age 60 or older, you should have a comprehensive dilated eye exam at least once a year. If you are at increased risk for or have any age-related eye disease, you may need to see your eye care professional more often.

Other Tests to Ask About

You know your body better than anyone else. Always tell your doctor or nurse about any changes in your health. Ask them about being checked for any condition you are concerned about, not just the ones here. If you are wondering about Alzheimer's disease or skin cancer, for example, ask about them.

Section 8.3

Recommended Screenings for Seniors – Women

Text in this section is excerpted from "Health Screenings and Immunizations," National Institutes of Health (NIH), December, 2014.

BRCA 1 and 2 Genes

If you have a family member with breast, ovarian, or peritoneal cancer, talk with your doctor or nurse about your family history. Women with a strong family history of certain cancers may benefit from genetic counseling and BRCA genetic testing.

Breast Cancer

Talk with your health care team about whether you need a mammogram.

Cervical Cancer

Get a Pap smear every 3 years or get a combination Pap smear and human papilloma virus (HPV) test every 5 years until age 65. If you are older than 65 or have had a hysterectomy, talk with your doctor or nurse about whether you still need to be screened.

Colon Cancer

Between the ages of 50 and 75, get a screening test for colorectal cancer. Several tests – for example, a stool test or a colonoscopy – can detect this cancer. Your health care team can help you decide which is best for you. If you are between the ages of 76 and 85, talk with your doctor or nurse about whether you should continue to be screened.

Depression

Your emotional health is as important as your physical health. Talk to your health care team about being screened for depression, especially if during the last 2 weeks:

- you have felt down, sad, or hopeless.
- you have felt little interest or pleasure in doing things.

Diabetes

Ask your doctor if you should be screened for diabetes.

Diabetes can cause problems with your heart, brain, eyes, feet, kidneys, nerves, and other body parts.

Hepatitis C Virus (HCV)

Get screened one time for HCV infection if

- you were born between 1945 and 1965
- you have ever injected drugs
- you received a blood transfusion before 1992.

If you currently are an injection drug user, you should be screened regularly.

High Blood Cholesterol

Have your blood cholesterol checked regularly with a blood test if

- you use tobacco.
- you are overweight or obese.
- you have a personal history of heart disease or blocked arteries.
- a male relative in your family had a heart attack before age 50 or a female relative, before age 60.
- you have diabetes.
- you have high blood pressure.

High blood cholesterol increases your chance of heart disease, stroke, and poor circulation.

High Blood Pressure

Have your blood pressure checked at least every 2 years. High blood pressure can cause strokes, heart attacks, kidney and eye problems, and heart failure.

HIV

If you are 65 or younger, get screened for HIV. If you are older than 65, talk to your doctor or nurse about whether you should be screened.

Lung Cancer

Talk to your doctor or nurse about getting screened for lung cancer if you are between the ages of 55 and 80, have a 30 pack-year smoking history, and smoke now or have quit within the past 15 years. (Your pack-year history is the number of packs of cigarettes smoked per day times the number of years you have smoked.) Know that quitting smoking is the best thing you can do for your health.

Osteoporosis (Bone Thinning)

Have a screening test at age 65 to make sure your bones are strong. The most common test is a DEXA scan – a low-dose X-ray of the spine and hip. If you are younger than 65 and at high risk for bone fractures, you should also be screened. Talk with your health care team about your risk for bone fractures.

Overweight and Obesity

The best way to learn if you are overweight or obese is to find your body mass index (BMI).

A BMI between 18.5 and 25 indicates a normal weight. Persons with a BMI of 30 or higher may be obese. If you are obese, talk to your doctor or nurse about getting intensive counseling and help with changing your behaviors to lose weight. Overweight and obesity can lead to diabetes and cardiovascular disease.

Sexually Transmitted Infections

Talk to your doctor or nurse about whether you should be screened for sexually transmitted infections, such as gonorrhea and chlamydia.

Vision Disorders

If you are age 60 or older, you should have a comprehensive dilated eye exam at least once a year. If you are at increased risk for or have any age-related eye disease, you may need to see your eye care professional more often.

Other Tests to Ask About

You know your body better than anyone else. Always tell your doctor or nurse about any changes in your health. Ask them about being checked for any condition you are concerned about, not just the ones listed here. If you are wondering about Alzheimer's disease, skin cancer, or hearing loss, for example, ask about them.

Section 8.4

Get a Bone Density Test

Text in this section is excerpted from "Get a Bone Density Test," Office of Disease Prevention and Health Promotion (ODPHP), July 15, 2015.

The Basics

A bone density test measures how strong your bones are. The test will tell you if you have osteoporosis, or weak bones. If your bones are weak, they're more likely to break.

- If you are a woman age 65 or older, schedule a bone density test.

- If you are a woman age 50 to 64, ask your doctor if you need a bone density test.

If you are at risk for osteoporosis, your doctor or nurse may recommend getting a bone density test every 2 years.

Men can get osteoporosis, too. If you are a man over age 65 and you are concerned about your bone strength, talk with your doctor or nurse.

What happens during a bone density test?

A bone density test is like an X-ray or scan of your body. A bone density test doesn't hurt. It only takes about 15 minutes.

What is osteoporosis?

Osteoporosis is a bone disease. It means your bones are weak and more likely to break. People with osteoporosis most often break bones in the hip, spine, and wrist.

There are no signs or symptoms of osteoporosis. You might not know you have the disease until you break a bone. That's why it's so important to get a bone density test to measure your bone strength.

Am I at risk for osteoporosis?

Anyone can get osteoporosis, but it's most common in older women. The older you are, the greater your risk for osteoporosis.

These things can also increase your risk for osteoporosis:

- Not getting enough calcium and Vitamin D

- Taking certain medicines

- Smoking cigarettes or drinking too much alcohol

- Not getting enough physical activity

What if I have osteoporosis?

If you have osteoporosis, you can still slow down bone loss. Finding and treating it early can keep you healthier and more active – and lower your chances of breaking a bone.

Depending on the results of your bone density test, you may need to:

- Add more calcium and vitamin D to your diet

- Exercise more to strengthen your bones

- Take medicine to stop bone loss

Your doctor can tell you what steps are right for you. It doesn't matter how old you are – it's not too late to stop bone loss!

Take Action!

Take these steps to protect your bone health.

Schedule a bone density test.

Ask your doctor if you are at risk for osteoporosis. Find out when to start getting bone density tests.

What about cost?

Screening for osteoporosis is covered under the Affordable Care Act, the health care reform law passed in 2010. Depending on your insurance plan, you may be able to get screened at no cost to you.

- If you have private insurance, check with your insurance provider to find out what's included in your plan. Ask what's covered under the Affordable Care Act.

- If you have Medicare, find out about Medicare coverage for bone density tests.

- If you don't have health insurance, you can still get a bone density test.

Get enough calcium.

Getting enough calcium helps keep your bones strong. Good sources of calcium include:

- Low-fat or fat-free milk, cheese, and yogurt

- Almonds

- Broccoli and greens

- Tofu with added calcium

- Orange juice with added calcium

- Calcium pills

Get enough vitamin D.

Vitamin D helps your body absorb (take in) calcium. You need both vitamin D and calcium for strong bones.

Your body makes vitamin D when you are out in the sun. You can also get vitamin D from:

- Salmon or tuna
- Fat-free or low-fat milk and yogurt with added vitamin D
- Breakfast cereals and juices with added vitamin D
- Vitamin D pills

Stay away from cigarettes and alcohol.

Smoking cigarettes and drinking too much alcohol can weaken your bones.

- Learn more about how to quit smoking.
- If you drink alcohol, drink only in moderation. This means no more than 1 drink a day for women and no more than 2 drinks a day for men.

Take steps to prevent falls.

Falls can be especially serious for people with weak bones. You can make small changes to lower your risk of falling, like doing exercises that improve your balance. For example, try walking backwards or standing from a sitting position.

Get active.

Physical activity can help slow down bone loss. Weight-bearing activities (like running and jumping jacks) help keep your bones strong.

- Aim for 2 hours and 30 minutes a week of moderate aerobic activity. If you are new to exercise, start with 10 minutes of activity at a time.
- Do strengthening activities at least 2 days a week. These include lifting weights or using resistance bands (long rubber strips that stretch).

- Find an exercise buddy. You will be more likely to stick with it if you exercise with a friend.

  If you have a health condition or a disability, be as active as you can be. Your doctor can help you choose activities that are right for you.

Find an activity that works for you.

Check with your local community or senior center to find fun, low-cost or free exercise options. Try a new activity, like:

- Aerobics

- Tai chi ("ty chee")—A Chinese mind-body exercise that involves moving slowly and gently

- Yoga

- Weight training

- Walking with friends

Section 8.5

Get Your Vision Tested

Text in this section is excerpted from "Get Your Eyes Tested," Office of Disease Prevention and Health Promotion (ODPHP), August 4, 2015.

The Basics

Have your eyes tested (examined) regularly to help find problems early, when they may be easier to treat. The doctor will also do tests to make sure you are seeing as clearly as possible.

How often do I need an eye exam?

How often you need an eye exam depends on your risk for eye disease. Talk to your doctor about how often to get your eyes tested.

Get an eye exam every 1 to 2 years if you:

- Are over age 60

- Are African American and over age 40

- Have a family history of glaucoma

People with diabetes need eye exams more often.
If you have diabetes, get your eyes tested at least once a year.

What happens during an eye exam?

- The doctor will ask you questions about your health and vision.

- You will read charts with letters and numbers so the doctor can check your vision.

- The doctor will do tests to look for problems with your eyes, including glaucoma.

- The doctor will put drops in your eyes to dilate (enlarge) your pupils. A dilated eye exam is the only way to find some types of eye disease.

Am I at risk for a vision problem?

As you get older, your eyes change. This increases your chance of developing a vision problem. You may be at higher risk if one of your parents had a vision problem, like needing to wear glasses.

Common vision problems are:

- Nearsightedness – when far away objects are blurry

- Farsightedness – when far away objects are easier to see than near ones

- Astigmatism – a condition that makes it hard to see fine details

- Presbyopia ("prez-bee-OH-bee-uh") – problems seeing things up close

Am I at risk for eye disease?

Getting older increases your risk of certain eye diseases. You may be at higher risk if you have diabetes or high blood pressure – or if you have a family member with diabetes or an eye disease.

Eye diseases like glaucoma can lead to vision loss and blindness if they aren't caught and treated early.

Depending on your age and medical history, the doctor may look for eye problems that are common in older adults, including:

- Cataracts

- Glaucoma

- Age-related macular degeneration (or AMD)

- Diabetic eye disease

- Low vision

What's the difference between a vision screening and an eye exam?

A vision screening is a short checkup for your eyes. It usually takes place during a regular doctor visit. Vision screenings can only find certain eye problems.

An eye exam takes more time than a vision screening, and it's the only way to find some types of eye disease.

These two kinds of doctors can perform eye exams:

1. Optometrist

2. Ophthalmologist

Take Action!

Protect your vision. Get regular eye exams so you can find problems early, when they may be easier to treat.

Schedule an eye exam.

Ask your doctor or health center for the name of an eye care professional.

When you go for your exam, be sure to:

- Ask the doctor for a dilated eye exam.

- Tell the doctor if anyone in your family has eye problems or diabetes.

What about cost?

Check with your insurance plan about costs and co-payments. Medicare covers eye exams for:

- People with diabetes

- People who are at high risk for glaucoma
- Some people who have age-related macular degeneration

If you don't have insurance, look for free or low-cost eye care programs where you live.

Tell a doctor about problems.

See an eye doctor right away if you have any of these problems:

- Sudden loss of vision
- Flashes of light
- Tiny spots that float across your eye
- Eye pain
- Redness or swelling

Get regular physical exams.

Get regular checkups to help you stay healthy. Ask your doctor or nurse how you can prevent type 2 diabetes and high blood pressure. These diseases can cause eye problems if they aren't treated.

Lower your risk of falling.

Poor vision or the wrong glasses can increase your risk of falling. One in 3 older adults will fall each year. Falling can cause serious injuries and health problems, especially for people over age 64.

Section 8.6

Get Your Hearing Checked

Text in this section is excerpted from "Get Your Hearing Checked,"
Office of Disease Prevention and Health Promotion (ODPHP),
July 14, 2015.

The Basics

If you are worried that you might have hearing loss, you aren't alone. Many people lose their hearing slowly as they age.

- 1 in 3 Americans between ages 65 and 74 has a hearing problem.

- Almost 1 in 2 Americans over age 75 has a hearing problem.

Start by asking your doctor for a hearing test. Depending on your test results, your doctor may refer you to a hearing specialist.

Hearing problems are serious.

Hearing loss can be frustrating and even dangerous. If you have hearing loss, you may:

- Have trouble hearing doorbells or alarms

- Miss important directions or warnings

- Feel lonely or depressed

Hearing problems can get worse if they aren't treated. That's why it's important to get your hearing checked.

If you find out you have a hearing problem, you can take steps to deal with it before it gets worse.

How do I know if I have hearing loss?

- Do you often ask people to repeat themselves?

- Do you hear ringing in your ears?

- Do people say your TV is too loud?

- Do you have trouble hearing on the telephone?
- Do you have trouble hearing when there's noise in the background?

If you answered yes to some of these questions, you may have hearing loss.

How is hearing loss treated?

There are many products that can help with hearing loss:

- Hearing aids you wear in or behind your ear
- Special phones that make sounds louder
- Tools to help you hear in places like a classroom or theater (called assistive listening devices)
- TVs that also show text (called closed captioning)
- Flashing lights to let you know when an alarm or doorbell is ringing

If you think you have hearing loss, start by seeing a doctor. Find out which treatment options are right for you.

Take Action!

Take steps to find out if you have hearing loss.

Ask your doctor about a hearing test.

If you are worried about your hearing, talk to a doctor. Call your doctor or health center and make an appointment for a hearing test.

What about cost?

Private health insurance or Medicare may cover the cost of a hearing test. Check with your insurance provider to find out if you are covered.

You can still get some screening tests even if you don't have insurance.

Talk to your friends and family.

If you have trouble hearing, your friends and family need to know. They can make small changes to help you hear better when they talk. Ask them to:

- Find a quiet place to talk where there isn't a lot of background noise

- Face you and talk clearly

- Speak slowly

- Keep their hands away from their mouths while they talk

- Avoid eating or chewing gum while talking with you

- Repeat what they said if you didn't hear it the first time

- Write down important information for you

Protect your ears from loud noises.

Wear earplugs or special earmuffs if you need to be around loud noises, like at a construction site or concert. This can help prevent damage to your hearing.

Section 8.7

Recommended Immunizations for Seniors

Text in this section is excerpted from "Health Screenings and Immunizations," National Institutes of Health (NIH), December 2014.

Vaccines, Vaccinations, and Immunizations

Understanding the difference between vaccines, vaccinations, and immunizations can be tricky. Below is an easy guide that explains how these terms are used.

- A vaccine is a product that produces immunity from a disease and can be administered through needle injections, by mouth, or by aerosol.

- A vaccination is the injection of a killed or weakened organism that produces immunity in the body against that organism.

- An immunization is the process by which a person or animal becomes protected from a disease. This term is often used interchangeably with vaccination or inoculation.

How Vaccines Work

Vaccines contain the same germs that cause disease. (For example, measles vaccine contains measles virus.) But they have been either killed or weakened to the point that they don't make you sick. Some vaccines contain only a part of the disease germ.

A vaccine stimulates your immune system to produce antibodies, exactly like it would if you were exposed to the disease. After getting vaccinated, you develop immunity to that disease without having to get the disease first.

This is what makes vaccines such powerful medicine. Unlike most medicines, which treat or cure diseases, vaccines prevent them.

Immunizations for Adults 50+

Here is a list of immunizations adults 50 and older should consider.

- Get a flu shot every year. Over 60 percent of seasonal flu-related hospitalizations occur in people 65 years and older.

- Get a shot for tetanus, diphtheria, and whooping cough. Get a tetanus booster if it has been more than 10 years since your last shot.

- If you are 60 or older, get a shot to prevent shingles. Even if you have had shingles, you can still get the shingles vaccine to help prevent future occurrences of the disease.

- People 65 years or older need a series of two different vaccines for pneumococcal disease. Talk with your health care team about how to schedule them. Be sure to let the team know if you have ever had a pneumococcal vaccine before.

Talk with your health care team about whether you need other vaccinations.

Chapter 9

Genetic Testing

Chapter Contents

Section 9.1

Frequently Asked Questions about Genetic Testing

Text in this section is excerpted from "Genetic Testing," Genetics
Home Reference (GHR), September 1, 2015.

What is genetic testing?

Genetic testing is a type of medical test that identifies changes
in chromosomes, genes, or proteins. The results of a genetic test can
confirm or rule out a suspected genetic condition or help determine a
person's chance of developing or passing on a genetic disorder. More
than 1,000 genetic tests are currently in use, and more are being
developed.

Several methods can be used for genetic testing:

- Molecular genetic tests (or gene tests) study single genes or
  short lengths of DNA to identify variations or mutations that
  lead to a genetic disorder.

- Chromosomal genetic tests analyze whole chromosomes or long
  lengths of DNA to see if there are large genetic changes, such as
  an extra copy of a chromosome, that cause a genetic condition.

- Biochemical genetic tests study the amount or activity level of
  proteins; abnormalities in either can indicate changes to the
  DNA that result in a genetic disorder.

Genetic testing is voluntary. Because testing has benefits as well
as limitations and risks, the decision about whether to be tested is a
personal and complex one. A geneticist or genetic counselor can help
by providing information about the pros and cons of the test and dis-
cussing the social and emotional aspects of testing.

What are the types of genetic tests?

Genetic testing can provide information about a person's genes and
chromosomes. Available types of testing include:

184

Newborn screening

Newborn screening is used just after birth to identify genetic disorders that can be treated early in life. Millions of babies are tested each year in the United States. All states currently test infants for phenylketonuria (a genetic disorder that causes intellectual disability if left untreated) and congenital hypothyroidism (a disorder of the thyroid gland). Most states also test for other genetic disorders.

Diagnostic testing

Diagnostic testing is used to identify or rule out a specific genetic or chromosomal condition. In many cases, genetic testing is used to confirm a diagnosis when a particular condition is suspected based on physical signs and symptoms. Diagnostic testing can be performed before birth or at any time during a person's life, but is not available for all genes or all genetic conditions. The results of a diagnostic test can influence a person's choices about health care and the management of the disorder.

Carrier testing

Carrier testing is used to identify people who carry one copy of a gene mutation that, when present in two copies, causes a genetic disorder. This type of testing is offered to individuals who have a family history of a genetic disorder and to people in certain ethnic groups with an increased risk of specific genetic conditions. If both parents are tested, the test can provide information about a couple's risk of having a child with a genetic condition.

Prenatal testing

Prenatal testing is used to detect changes in a fetus's genes or chromosomes before birth. This type of testing is offered during pregnancy if there is an increased risk that the baby will have a genetic or chromosomal disorder. In some cases, prenatal testing can lessen a couple's uncertainty or help them make decisions about a pregnancy. It cannot identify all possible inherited disorders and birth defects, however.

Preimplantation testing

Preimplantation testing, also called preimplantation genetic diagnosis (PGD), is a specialized technique that can reduce the risk of having a child with a particular genetic or chromosomal disorder. It is used to detect genetic changes in embryos that were created using

185

assisted reproductive techniques such as in-vitro fertilization. In-vitro fertilization involves removing egg cells from a woman's ovaries and fertilizing them with sperm cells outside the body. To perform preimplantation testing, a small number of cells are taken from these embryos and tested for certain genetic changes. Only embryos without these changes are implanted in the uterus to initiate a pregnancy.

Predictive and presymptomatic testing

Predictive and presymptomatic types of testing are used to detect gene mutations associated with disorders that appear after birth, often later in life. These tests can be helpful to people who have a family member with a genetic disorder, but who have no features of the disorder themselves at the time of testing. Predictive testing can identify mutations that increase a person's risk of developing disorders with a genetic basis, such as certain types of cancer. Presymptomatic testing can determine whether a person will develop a genetic disorder, such as hereditary hemochromatosis (an iron overload disorder), before any signs or symptoms appear. The results of predictive and presymptomatic testing can provide information about a person's risk of developing a specific disorder and help with making decisions about medical care.

Forensic testing

Forensic testing uses DNA sequences to identify an individual for legal purposes. Unlike the tests described above, forensic testing is not used to detect gene mutations associated with disease. This type of testing can identify crime or catastrophe victims, rule out or implicate a crime suspect, or establish biological relationships between people (for example, paternity).

How is genetic testing done?

Once a person decides to proceed with genetic testing, a medical geneticist, primary care doctor, specialist, or nurse practitioner can order the test. Genetic testing is often done as part of a genetic consultation.

Genetic tests are performed on a sample of blood, hair, skin, amniotic fluid (the fluid that surrounds a fetus during pregnancy), or other tissue. For example, a procedure called a buccal smear uses a small brush or cotton swab to collect a sample of cells from the inside surface of the cheek. The sample is sent to a laboratory where technicians look for specific changes in chromosomes, DNA, or proteins, depending on the suspected disorder. The laboratory reports the test results in writing to a person's doctor or genetic counselor, or directly to the patient if requested.

Newborn screening tests are done on a small blood sample, which is taken by pricking the baby's heel. Unlike other types of genetic testing, a parent will usually only receive the result if it is positive. If the test result is positive, additional testing is needed to determine whether the baby has a genetic disorder.

Before a person has a genetic test, it is important that he or she understands the testing procedure, the benefits and limitations of the test, and the possible consequences of the test results. The process of educating a person about the test and obtaining permission is called informed consent.

What is informed consent?

Before a person has a genetic test, it is important that he or she fully understands the testing procedure, the benefits and limitations of the test, and the possible consequences of the test results. The process of educating a person about the test and obtaining permission to carry out testing is called informed consent. "Informed" means that the person has enough information to make an educated decision about testing; "consent" refers to a person's voluntary agreement to have the test done.

In general, informed consent can only be given by adults who are competent to make medical decisions for themselves. For children and others who are unable to make their own medical decisions (such as people with impaired mental status), informed consent can be given by a parent, guardian, or other person legally responsible for making decisions on that person's behalf.

Informed consent for genetic testing is generally obtained by a doctor or genetic counselor during an office visit. The healthcare provider will discuss the test and answer any questions. If the person wishes to have the test, he or she will then usually read and sign a consent form.

Several factors are commonly included on an informed consent form:

- A general description of the test, including the purpose of the test and the condition for which the testing is being performed.

- How the test will be carried out (for example, a blood sample).

- What the test results mean, including positive and negative results, and the potential for uninformative results or incorrect results such as false positives or false negatives.

- Any physical or emotional risks associated with the test.

- Whether the results can be used for research purposes.

- Whether the results might provide information about other family members' health, including the risk of developing a particular condition or the possibility of having affected children.

- How and to whom test results will be reported and under what circumstances results can be disclosed (for example, to health insurance providers).

- What will happen to the test specimen after the test is complete.

- Acknowledgement that the person requesting testing has had the opportunity to discuss the test with a healthcare professional.

- The individual's signature, and possibly that of a witness.

The elements of informed consent may vary, because some states have laws that specify factors that must be included. (For example, some states require disclosure that the test specimen will be destroyed within a certain period of time after the test is complete.)

Informed consent is not a contract, so a person can change his or her mind at any time after giving initial consent. A person may choose not to go through with genetic testing even after the test sample has been collected. A person simply needs to notify the healthcare provider if he or she decides not to continue with the testing process.

What do the results of genetic tests mean?

The results of genetic tests are not always straightforward, which often makes them challenging to interpret and explain. Therefore, it is important for patients and their families to ask questions about the potential meaning of genetic test results both before and after the test is performed. When interpreting test results, healthcare professionals consider a person's medical history, family history, and the type of genetic test that was done.

A positive test result means that the laboratory found a change in a particular gene, chromosome, or protein of interest. Depending on the purpose of the test, this result may confirm a diagnosis, indicate that a person is a carrier of a particular genetic mutation, identify an increased risk of developing a disease (such as cancer) in the future, or suggest a need for further testing. Because family members have some genetic material in common, a positive test result may also have implications for certain blood relatives of the person undergoing testing. It is important to note that a positive result of a predictive or presymptomatic genetic test usually cannot establish the exact risk of developing a disorder. Also, health professionals typically cannot use a positive test result to predict the course or severity of a condition.

A negative test result means that the laboratory did not find a change in the gene, chromosome, or protein under consideration. This result can indicate that a person is not affected by a particular disorder, is not a carrier of a specific genetic mutation, or does not have an increased risk of developing a certain disease. It is possible, however, that the test missed a disease-causing genetic alteration because many tests cannot detect all genetic changes that can cause a particular disorder. Further testing may be required to confirm a negative result.

In some cases, a negative result might not give any useful information. This type of result is called uninformative, indeterminate, inconclusive, or ambiguous. Uninformative test results sometimes occur because everyone has common, natural variations in their DNA, called polymorphisms that do not affect health. If a genetic test finds a change in DNA that has not been associated with a disorder in other people, it can be difficult to tell whether it is a natural polymorphism or a disease-causing mutation. An uninformative result cannot confirm or rule out a specific diagnosis, and it cannot indicate whether a person has an increased risk of developing a disorder. In some cases, testing other affected and unaffected family members can help clarify this type of result.

What is the cost of genetic testing, and how long does it take to get the results?

The cost of genetic testing can range from under $100 to more than $2,000, depending on the nature and complexity of the test. The cost increases if more than one test is necessary or if multiple family members must be tested to obtain a meaningful result. For newborn screening, costs vary by state. Some states cover part of the total cost, but most charge a fee of $15 to $60 per infant.

From the date that a sample is taken, it may take a few weeks to several months to receive the test results. Results for prenatal testing are usually available more quickly because time is an important consideration in making decisions about a pregnancy. The doctor or genetic counselor who orders a particular test can provide specific information about the cost and time frame associated with that test.

Will health insurance cover the costs of genetic testing?

In many cases, health insurance plans will cover the costs of genetic testing when it is recommended by a person's doctor. Health insurance providers have different policies about which tests are covered, however. A person interested in submitting the costs of testing may wish to contact his or her insurance company beforehand to ask about coverage.

Some people may choose not to use their insurance to pay for testing because the results of a genetic test can affect a person's health insurance coverage. Instead, they may opt to pay out-of-pocket for the test. People considering genetic testing may want to find out more about their state's privacy protection laws before they ask their insurance company to cover the costs.

What are the benefits of genetic testing?

Genetic testing has potential benefits whether the results are positive or negative for a gene mutation. Test results can provide a sense of relief from uncertainty and help people make informed decisions about managing their health care. For example, a negative result can eliminate the need for unnecessary checkups and screening tests in some cases. A positive result can direct a person toward available prevention, monitoring, and treatment options. Some test results can also help people make decisions about having children. Newborn screening can identify genetic disorders early in life so treatment can be started as early as possible.

What are the risks and limitations of genetic testing?

The physical risks associated with most genetic tests are very small, particularly for those tests that require only a blood sample or buccal smear (a procedure that samples cells from the inside surface of the cheek). The procedures used for prenatal testing carry a small but real risk of losing the pregnancy (miscarriage) because they require a sample of amniotic fluid or tissue from around the fetus.

Many of the risks associated with genetic testing involve the emotional, social, or financial consequences of the test results. People may feel angry, depressed, anxious, or guilty about their results. In some cases, genetic testing creates tension within a family because the results can reveal information about other family members in addition to the person who is tested. The possibility of genetic discrimination in employment or insurance is also a concern.

Genetic testing can provide only limited information about an inherited condition. The test often can't determine if a person will show symptoms of a disorder, how severe the symptoms will be, or whether the disorder will progress over time. Another major limitation is the lack of treatment strategies for many genetic disorders once they are diagnosed.

A genetics professional can explain in detail the benefits, risks, and limitations of a particular test. It is important that any person who is considering genetic testing understand and weigh these factors before making a decision.

How does genetic testing in a research setting differ from clinical genetic testing?

The main differences between clinical genetic testing and research testing are the purpose of the test and who receives the results. The goals of research testing include finding unknown genes, learning how genes work, developing tests for future clinical use, and advancing our understanding of genetic conditions. The results of testing done as part of a research study are usually not available to patients or their healthcare providers. Clinical testing, on the other hand, is done to find out about an inherited disorder in an individual patient or family. People receive the results of a clinical test and can use them to help them make decisions about medical care or reproductive issues.

It is important for people considering genetic testing to know whether the test is available on a clinical or research basis. Clinical and research testing both involve a process of informed consent in which patients learn about the testing procedure, the risks and benefits of the test, and the potential consequences of testing.

Section 9.2

Inheriting Genetic Conditions

Text in this section is excerpted from "Inheriting Genetic Conditions,"
Genetics Home Reference (GHR), September 1, 2015.

What does it mean if a disorder seems to run in my family?

A particular disorder might be described as "running in a family" if more than one person in the family has the condition. Some disorders that affect multiple family members are caused by gene mutations, which can be inherited (passed down from parent to child). Other conditions that appear to run in families are not caused by mutations in single genes. Instead, environmental factors such as dietary habits or a combination of genetic and environmental factors are responsible for these disorders.

It is not always easy to determine whether a condition in a family is inherited. A genetics professional can use a person's family history (a record of health information about a person's immediate and extended family) to help determine whether a disorder has a genetic component. He or she will ask about the health of people from several generations of the family, usually first-, second-, and third-degree relatives.

Why is it important to know my family medical history?

A family medical history is a record of health information about a person and his or her close relatives. A complete record includes information from three generations of relatives, including children, brothers and sisters, parents, aunts and uncles, nieces and nephews, grandparents, and cousins.

Table 9.1. Degrees of relationship

Degrees of relationship	Examples
First-degree relatives	Parents, children, brothers, and sisters
Second-degree relatives	Grandparents, aunts and uncles, nieces and nephews, and grandchildren
Third-degree relatives	First cousin

Families have many factors in common, including their genes, environment, and lifestyle. Together, these factors can give clues to medical conditions that may run in a family. By noticing patterns of disorders among relatives, healthcare professionals can determine whether an individual, other family members, or future generations may be at an increased risk of developing a particular condition.

A family medical history can identify people with a higher-than-usual chance of having common disorders, such as heart disease, high blood pressure, stroke, certain cancers, and diabetes. These complex disorders are influenced by a combination of genetic factors, environmental conditions, and lifestyle choices. A family history also can provide information about the risk of rarer conditions caused by mutations in a single gene, such as cystic fibrosis and sickle cell anemia.

While a family medical history provides information about the risk of specific health concerns, having relatives with a medical condition does not mean that an individual will definitely develop that condition. On the other hand, a person with no family history of a disorder may still be at risk of developing that disorder.

Knowing one's family medical history allows a person to take steps to reduce his or her risk. For people at an increased risk of certain cancers, healthcare professionals may recommend more frequent screening (such as mammography or colonoscopy) starting at an earlier age. Healthcare providers may also encourage regular checkups or testing for people with a medical condition that runs in their family. Additionally, lifestyle changes such as adopting a healthier diet, getting regular exercise, and quitting smoking help many people lower their chances of developing heart disease and other common illnesses.

The easiest way to get information about family medical history is to talk to relatives about their health. Have they had any medical problems, and when did they occur? A family gathering could be a good time to discuss these issues. Additionally, obtaining medical records and other documents (such as obituaries and death certificates) can help complete a family medical history. It is important to keep this information up-to-date and to share it with a healthcare professional regularly.

What are the different ways in which a genetic condition can be inherited?

Some genetic conditions are caused by mutations in a single gene. These conditions are usually inherited in one of several straightforward patterns, depending on the gene involved:

Many other disorders are caused by a combination of the effects of multiple genes or by interactions between genes and the environment. Such disorders are more difficult to analyze because their genetic causes are often unclear, and they do not follow the patterns of inheritance described above. Examples of conditions caused by multiple genes or gene/environment interactions include heart disease, diabetes, schizophrenia, and certain types of cancer.

Disorders caused by changes in the number or structure of chromosomes do not follow the straightforward patterns of inheritance listed above.

If a genetic disorder runs in my family, what are the chances that my children will have the condition?

When a genetic disorder is diagnosed in a family, family members often want to know the likelihood that they or their children will develop the condition. This can be difficult to predict in some cases because many factors influence a person's chances of developing a genetic condition. One important factor is how the condition is inherited. For example:

- Autosomal dominant inheritance: A person affected by an autosomal dominant disorder has a 50 percent chance of passing the mutated gene to each child. The chance that a child will not inherit the mutated gene is also 50 percent

- Autosomal recessive inheritance: Two unaffected people who each carry one copy of the mutated gene for an autosomal recessive disorder (carriers) have a 25 percent chance with each pregnancy of having a child affected by the disorder. The chance with each pregnancy of having an unaffected child who is a carrier of the disorder is 50 percent, and the chance that a child will not have the disorder and will not be a carrier is 25 percent.

- X-linked dominant inheritance: The chance of passing on an X-linked dominant condition differs between men and women because men have one X chromosome and one Y chromosome, while women have two X chromosomes. A man passes on his Y chromosome to all of his sons and his X chromosome to all of his daughters. Therefore, the sons of a man with an X-linked dominant disorder will not be affected, but all of his daughters will inherit the condition. A woman passes on one or the other of her X chromosomes to each child. Therefore, a woman with an

Table 9.2. Patterns of inheritance

Inheritance pattern	Description	Examples
Autosomal dominant	One mutated copy of the gene in each cell is sufficient for a person to be affected by an autosomal dominant disorder. Each affected person usually has one affected parent (illustration). Autosomal dominant disorders tend to occur in every generation of an affected family.	Huntington disease, neurofibromatosis type 1
Autosomal recessive	Two mutated copies of the gene are present in each cell when a person has an autosomal recessive disorder. An affected person usually has unaffected parents who each carry a single copy of the mutated gene (and are referred to as carriers) (illustration). Autosomal recessive disorders are typically not seen in every generation of an affected family.	cystic fibrosis, sickle cell anemia
X-linked dominant	X-linked dominant disorders are caused by mutations in genes on the X chromosome. Females are more frequently affected than males, and the chance of passing on an X-linked dominant disorder differs between men (illustration) and women (illustration). Families with an X-linked dominant disorder often have both affected males and affected females in each generation. A characteristic of X-linked inheritance is that fathers cannot pass X-linked traits to their sons (no male-to-male transmission).	fragile X syndrome
X-linked recessive	X-linked recessive disorders are also caused by mutations in genes on the X chromosome. Males are more frequently affected than females, and the chance of passing on the disorder differs between men (illustration) and women (illustration). Families with an X-linked recessive disorder often have affected males, but rarely affected females, in each generation. A characteristic of X-linked inheritance is that fathers cannot pass X-linked traits to their sons (no male-to-male transmission).	hemophilia, Fabry disease

Table 9.2. Continued

Inheritance pattern	Description	Examples
Codominant	In codominant inheritance, two different versions (alleles) of a gene can be expressed, and each version makes a slightly different protein (illustration). Both alleles influence the genetic trait or determine the characteristics of the genetic condition.	ABO blood group, alpha-1 antitrypsin deficiency
Mitochondrial	This type of inheritance, also known as maternal inheritance, applies to genes in mitochondrial DNA. Mitochondria, which are structures in each cell that convert molecules into energy, each contain a small amount of DNA. Because only egg cells contribute mitochondria to the developing embryo, only females can pass on mitochondrial mutations to their children (illustration). Disorders resulting from mutations in mitochondrial DNA can appear in every generation of a family and can affect both males and females, but fathers do not pass these disorders to their children.	Leber hereditary optic neuropathy (LHON)

X-linked dominant disorder has a 50 percent chance of having an affected daughter or son with each pregnancy.

- X-linked recessive inheritance: Because of the difference in sex chromosomes, the probability of passing on an X-linked recessive disorder also differs between men and women. The sons of a man with an X-linked recessive disorder will not be affected, and his daughters will carry one copy of the mutated gene. With each pregnancy, a woman who carries an X-linked recessive disorder has a 50 percent chance of having sons who are affected and a 50 percent chance of having daughters who carry one copy of the mutated gene.

- Codominant inheritance: In codominant inheritance, each parent contributes a different version of a particular gene, and both versions influence the resulting genetic trait. The chance of developing a genetic condition with codominant inheritance, and the characteristic features of that condition, depend on which versions of the gene are passed from parents to their child.

- Mitochondrial inheritance: Mitochondria, which are the energy-producing centers inside cells, each contain a small amount of DNA. Disorders with mitochondrial inheritance result from mutations in mitochondrial DNA. Although these disorders can affect both males and females, only females can pass mutations in mitochondrial DNA to their children. A woman with a disorder caused by changes in mitochondrial DNA will pass the mutation to all of her daughters and sons, but the children of a man with such a disorder will not inherit the mutation.

It is important to note that the chance of passing on a genetic condition applies equally to each pregnancy. For example, if a couple has a child with an autosomal recessive disorder, the chance of having another child with the disorder is still 25 percent (or 1 in 4). Having one child with a disorder does not "protect" future children from inheriting the condition. Conversely, having a child without the condition does not mean that future children will definitely be affected.

Although the chances of inheriting a genetic condition appear straightforward, factors such as a person's family history and the results of genetic testing can sometimes modify those chances. In addition, some people with a disease-causing mutation never develop any health problems or may experience only mild symptoms of the disorder. If a disease that runs in a family does not have a clear-cut inheritance pattern, predicting the likelihood that a person will develop the condition can be particularly difficult.

Estimating the chance of developing or passing on a genetic disorder can be complex. Genetics professionals can help people understand these chances and help them make informed decisions about their health.

Chapter 10

Screening Tests for Immigrants and Refugees

Medical Screening: General Information

What is CDC's role in medical screening?

The Division of Global Migration and Quarantine, CDC, provides the technical instructions and guidance to physicians conducting the medical examination for immigration. These instructions are developed in accordance with Section 212(a)(1)(A) of the INA, which states those classes of aliens ineligible for visas or admission based on health-related grounds. The health-related grounds include those aliens who have a communicable disease of public health significance, who fail to present documentation of having received vaccination against vaccine-preventable diseases (immigrants only), who have or have had a physical or mental disorder with associated harmful behavior, and who are drug abusers or addicts.

Who performs the medical examination?

Outside the United States, medical examinations are performed by physicians called panel physicians, who are selected by Department of State Consular Officials. In the United States, medical examinations are performed by physicians called civil surgeons, who are designated by district directors of the USCIS.

Text in this chapter is excerpted from "CDC Domestic Refugee Health Program," Centers for Disease Control and Prevention (CDC), July 31, 2014.

What is a panel physician?

A panel physician is a physician outside the United States who performs the medical examinations for refugees and individuals applying for an immigrant visa. These physicians are selected by Department of State Consular Officials.

What is a civil surgeon?

A civil surgeon is a physician who performs medical examinations in the United States for aliens applying for adjustment of their immigration status to that of permanent resident. These physicians are designated by district directors of the U.S. Citizenship and Immigration Service.

Who is required to have a medical examination?

A medical examination is mandatory for all refugees coming to the United States and all applicants outside the United States applying for an immigrant visa. Aliens in the United States who apply for adjustment of their immigration status to that of permanent resident are also required to be medically examined. Aliens applying for non-immigrant visas (temporary admission) may be required to undergo a medical examination at the discretion of the consular officer overseas or immigration officer at the U.S. port of entry, if there is reason to suspect that an inadmissible health-related condition exists. Asylees are not required to have a medical examination.

What is the required overseas medical screening for a refugee?

Overseas, U.S.-bound refugees must undergo a medical examination as part of the visa application process. The purpose of the medical examination is to identify the presence or absence of certain physical or mental disorders that could result in ineligibility for admission to (or exclusion from) the United States under the provisions of the Immigration and Nationality Act. Waivers of ineligibility are available for certain medical grounds of inadmissibility.

How long are laboratory results valid for?

The 1991 Technical Instructions for Medical Examination of Aliens do not address the validity of laboratory results. However, the physician who performs the exam is required to ensure that all medical tests are properly conducted and that test results are in fact those of the applicant and are current. A standard medical examination is valid for immigration purposes for one year from the date of the physician's signature.

What is the allowable time interval between the overseas examination (validity period) and U.S. arrival?

The allowable time interval between the completion of the overseas examination and U.S. arrival is 12 months. If the applicant has a Class A or TB classification, the interval is 6 months. For Hmong and Burmese refugees resettling from Thailand, the allowable time interval between the overseas examination and U.S. arrival is 3 months, regardless of whether the refugee has a TB classification. For Class B1 refugees, the 3-month interval begins when the culture results are reported; culture results are usually reported within 8 weeks of sputum collection.

Medical Screening: STDs

What STD screening tests are done overseas on refugees?

The sexually transmitted diseases that are screened/tested for are HIV, syphilis, chancroid, gonorrhea, granuloma inguinale, and lymphogranuloma venereum. The medical history and physical examination must include a search for symptoms or lesions consistent with these diseases. Further testing should be done as necessary to confirm a suspected diagnosis. Routine laboratory testing is performed only for HIV and syphilis.

At what age are refugees screened overseas for syphilis and HIV?

All applicants 15 years of age or older must be tested for evidence of syphilis and HIV infection. Applicants under the age of 15 must be tested for HIV if there is reason to suspect HIV infection (e.g., a child with hemophilia or a child whose mother or father is HIV positive). Applicants under the age of 15 must be tested for syphilis if there is reason to suspect infection with syphilis.

Are hepatitis panels routinely done on all refugees overseas?

Hepatitis panels are not routinely done on refugees overseas.

If an overseas blood screening reveals syphilis, what procedure are the overseas panel physicians following to assess whether the condition is actually syphilis and not another treponemal infection?

If the screening test is positive, a confirmatory test must be done. The applicant must be treated by using a standard treatment regimen before he/she can travel to the United States. Once the recommended treatment is completed, syphilis is no longer considered a Class A condition.

Post-treatment, the syphilis would be considered a Class B condition only if the applicant has some residual disability (e.g., an individual treated for neurosyphilis who has a residual neurologic abnormality).

Medical Screening: Vaccinations

Who is required to have vaccinations as part of the medical screening?

On September 30, 1996, the U.S. Congress amended the Immigration and Nationality Act by adding to the health-related grounds of inadmissibility a new subsection, "Proof of Vaccination Requirements for Immigrants." This new subsection requires any person who seeks an immigrant visa to show proof of having received vaccination against vaccine-preventable diseases, as recommended by the U.S. Advisory Committee on Immunization Practices.

The U.S. Immigration and Naturalization Service – now Department of Homeland Security, United States Citizenship and Immigrant Service – has determined that the vaccination requirements do not apply to refugees and nonimmigrants at the time of their initial admission to the United States. However, refugees and V (spouses or children of permanent residents) and K (fiancé(e) of permanent resident) visa holders in the U.S. must comply with the vaccination requirements when they apply for adjustment of status to Legal Permanent Resident; for refugees this application occurs one year after arrival in the United States.

Are asylees required to have vaccinations?

No, asylees are not required to have any vaccinations. However, asylees must comply with the vaccination requirements if they apply for adjustment of status to Legal Permanent Resident.

What is the Advisory Committee on Immunization Practices (ACIP)?

The ACIP is a committee appointed by the Secretary of the U.S. Department of Health and Human Services to provide federal recommendations on the routine administration of and schedules for vaccines.

Medical Screening: Domestic

Is there domestic guidance for states performing refugee health assessments for newly arrived refugees?

Currently, the guidance for states for the domestic follow-up examination for newly arrived refugees is the 1995 ORR Medical Screening

Protocol (State Letter 95-37). Many states have added requirements in addition to the ORR protocol. The Department of Health and Human Services is now drafting guidance for an expanded domestic protocol for states.

Is the post-arrival medical screening mandatory for immigrants and refugees who have B1 or B2 tuberculosis classifications?

The post-arrival medical screening for immigrants and refugees with TB conditions is not mandatory, but it is highly recommended that the assessment be done. Any follow-up examination should be completed within 30 days post-arrival.

What are the post-arrival requirements for health assessments of HIV-positive refugees?

The health-care provider should perform an initial evaluation, counseling, and follow-up for the refugee. The post-arrival HIV(+) health assessment is procedurally distinct from the standard post-arrival health assessment. CDC should receive a copy of a letter from the health-care provider stating that the refugee has received an initial evaluation.

Notifications and the Electronic Disease Notification (EDN) System

What are the DS forms?

The DS forms are Department of State forms used to collect the medical screening results from the overseas examinations. All immigrant visa and refugee applicants must undergo a physical examination and mental status assessment as part of their application process. The panel physicians complete these forms overseas, and the refugee carries copies to the United States. After processing the documents of the refugee or immigrant at the Port of Entry, the CDC Quarantine Station sends the DS forms to the state or local health department at the refugee's or immigrant's destination.

What is EDN?

The Electronic Disease Notification (EDN) system is a Web-based system that improves and automates the process that notifies state or local health officials of the arrival of immigrants with notifiable conditions and refugees to their jurisdictions. EDN provides relevant overseas medical screening and treatment information for stateside follow-up. EDN was launched on March 20, 2006 and as of July 2007 has been deployed to 18 states.

Part Three

Laboratory Tests

Chapter 11

Understanding Laboratory Tests

What are lab tests?

Laboratory tests are medical procedures that involve testing samples of blood, urine, or other tissues or substances in the body.

Why does your doctor use lab tests?

Your doctor uses laboratory tests to help:

- identify changes in your health condition before any symptoms occur
- diagnose a disease or condition before you have symptoms
- plan your treatment for a disease or condition
- evaluate your response to a treatment or
- monitor the course of a disease over time

How are lab tests analyzed?

After your doctor collects a sample from your body, it is sent to a laboratory. Laboratories perform tests on the sample to see if it reacts

Text in this chapter is excerpted from "Laboratory Tests," U.S. Food and Drug Administration (FDA), June 5, 2014.

to different substances. Depending on the test, a reaction may mean you do have a particular condition or it may mean that you do not have the particular condition. Sometimes laboratories compare your results to results obtained from previous tests, to see if there has been a change in your condition.

What do lab tests show?

Lab tests show whether or not your results fall within normal ranges. Normal test values are usually given as a range, rather than as a specific number, because normal values vary from person to person. What is normal for one person may not be normal for another person.

Some laboratory tests are precise, reliable indicators of specific health problems, while others provide more general information that gives doctors clues to your possible health problems. Information obtained from laboratory tests may help doctors decide whether other tests or procedures are needed to make a diagnosis or to develop or revise a previous treatment plan. All laboratory test results must be interpreted within the context of your overall health and should be used along with other exams or tests.

What factors affect your lab test results?

Many factors can affect test results, including:

- sex
- age
- race
- medical history
- general health
- specific foods
- drugs you are taking
- how closely your follow preparatory instructions
- variations in laboratory techniques
- variation from one laboratory to another

Chapter 12

Lead Screening Test

Lead – An Introduction

Lead is a naturally occurring element found in small amounts in the earth's crust. While it has some beneficial uses, it can be toxic to humans and animals causing of health effects.

Where is Lead Found?

Lead can be found in all parts of our environment – the air, the soil, the water, and even inside our homes. Much of our exposure comes from human activities including the use of fossil fuels including past use of leaded gasoline, some types of industrial facilities, and past use of lead-based paint in homes. Lead and lead compounds have been used in a wide variety of products found in and around our homes, including paint, ceramics, pipes and plumbing materials, solders, gasoline, batteries, ammunition, and cosmetics.

Lead may enter the environment from these past and current uses. Lead can also be emitted into the environment from industrial sources and contaminated sites, such as former lead smelters. While natural levels of lead in soil range between 50 and 400 parts per million, mining, smelting, and refining activities have resulted in substantial

This chapter includes excerpts from "Human Health and Lead," United States Environmental Protection Agency (EPA), November 26, 2013; and text from "Rapid Lead Screening Test," U.S. Food and Drug Administration (FDA), June 5, 2014.

increases in lead levels in the environment, especially near mining and smelting sites.

When lead is released to the air from industrial sources or vehicles, it may travel long distances before settling to the ground, where it usually sticks to soil particles. Lead may move from soil into ground water depending on the type of lead compound and the characteristics of the soil.

Federal and state regulatory standards have helped to minimize or eliminate the amount of lead in air, drinking water, soil, consumer products, food, and occupational settings.

Who are at Risk?

Children

Lead is particularly dangerous to children because their growing bodies absorb more lead than adults do and their brains and nervous systems are more sensitive to the damaging effects of lead. Babies and young children can also be more highly exposed to lead because they often put their hands and other objects that can have lead from dust or soil on them into their mouths. Children may also be exposed to lead by eating and drinking food or water containing lead or from dishes or glasses that contain lead, inhaling lead dust from lead-based paint or lead-contaminated soil or from playing with toys with lead paint.

Adults, Including Pregnant Women

Adults may be exposed to lead by eating and drinking food or water containing lead or from dishes or glasses that contain lead. They may also breath lead dust by spending time in areas where lead-based paint is deteriorating, and during renovation or repair work that disturbs painted surfaces in older homes and buildings. Working in a job or engaging in hobbies where lead is used, such as making stained glass, can increase exposure as can certain folk remedies containing lead. A pregnant woman's exposure to lead from these sources is of particular concern because it can result in exposure to her developing baby.

What are the Health Effects of Lead?

Lead can affect almost every organ and system in your body. Children six years old and younger are most susceptible to the effects of lead.

Children

Even low levels of lead in the blood of children can result in:

- Behavior and learning problems
- Lower IQ and Hyperactivity
- Slowed growth
- Hearing Problems
- Anemia

In rare cases, ingestion of lead can cause seizures, coma and even death.

Pregnant Women

Lead can accumulate in our bodies over time, where it is stored in bones along with calcium. During pregnancy, lead is released from bones as maternal calcium and is used to help form the bones of the fetus. This is particularly true if a woman does not have enough dietary calcium. Lead can also cross the placental barrier exposing the fetus the lead. This can result in serious effects to the mother and her developing fetus, including:

- Reduced growth of the fetus
- Premature birth

Other Adults

Lead is also harmful to other adults. Adults exposed to lead can suffer from:

- Cardiovascular effects, increased blood pressure and incidence of hypertension
- Decreased kidney function
- Reproductive problems (in both men and women)

Lower Your Chances of Exposure to Lead

Simple steps like keeping your home clean and well-maintained will go a long way in preventing lead exposure. You can lower the chances of exposure to lead in your home, both now and in the future, by taking these steps:

- Inspect and maintain all painted surfaces to prevent paint deterioration

- Address water damage quickly and completely

- Keep your home clean and dust-free

- Clean around painted areas where friction can generate dust, such as doors, windows, and drawers. Wipe these areas with a wet sponge or rag to remove paint chips or dust

- Use only cold water to prepare food and drinks

- Flush water outlets used for drinking or food preparation

- Clean debris out of outlet screens or faucet aerators on a regular basis

- Wash children's hands, bottles, pacifiers and toys often

- Teach children to wipe and remove their shoes and wash hands after playing outdoors

- Ensure that your family members eat well-balanced meals. Children with healthy diets absorb less lead.

What do I do if I think my child or I have been exposed to lead?

Talk to your pediatrician, general physician, or local health agency about what you can do. Your doctor can do a simple blood test to check you or your child for lead exposure. You may also want to test your home for sources of lead.

Rapid Lead Screening Test

There is now a test that provides immediate results on lead levels in children and adults that can be used at thousands of places nationwide, including health clinics, mobile healthcare units and doctors' offices. Broader availability and easier access to this test means lead exposure can be detected and treated earlier before the damaging effects of lead poisoning occur.

U.S. Department of Health and Human Services is allowing the LeadCare II Blood Lead Test System, made by ESA Biosciences (Chelmsford, Mass.), to be used at more than 115,000 certified point-of-care settings because the company proved to the U.S. Food and Drug Administration (FDA) that the test is simple, accurate and poses very little risk of harm to a patient. The test was only available for use in certain laboratories and patients oftentimes had to wait several days or more to find out their results. Doctors have said that it is sometimes difficult to reach patients to give them their results or to discuss treatment options when they have elevated blood lead levels.

The Centers for Disease Control and Prevention (CDC) has found that more than 300,000 children under age six each year have blood levels that exceed 10μg/dL, the threshold used to indicate lead poisoning. The American Academy of Pediatrics (AAP) estimates one out of four homes with children under age six has lead contamination. The CDC and AAP recommend screening children at ages one and two who live in high-risk homes.

Lead poisoning in children typically results from drinking water from corroding plumbing, and inhaling or ingesting dust from deteriorating lead-based paint. Symptoms of lead poisoning include headaches, stomach cramps, fatigue, memory loss, high blood pressure, and seizures. Lead poisoning in children has been linked to learning disabilities and developmental delays.

The LeadCare II Blood Test System measures lead in blood samples using a finger stick or taking a blood sample from a person's vein, and gives results in as little as three minutes. The rapid result means a second sample for further testing can be obtained quickly if needed, reducing the need for a follow-up visit.

Chapter 13

Common Blood Tests

What are Blood Tests?

Blood tests help doctors check for certain diseases and conditions. They also help check the function of your organs and show how well treatments are working.

Specifically, blood tests can help doctors:

- Evaluate how well organs—such as the kidneys, liver, thyroid, and heart—are working

- Diagnose diseases and conditions such as cancer, HIV/AIDS, diabetes, anemia (uh-NEE-me-eh), and coronary heart disease

- Find out whether you have risk factors for heart disease

- Check whether medicines you're taking are working

- Assess how well your blood is clotting

Overview

Blood tests are very common. When you have routine checkups, your doctor may recommend blood tests to see how your body is working.

Many blood tests don't require any special preparations. For some, you may need to fast (not eat any food) for 8 to 12 hours before the test. Your doctor will let you know how to prepare for blood tests.

Text in this chapter is excerpted from "Blood Tests," National Heart, Lung, and Blood Institute (NHLBI), January 6, 2012.

During a blood test, a small sample of blood is taken from your body. It's usually drawn from a vein in your arm using a needle. A finger prick also might be used.

The procedure usually is quick and easy, although it may cause some short-term discomfort. Most people don't have serious reactions to having blood drawn.

Laboratory (lab) workers draw the blood and analyze it. They use either whole blood to count blood cells, or they separate the blood cells from the fluid that contains them. This fluid is called plasma or serum.

The fluid is used to measure different substances in the blood. The results can help detect health problems in early stages, when treatments or lifestyle changes may work best.

Doctors can't diagnose many diseases and medical problems with blood tests alone. Your doctor may consider other factors to confirm a diagnosis. These factors can include your signs and symptoms, your medical history, your vital signs (blood pressure, breathing, pulse, and temperature), and results from other tests and procedures.

Outlook

Blood tests have few risks. Most complications are minor and go away shortly after the tests are done.

Types of Blood Tests

Some of the most common blood tests are:

- A complete blood count (CBC)
- Blood chemistry tests
- Blood enzyme tests
- Blood tests to assess heart disease risk

Complete Blood Count

The CBC is one of the most common blood tests. It's often done as part of a routine checkup.

The CBC can help detect blood diseases and disorders, such as anemia, infections, clotting problems, blood cancers, and immune system disorders. This test measures many different parts of your blood, as discussed in the following paragraphs.

Red Blood Cells

Red blood cells carry oxygen from your lungs to the rest of your body. Abnormal red blood cell levels may be a sign of anemia, dehydration (too little fluid in the body), bleeding, or another disorder.

White Blood Cells

White blood cells are part of your immune system, which fights infections and diseases. Abnormal white blood cell levels may be a sign of infection, blood cancer, or an immune system disorder.

A CBC measures the overall number of white blood cells in your blood. A CBC with differential looks at the amounts of different types of white blood cells in your blood.

Platelets

Platelets (PLATE-lets) are blood cell fragments that help your blood clot. They stick together to seal cuts or breaks on blood vessel walls and stop bleeding.

Abnormal platelet levels may be a sign of a bleeding disorder (not enough clotting) or a thrombotic disorder (too much clotting).

Hemoglobin

Hemoglobin (HEE-muh-glow-bin) is an iron-rich protein in red blood cells that carries oxygen. Abnormal hemoglobin levels may be a sign of anemia, sickle cell anemia, thalassemia (thal-a-SE-me-ah), or other blood disorders.

If you have diabetes, excess glucose in your blood can attach to hemoglobin and raise the level of hemoglobin A1c.

Hematocrit

Hematocrit (hee-MAT-oh-crit) is a measure of how much space red blood cells take up in your blood. A high hematocrit level might mean you're dehydrated. A low hematocrit level might mean you have anemia. Abnormal hematocrit levels also may be a sign of a blood or bone marrow disorder.

Mean Corpuscular Volume

Mean corpuscular volume (MCV) is a measure of the average size of your red blood cells. Abnormal MCV levels may be a sign of anemia or thalassemia.

Blood Chemistry Tests / Basic Metabolic Panel

The basic metabolic panel (BMP) is a group of tests that measures different chemicals in the blood. These tests usually are done on the fluid (plasma) part of blood. The tests can give doctors information about your muscles (including the heart), bones, and organs, such as the kidneys and liver.

The BMP includes blood glucose, calcium, and electrolyte tests, as well as blood tests that measure kidney function. Some of these tests require you to fast (not eat any food) before the test, and others don't. Your doctor will tell you how to prepare for the test(s) you're having.

Blood Glucose

Glucose is a type of sugar that the body uses for energy. Abnormal glucose levels in your blood may be a sign of diabetes.

For some blood glucose tests, you have to fast before your blood is drawn. Other blood glucose tests are done after a meal or at any time with no preparation.

Calcium

Calcium is an important mineral in the body. Abnormal calcium levels in the blood may be a sign of kidney problems, bone disease, thyroid disease, cancer, malnutrition, or another disorder.

Electrolytes

Electrolytes are minerals that help maintain fluid levels and acid-base balance in the body. They include sodium, potassium, bicarbonate, and chloride.

Abnormal electrolyte levels may be a sign of dehydration, kidney disease, liver disease, heart failure, high blood pressure, or other disorders.

Kidneys

Blood tests for kidney function measure levels of blood urea nitrogen (BUN) and creatinine. Both of these are waste products that the kidneys filter out of the body. Abnormal BUN and creatinine levels may be signs of a kidney disease or disorder.

Blood Enzyme Tests

Enzymes are chemicals that help control chemical reactions in your body. There are many blood enzyme tests. This section focuses on blood enzyme tests used to check for heart attack. These include troponin and creatine kinase (CK) tests.

Troponin

Troponin is a muscle protein that helps your muscles contract. When muscle or heart cells are injured, troponin leaks out, and its levels in your blood rise.

For example, blood levels of troponin rise when you have a heart attack. For this reason, doctors often order troponin tests when patients have chest pain or other heart attack signs and symptoms.

Creatine Kinase

A blood product called CK-MB is released when the heart muscle is damaged. High levels of CK-MB in the blood can mean that you've had a heart attack.

Blood Tests To Assess Heart Disease Risk

A lipoprotein panel is a blood test that can help show whether you're at risk for coronary heart disease (CHD). This test looks at substances in your blood that carry cholesterol.

A lipoprotein panel gives information about your:

- Total cholesterol.
- LDL ("bad") cholesterol. This is the main source of cholesterol buildup and blockages in the arteries. (For more information about blockages in the arteries, go to the Diseases and Conditions Index Atherosclerosis article.)
- HDL ("good") cholesterol. This type of cholesterol helps decrease blockages in the arteries.
- Triglycerides. Triglycerides are a type of fat in your blood.

A lipoprotein panel measures the levels of LDL and HDL cholesterol and triglycerides in your blood. Abnormal cholesterol and triglyceride levels may be signs of increased risk for CHD.

Most people will need to fast for 9 to 12 hours before a lipoprotein panel.

Blood Clotting Tests

Blood clotting tests sometimes are called a coagulation panel. These tests check proteins in your blood that affect the blood clotting process.

Abnormal test results might suggest that you're at risk of bleeding or developing clots in your blood vessels.

Your doctor may recommend these tests if he or she thinks you have a disorder or disease related to blood clotting.

Blood clotting tests also are used to monitor people who are taking medicines to lower the risk of blood clots. Warfarin and heparin are two examples of such medicines.

Chapter 14

Biopsies

Chapter Contents

Section 14.1

Breast Biopsy

Text in this section is excerpted from "Understanding Breast
Changes: A Health Guide for Women," National Cancer Institute
(NCI), April 23, 2015.

A breast biopsy is a procedure to remove a sample of breast cells
or tissue, or an entire lump. A pathologist then looks at the sample
under a microscope to check for signs of disease. A biopsy is the only
way to find out if cells are cancer. Biopsies are usually done in an
office or a clinic on an outpatient basis. This means you will go home
the same day as the procedure. Local anesthesia is used for some
biopsies. This means you will be awake, but you won't feel pain in
your breast during the procedure. General anesthesia is often used
for a surgical biopsy.

This means that you will be asleep and won't wake up during the
procedure. Common types of breast biopsies include:

- **Fine-needle aspiration biopsy:** A fine-needle aspiration
  biopsy is a simple procedure that takes only a few minutes. Your
  health care provider inserts a thin needle into the breast to take
  out fluid and cells.

- **Core biopsy:** A core biopsy, also called a core needle biopsy,
  uses a needle to remove small pieces or cores of breast tissue.
  The samples are about the size of a grain of rice. You may have a
  bruise, but usually not a scar.

- **Vacuum-assisted biopsy:** A vacuum-assisted biopsy uses a
  probe, connected to a vacuum device, to remove a small sample of breast tissue. The small cut made in the breast is much
  smaller than with surgical biopsy. This procedure causes very
  little scarring, and no stitches are needed.

- **Surgical biopsy:** A surgical biopsy is an operation to remove
  part, or all, of a lump so it can be looked at under a microscope to check for signs of disease. Sometimes a doctor will do
  a surgical biopsy as the first step. Other times, a doctor may

do a surgical biopsy if the results of a needle biopsy do not give enough information. When only a sample of breast tissue is removed, it's called an incisional biopsy. When the entire lump or suspicious area is removed, it's called an excisional biopsy.

Section 14.2

Liver Biopsy

Text in this section is excerpted from "Liver Biopsy," National Institute of Diabetes and Digestive and Kidney Diseases (NIDDK), May 7, 2014.

What is a liver biopsy?

A liver biopsy is a procedure that involves taking a small piece of liver tissue for examination with a microscope for signs of damage or disease. The three types of liver biopsy are the following:

- Percutaneous biopsy—the most common type of liver biopsy—involves inserting a hollow needle through the abdomen into the liver. The abdomen is the area between the chest and hips.

- Transvenous biopsy involves making a small incision in the neck and inserting a needle through a hollow tube called a sheath through the jugular vein to the liver.

- Laparoscopic biopsy involves inserting a laparoscope, a thin tube with a tiny video camera attached, through a small incision to look inside the body to view the surface of organs. The health care provider will insert a needle through a plastic, tube-like instrument called a cannula to remove the liver tissue sample.

What is the liver and what does it do?

The liver is the body's largest internal organ. The liver is called the body's metabolic factory because of the important role it plays in metabolism—the way cells change food into energy after food is digested and absorbed into the blood. The liver has many functions, including

- taking up, storing, and processing nutrients from food—including fat, sugar, and protein—and delivering them to the rest of the body when needed

- making new proteins, such as clotting factors and immune factors

- producing bile, which helps the body absorb fats, cholesterol, and fat-soluble vitamins

- removing waste products the kidneys cannot remove, such as fats, cholesterol, toxins, and medications

A healthy liver is necessary for survival. The liver can regenerate most of its own cells when they become damaged.

The liver, the body's largest internal organ, has many important functions.

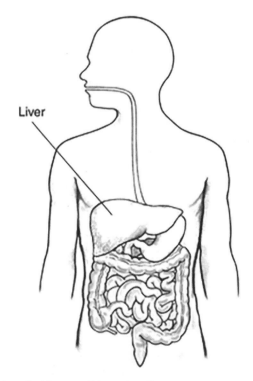

Figure 14.1. *Liver in Human Digestive Tract*

Why is a liver biopsy performed?

A health care provider will perform a liver biopsy to

- diagnose liver diseases that cannot be diagnosed with blood or imaging tests
- estimate the degree of liver damage, a process called staging
- help determine the best treatment for liver damage or disease

How does a person prepare for a liver biopsy?

A person prepares for a liver biopsy by

- talking with a health care provider
- having blood tests
- arranging for a ride home
- fasting before the procedure

Talking with a health care provider. People should talk with their health care provider about medical conditions they have and all prescribed and over-the-counter medications, vitamins, and supplements they take, including

- antibiotics
- antidepressants
- aspirin
- asthma medications
- blood pressure medications
- blood thinners
- diabetes medications
- dietary supplements
- nonsteroidal anti-inflammatory drugs such as ibuprofen and naproxen

The health care provider may tell the person to stop taking medications temporarily that affect blood clotting or interact with anesthesia, which people sometimes receive during a liver biopsy.

Having blood tests. A person will have a test to show how well his or her blood clots. A person will have a test to show how well his or her blood clots. A technician or nurse draws a blood sample during an office visit or at a commercial facility and sends the sample to a lab for analysis. People with severe liver disease often have blood-clotting problems that can increase their chance of bleeding after the biopsy. A health care provider may give the person a medication called clotting factor concentrates just before a liver biopsy to reduce the chance of bleeding.

Arranging for a ride home after the procedure. For safety reasons, most people cannot drive home after the procedure. A health care provider will ask a person to make advance arrangements for getting home after the procedure.

Fasting before the procedure. A health care provider will ask a person not to eat or drink for 8 hours before the procedure if the provider anticipates using anesthesia or sedation.

How is a liver biopsy performed?

A health care provider performs the liver biopsy at a hospital or an outpatient center and determines which type of biopsy is best for the person.

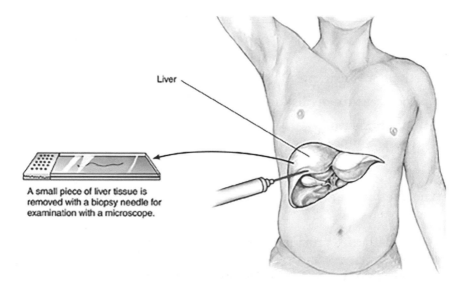

Liver

A small piece of liver tissue is removed with a biopsy needle for examination with a microscope.

Figure 14.2. *Percutaneous Liver Biopsy*

A person lies face up on a table and rests the right hand above the head. A health care provider gives the person a local anesthetic on the area where he or she will insert the biopsy needle. If needed, the health care provider will give the person sedatives and pain medication.

The health care provider either taps on the abdomen to locate the liver or uses one of the following imaging techniques:

- **Ultrasound**. Ultrasound uses a device, called a transducer that bounces safe, painless sound waves off organs to create an image of their structure.

- **Computerized tomography (CT) scan**. A CT scan uses a combination of X rays and computer technology to create images. For a CT scan, a technician may give the person a solution to drink and an injection of a special dye, called contrast medium. CT scans require the person to lie on a table that slides into a tunnel-shaped device where the technician takes the X rayss.

Research has shown fewer complications after biopsy when health care providers use ultrasound to locate the liver compared with tapping on the abdomen. Health care providers may select ultrasound over a CT scan because it is quicker and less expensive, and can show the biopsy needle in real time.

The health care provider will

- make a small incision in the right side of the person's abdomen, either toward the bottom of or just below the rib cage

- insert the biopsy needle

- ask the person to exhale and hold his or her breath while the health care provider inserts the needle and quickly removes a sample of liver tissue

- insert and remove the needle several times if multiple samples are needed

- place a bandage over the incision

After the biopsy, the person must lie on his or her right side for up to 2 hours to reduce the chance of bleeding. Medical staff monitor the person for signs of bleeding for 2 to 4 more hours.

Transvenous Liver Biopsy

When a person's blood clots slowly or the person has ascites—a buildup of fluid in the abdomen—the health care provider may perform a transvenous liver biopsy.

For this procedure, the person lies face up on an X-ray table, and a health care provider applies local anesthetic to one side of the neck. The health care provider will give sedatives and pain medication if the person needs them.

The health care provider will

- make a small incision in the neck.

- insert a sheath into the jugular vein and thread the sheath down the jugular vein, along the side of the heart, and into one of the veins in the liver.

- inject contrast medium into the sheath and take an X rays. The contrast medium makes the blood vessels and the location of the sheath clearly visible on the X-ray images.

- thread a biopsy needle through the sheath and into the liver and quickly remove a liver tissue sample.

- insert and remove the biopsy needle several times if multiple samples are needed.

- carefully withdraw the sheath and close the incision with a bandage.

Medical staff monitor the person for 4 to 6 hours afterwards for signs of bleeding.

Laparoscopic Liver Biopsy

Health care providers use this type of biopsy to obtain a tissue sample from a specific area or from multiple areas of the liver, or when the risk of spreading cancer or infection exists. A health care provider may take a liver tissue sample during laparoscopic surgery performed for other reasons, including liver surgery.

The person lies on his or her back on an operating table. A nurse or technician will insert an intravenous (IV) needle into the person's arm to give anesthesia

The health care provider will

- make a small incision in the abdomen, just below the rib cage

- insert a cannula into the incision and fill the abdomen with gas to provide space to work inside the abdominal cavity and to see the liver

- insert a biopsy needle through the cannula and into the liver and quickly remove a liver tissue sample

- insert and remove the biopsy needle several times if multiple samples are needed

- remove the cannula and close the incisions with dissolvable stitches

The health care provider can easily spot any bleeding from the procedure with the camera on the laparoscope and treat it using an electric probe. The person stays at the hospital or an outpatient center for a few hours while the anesthesia wears off.

What can a person expect after a liver biopsy?

After a liver biopsy, a person can expect

- full recovery in 1 to 2 days.

- to avoid intense activity, exercise, or heavy lifting for up to 1 week.

- soreness around the biopsy or incision site for about a week. Acetaminophen (Tylenol) or other pain medications that do not interfere with blood clotting may help. People should check with their health care provider before taking any pain medications.

- a member of the health care team to review the discharge instructions with the person—or with an accompanying friend or family member if the person is still groggy—and provide a written copy. The person should follow all instructions given.

Liver biopsy results take a few days to come back. The liver sample goes to a pathology lab where a technician stains the tissue. Staining highlights important details within the liver tissue and helps identify any signs of liver disease. The pathologist—a doctor who specializes in diagnosing diseases—looks at the tissue with a microscope and sends a report to the person's health care provider.

What are the risks of liver biopsy?

The risks of a liver biopsy include

- pain and bruising at the biopsy or incision site—the most common complication after a liver biopsy. Most people experience mild pain that does not require medication; however, some people need medications to relieve the pain.

229

- prolonged bleeding from the biopsy or incision site or internal bleeding. A person may require hospitalization, transfusions, and sometimes surgery or another procedure to stop the bleeding.

- infection of the biopsy site or incision site that may cause sepsis. Sepsis is an illness in which the body has a severe response to bacteria or a virus.

- pneumothorax, also called collapsed lung, which occurs when air or gas builds up in the pleural space. The pleural space is thin layers of tissue that wrap around the outside of the lungs and line the inside of the chest cavity. Pneumothorax may happen when the biopsy needle punctures the pleural space.

- hemothorax, or the buildup of blood in the pleural space.

- puncture of other organs.

Section 14.3

Other Biopsies

This section includes excerpts from "Lymphedema and Breast Cancer Surgery," National Cancer Institute (NCI), March 1, 2013; text from "Thyroid Cancer Treatment (PDQ®)," National Cancer Institute (NCI), June 17, 2015; text from "Non-Small Cell Lung Cancer Treatment (PDQ®)," National Cancer Institute (NCI), May 12, 2015; text from "Skin Cancer Treatment (PDQ®)," National Cancer Institute (NCI), April 2, 2015; and text from "Adult Acute Lymphoblastic Leukemia Treatment (PDQ®)," National Cancer Institute (NCI), June 18, 2015.

Sentinel Lymph Node Biopsy is a type of surgery in which the surgeon removes a few lymph nodes for testing. First, the surgeon injects a dye, a radioactive tracer, or both into the breast near the tumor. This helps the surgeon see which lymph nodes the lymph from that area of the breast flows to first. Then, he or she removes the node or nodes that contain the dye or radioactive tracer to see if they have cancer. If they do not contain cancer, it is not likely that the other nodes under the arm have cancer. This means that the surgeon usually doesn't have to remove any other lymph nodes.

Fewer lymph nodes are removed with sentinel lymph node biopsy than with standard lymph node surgery. Having fewer lymph nodes removed helps lower the chances that you will develop lymphedema and other problems caused by damage to lymph vessels and lymph nodes.

Fine-needle aspiration biopsy of the thyroid: The removal of thyroid tissue using a thin needle. The needle is inserted through the skin into the thyroid. Several tissue samples are removed from different parts of the thyroid. A pathologist views the tissue samples under a microscope to look for cancer cells. Because the type of thyroid cancer can be hard to diagnose, patients should ask to have biopsy samples checked by a pathologist who has experience diagnosing thyroid cancer.

Fine-needle aspiration (FNA) biopsy of the lung: The removal of tissue or fluid from the lung using a thin needle. A CT scan, ultrasound, or other imaging procedure is used to locate the abnormal tissue or fluid in the lung. A small incision may be made in the skin where the biopsy needle is inserted into the abnormal tissue or fluid. A sample is removed with the needle and sent to the laboratory. A pathologist then views the sample under a microscope to look for cancer cells. A chest X-ray is done after the procedure to make sure no air is leaking from the lung into the chest.

Skin biopsy: All or part of the abnormal-looking growth is cut from the skin and viewed under a microscope by a pathologist to check for signs of cancer. There are four main types of skin biopsies:

- Shave biopsy: A sterile razor blade is used to "shave-off" the abnormal-looking growth.

- Punch biopsy: A special instrument called a punch or a trephine is used to remove a circle of tissue from the abnormal-looking growth.

- Incisional biopsy: A scalpel is used to remove part of a growth.

- Excisional biopsy: A scalpel is used to remove the entire growth.

Bone marrow aspiration and biopsy: The removal of bone marrow, blood, and a small piece of bone by inserting a hollow needle into the hipbone or breastbone. A pathologist views the bone marrow, blood, and bone under a microscope to look for abnormal cells.

The following tests may be done on the samples of blood or bone marrow tissue that are removed:

- **Cytogenetic analysis:** A laboratory test in which the cells in a sample of blood or bone marrow are looked at under a microscope to find out if there are certain changes in the chromosomes in the lymphocytes. For example, sometimes in ALL, part of one chromosome is moved to another chromosome. This is called the Philadelphia chromosome. Other tests, such as fluorescence in situ hybridization (FISH), may also be done to look for certain changes in the chromosomes.

- **Immunophenotyping:** A process used to identify cells, based on the types of antigens or markers on the surface of the cell. This process is used to diagnose the subtype of ALL by comparing the cancer cells to normal cells of the immune system. For example, a cytochemistry study may test the cells in a sample of tissue using chemicals (dyes) to look for certain changes in the sample. A chemical may cause a color change in one type of leukemia cell but not in another type of leukemia cell.

Chapter 15

Bone Marrow Tests

What Are Bone Marrow Tests?

Bone marrow tests are used to check whether your bone marrow is healthy. These tests also show whether your bone marrow is making normal amounts of blood cells.

Bone marrow is the sponge-like tissue inside the bones. It contains stem cells that develop into the three types of blood cells that the body needs:

- Red blood cells carry oxygen through the body.

- White blood cells fight infection.

- Platelets stop bleeding.

Another type of stem cell, called an embryonic stem cell, can develop into any type of cell in the body. These cells aren't found in bone marrow.

Overview

Doctors use bone marrow tests to diagnose blood and bone marrow diseases and conditions, including:

- Conditions in which a person produces too few or too many of certain types of blood cells (e.g., Aplastic anemia and agranulocytosis)

Text in this chapter is excerpted from "Bone Marrow Tests," National Heart, Lung, and Blood Institute (NHLBI), December 12, 2011. Reviewed September 2015.

- Problems with the structure of red blood cells (e.g., Megaloblastic anemia, iron deficiency anemia, sickle-cell anemia and spherocytic anemia)

- Bone marrow disorders, such as myelofibrosis

- Some cancers, such as leukemia, Hodgkin's disease, secondary cancer cell deposits, etc.

- Parasitic infections like visceral leishmaniasis

Bone marrow tests also help doctors figure out how severe a cancer is and how much it has spread in the body. The tests also are used to diagnose fevers and infections.

The two bone marrow tests are aspiration and biopsy.

Bone marrow aspiration usually is done first. For this test, your doctor removes a small amount of fluid bone marrow through a needle. He or she may have some idea of what the problem is, and the sample gives him or her useful information about the cells in the marrow. It is done in hip bone and sternum (breast bone).

A bone marrow trephine biopsy is a followup test. It's done when an aspiration doesn't give needed information. Or, it's done if your doctor wants to examine the bone marrow structure itself. For a bone marrow biopsy, your doctor removes a small amount of bone marrow tissue through a larger needle. It is usually done in the hip bone.

Outlook

Bleeding and infection are the most common risks of bone marrow tests, but they're rare. The tests are fairly simple, and they're safe for most people.

In some cases, these tests aren't safe for people who have certain bleeding disorders, such as hemophilia. Your doctor can tell you whether a bone marrow test is safe for you.

Who Needs Bone Marrow Tests?

Your doctor may recommend bone marrow tests if he or she thinks you have a blood or bone marrow disease or condition, such as:

- Myelodysplastic syndrome. This is a group of diseases in which your bone marrow doesn't make enough normal blood cells.

- Neutropenia. This is a condition in which you have a lower than normal number of white blood cells in your blood.

- Anemia. Anemia occurs if you have a lower than normal number of red blood cells. The condition also can occur if your red blood cells don't have enough of an iron-rich protein that carries oxygen from the lungs to the rest of the body.

- Aplastic anemia. This type of anemia occurs if your bone marrow doesn't make enough new blood cells (red blood cells, white blood cells, and platelets). Aplastic anemia is a rare, but serious condition.

- Myelofibrosis. This is a serious bone marrow disorder that disrupts normal production of blood cells and leads to severe anemia.

- Thrombocytopenia. This is a group of conditions in which your body doesn't make enough platelets and your blood doesn't clot as it should.

- Essential thrombocythemia. This is a disease in which your bone marrow makes too many blood cells, especially platelets.

- Leukemia. This is a cancer of the white blood cells. Types of leukemia include acute and chronic leukemias and multiple myeloma.

Your doctor also may recommend bone marrow tests if you have another type of cancer. Examples include breast cancer that has spread to the bone or Hodgkin's and non-Hodgkin's lymphomas (cancers of a certain type of white blood cell).

Bone marrow tests help show what stage the cancer is in. That is, the tests help doctors know how serious the cancer is and how much it has spread in the body.

Bone marrow tests also can show what's causing a fever, especially in cases of Pyrexia of unknown origin (P.U.O). . Doctors may recommend the tests for people who have diseases that affect the immune system. The tests also are used for patients who may have uncommon bacterial infections.

What to Expect before Bone Marrow Tests

Before having bone marrow tests, a doctor, nurse, or physician assistant will explain the testing process and procedure and answer questions you might have.

Let your health care team know:

- Whether you're allergic to any medicines

- Whether you have a bleeding disorder like haemophilia, Christmas disease.

- What medicines you're taking (you might have to stop taking some medicines, such as blood-thinning medicines, before having bone marrow tests)
- Whether you're pregnant

Before the tests, you may be given medicine to help you relax. This medicine makes you sleepy, so you likely won't be able to drive after the test. Thus, your health care team may advise you to arrange a ride home.

What to Expect during Bone Marrow Tests

Bone marrow tests usually take about 30 minutes. The tests can be done in a hospital, doctor's office, or other health care facility.

Bone marrow tests generally are done on the pelvic bone – posterior iliac crest in older children and medial surface of the tibia for young children. If your doctor uses that part of the pelvic bone, you'll lie on your side or stomach for the test. Aspiration might be done on the breastbone.

Precaution:

One or two days prior to bone marrow test, Vitamin K (1 mg) injection given and bleeding disorders will be ruled out.

Procedure:

Medicine will be used to numb the area where your doctor will insert the needle. Although you'll be awake during the tests, the medicine helps reduce pain

If you're very nervous or anxious, your doctor may give you medicine to help you relax or sleep. If so, your health care team will closely check your breathing, heart rate, and blood pressure during the tests.

The area on your body where your doctor will insert the needle is cleaned with iodine solution or spirit and draped with a cloth. Your doctor will see only the site where the needle is inserted. The iliac crest is grasped firmly and the bone-marrow aspiration needle with the trocar is introduced by applying firm boring movement. Once the needle enters the marrow, the needle remains fixed. A 20cc syringe is attached and firm suction is applied, till it draws about 0.2 to 0.3 ml of marrow. After the test, you might need stitches to close the cut.

For bone marrow aspiration, your doctor will insert the needle into the marrow and remove a sample of fluid bone marrow. You may feel a brief, sharp pain. The fluid that's removed from the bone marrow will be taken to a laboratory and studied under a microscope.

If your doctor decides to do a bone marrow biopsy, it will be done after the aspiration. For the biopsy, your doctor will use a needle to remove a sample of bone marrow tissue. Thin sections of this tissue will be studied under a microscope.

During both tests, it's important for you to remain still and as relaxed as possible (if you're awake).

What to Expect after Bone Marrow Tests

After the bone marrow tests, a nurse will hold a bandage on the site where the needle was inserted until the bleeding stops. Then he or she will put a smaller bandage on the site.

Most people can go home the same day as the tests. If you received medicine to help you relax during the tests, you may need to arrange a ride home.

After 24 hours, you can take off the bandage. Call your doctor if you develop a fever, have a lot of pain, or see redness, swelling, or discharge at the site. These are signs of infection.

Expect mild discomfort for about a week. Your doctor may tell you to take an over-the-counter pain medicine.

What Do Bone Marrow Tests Show?

Bone marrow tests show whether your bone marrow is making enough healthy blood cells. If it's not, the results can tell your doctor which cells are unhealthy and why.

Bone marrow tests are an important medical tool. They're used to diagnose many blood and bone marrow disorders, including anemia and certain kinds of cancer.

Bone marrow tests also are used to find out how severe cancer is and how much it has spread throughout the body. The tests also help doctors find the cause of fevers and infections.

Your doctor will combine information from your bone marrow tests with information from a physical exam, blood tests, and other tests, such as imaging scans and X-rays. This information will help your doctor diagnose your condition and plan how to treat it.

What Are the Risks of Bone Marrow Tests?

Bone marrow tests are safe for most people. Complications are rare, but can occur. For example, some people develop bleeding or infections.

To prevent bleeding from the site where the needle was inserted, don't do any heavy lifting or vigorous exercise for a few days after the tests.

To prevent infections, don't shower or bathe for the first day after the tests. After 24 hours, you can take off the bandage. Call your doctor if you develop a fever, have a lot of pain, or see redness, swelling, or discharge at the site. These are signs of infection.

Expect mild discomfort for about a week. Your doctor may tell you to take an over-the-counter pain medicine.

Bone marrow tests might not be safe for people who have certain bleeding disorders, such as hemophilia. Your doctor can tell you whether bone marrow tests are safe for you.

Clinical Trials

The National Heart, Lung, and Blood Institute (NHLBI) is strongly committed to supporting research aimed at preventing and treating heart, lung, and blood diseases and conditions and sleep disorders.

NHLBI-supported research has led to many advances in medical knowledge and care. Often, these advances depend on the willingness of volunteers to take part in clinical trials.

Clinical trials test new ways to prevent, diagnose, or treat various diseases and conditions. For example, new treatments for a disease or condition (such as medicines, medical devices, surgeries, or procedures) are tested in volunteers who have the illness. Testing shows whether a treatment is safe and effective in humans before it is made available for widespread use.

By taking part in a clinical trial, you can gain access to new treatments before they're widely available. You also will have the support of a team of health care providers, who will likely monitor your health closely. Even if you don't directly benefit from the results of a clinical trial, the information gathered can help others and add to scientific knowledge.

If you volunteer for a clinical trial, the research will be explained to you in detail. You'll learn about treatments and tests you may receive, and the benefits and risks they may pose. You'll also be given a chance to ask questions about the research. This process is called informed consent.

If you agree to take part in the trial, you'll be asked to sign an informed consent form. This form is not a contract. You have the right to withdraw from a study at any time, for any reason. Also, you have the right to learn about new risks or findings that emerge during the trial.

For more information about clinical trials related to bone marrow tests or blood or bone marrow diseases, talk with your doctor.

Chapter 16

Stool Tests

Chapter Contents

Section 16.1

Colorectal Cancer and Stool Test

Text in this section is excerpted from "Colorectal Cancer Tests
Save Lives," Centers for Disease Control and Prevention (CDC),
November 7, 2013.

Colorectal cancer (CRC) is the second leading cancer killer of men
and women in the US, following lung cancer. The US Preventive Services Task Force (USPSTF) recommends three CRC screening tests
that are effective at saving lives: colonoscopy, stool tests (guaiac fecal
occult blood test-FOBT or fecal immunochemical test-FIT), and sigmoidoscopy (now seldom done).

Testing saves lives, but only if people get tested. Studies show that
people who are able to pick the test they prefer are more likely to actually get the test done. Increasing the use of all recommended colorectal
cancer tests can save more lives and is cost-effective.

To increase testing, doctors, nurses, and health systems can:

- Offer all recommended test options with advice about each.

- Match patients with the test they are most likely to complete.

- Work with public health professionals to:

- Get more adults tested by hiring and training "patient navigators," who are staff that help people learn about, get scheduled
  for, and get procedures done like colonoscopy.

- Create ways to make it easier for people to get FOBT/FIT kits
  in places other than a doctor's office, like giving them out at flu
  shot clinics or mailing them to people's homes.

Problem

Not enough people are getting tested as needed.

About 23 million adults have never been tested.

- The people less likely to get tested are Hispanics, those aged
  50-64, men, American Indian or Alaska natives, those who don't
  live in a city, and people with lower education and income.

- People with lower education and income are less likely to get tested.

- About 2 of every 3 adults who have never been tested for CRC actually have a regular doctor and health insurance that could pay for the test. Providers and patients do not always know about or consider all of the available tests.

- The three main tests–colonoscopy, FOBT/FIT, and flexible sigmoidoscopy are all effective at finding cancer early.

- Doctors often recommend colonoscopy more than other tests. Scientific studies have shown that many people would prefer FOBT/FIT if their health care provider gave them that option.

Currently, most health care providers and systems are not set up to help more people get tested.

- Many people do not know they need to be tested and are not notified when it is time for them to be tested.

- Most health care systems rely on doctors to remember to offer CRC tests to their patients. Nurses and other office staff should also talk with patients about getting tested and doctors can be reminded to offer CRC testing whenever patients are due, whether they come in for a routine check-up or when they are sick.

- Health systems can make testing easier by:

- Mailing out FOBT/FIT kits that can be completed by the person at home and mailed back, then making sure everyone with a test that is not normal promptly gets a colonoscopy.

- Using a patient navigator to explain how to prepare for the test, how the test is done and to make sure people get to their appointments.

What Can Be Done

Federal government is

- Expanding insurance coverage of USPSTF recommended CRC tests at no cost to the patient through the Affordable Care Act.

- Supporting the use of patient navigators who work directly with people to help them get the preventive tests they need.

- Helping the Veterans Administration system's doctors and nurses increase and track CRC testing of its patients in its hospitals and clinics.

- Improving the delivery of preventive services by measuring CRC testing rates in health centers funded by the Health Resources and Services Administration (HRSA).

- Using existing CDC screening programs to improve cancer screening rates for everyone, whether insured or not.

- Identifying CRC screening as a Healthy People 2020 leading health indicator for clinical preventive services.

State and local public health can

- Work with those doctors, health systems and public health professionals who have already greatly increased CRC testing rates.

- Develop record systems to keep track of and notify those who need to be tested.

- Promote recommended testing options with the public.

- Use public health workers and patient navigators to increase testing rates in communities with low testing rates.

- Work with state Medicaid programs, primary care associations, and Medicare quality improvement organizations to help people get tested and make sure they get additional tests or treatment if needed.

Doctors, nurses, and health systems can

- Offer recommended test options, with advice about each.

- Match patients with the test they are most likely to complete.

- Use patient reminder systems to notify patients when it's time to get a screening test done.

- Make sure patients get their results quickly. If the test is not normal make sure they get the follow-up care they need.

- Use patient navigators to help patients get checked.

Everyone can

- Learn about testing options and get the test that is right for them.

- Know their own family history and any personal risks they may have for CRC.

- Encourage friends and family members to be tested for CRC.

- Contact their local health department to learn how they can get tested for CRC.

Section 16.2

Detection of Parasite Antigens

Text in this section is excerpted from "Stool Specimens," Centers for Disease Control and Prevention (CDC), November 29, 2013.

The diagnosis of human intestinal protozoa depends on microscopic detection of the various parasite stages in feces, duodenal fluid, or small intestine biopsy specimens. Since fecal examination is very labor-intensive and requires a skilled microscopist, antigen detection tests have been developed as alternatives using direct fluorescent antibody (DFA), enzyme immunoassay (EIA), and rapid, dipstick-like tests. Antigen detection methods can be performed quickly and do not require an experienced and skilled morphologist. Much work has been accomplished on the development of antigen detection tests, resulting in commercially available reagents for the intestinal parasites *Cryptosporidium* spp., *Entamoeba histolytica*, *Giardia duodenalis*, and *Trichomonas vaginalis*. In addition, antigen detection tests using blood or serum are available for **Plasmodium** and **Wuchereria bancrofti**.

Specimens for antigen detection

Fresh or preserved stool samples are the appropriate specimen for antigen detection testing with most kits, but refer to the recommended collection procedures included with each specific kit.

Amebiasis

EIA kits are commercially available for detection of fecal antigens for the diagnosis of intestinal amebiasis. Organisms of both the pathogenic *E. histolytica* and the nonpathogenic *Entamoeba dispar* strains are morphologically identical. These assays use monoclonal antibodies that detect the galactose-inhibitable adherence protein in the pathogenic *E. histolytica*. The primary drawback of these assays is the requirement for fresh, unpreserved stool specimens. Several EIA kits for antigen detection of the *E. histolytica/E. dispar* group are available in the U.S., but only the TechLab kit is specific for *E. histolytica*.

Cryptosporidiosis

Immunodetection of antigens on the surface of organisms in stool specimens, using monoclonal antibody-based DFA assays, is the current test of choice for diagnosis of cryptosporidiosis and provides increased sensitivity over modified acid-fast staining techniques. There are commercial products (DFA, IFA, EIA, and rapid tests) available in the United States for the diagnosis of cryptosporidiosis. Several kits are combined tests for *Cryptosporidium*, *Giardia*, and *E. histolytica*. Factors such as ease of use, technical skill and time, single versus batch testing, and test cost must be considered when determining the test of choice for individual laboratories. The most sensitive (99%) and specific (100%) method is reported to be the DFA test, which identifies oocysts in concentrated or unconcentrated fecal samples by using a fluorescein isothiocyanate (FITC)-labeled monoclonal antibody. A combined DFA test for the simultaneous detection of *Cryptosporidium* oocysts and *Giardia* cysts is available.

Some commercial EIA tests are available in the microplate format for the detection of *Cryptosporidium* antigens in fresh or frozen stool samples and also in stool specimens preserved in formalin, or sodium acetate-acetic acid-formalin (SAF) fixed stool specimens. Concentrated or polyvinyl alcohol-treated (PVA) samples are unsuitable for testing with available antigen detection EIA kits. The kits are reportedly superior to microscopy, especially acid-fast staining, and show good correlation with the DFA test. Kit sensitivities and specificities reportedly range from 93 to 100% when used in a clinical setting. Laboratories which use these EIA kits need to be aware of potential problems with false-positive results and take steps to monitor kit performance.

Rapid immunochromatographic assays are available for the combined antigen detection of either *Cryptosporidium* and *Giardia* or *Cryptosporidium*, *Giardia*, and *E. histolytica*. These offer the advantage of short test time and multiple results in one reaction device. Initial evaluations indicate comparable sensitivity and specificity to previously available tests.

The Meridian Merifluor DFA Kit for *Cryptosporidium* / *Giardia*, modified acid-fast stain for *Cryptosporidium* spp., or Wheatley's trichrome stain for *Giardia* spp. are used at CDC for routine identification of these parasites. These techniques can be used to confirm suspicious or discrepant diagnostic results.

Giardiasis

Detection of antigens on the surface of organisms in stool specimens is the current test of choice for diagnosis of giardiasis and provides increased sensitivity over more common microscopy techniques. Commercial products (DFA, EIAs, and rapid tests) are available in the United States for the immunodiagnosis of giardiasis. DFA assays may be purchased that employ FITC-labeled monoclonal antibody for detection of *Giardia* cysts alone or in a combined kit for the simultaneous detection of *Giardia* cysts and *Cryptosporidium* oocysts. The sensitivity and specificity of these kits were both 100% compared to those of microscopy. They may be used for quantitation of cysts and oocysts, and thus may be useful for epidemiologic and control studies.

Some commercial EIA tests are available in the microplate format for the detection of *Giardia* antigen in fresh or frozen stool samples and also in stool specimens preserved in formalin, MIF, or SAF fixatives. Concentrated or PVA samples are not suitable for testing with EIA kits. EIA kit sensitivity rates were recently reported as ranging from 94-100% while specificity rates were all 100%.

Rapid immunochromatographic assays are available for the combined antigen detection of either *Cryptosporidium* and *Giardia* or *Cryptosporidium*, *Giardia*, and *E. histolytica*. These offer the advantage of short test time and multiple results in one reaction device. Initial evaluations indicate comparable sensitivity and specificity to previously available tests.

The Meridian Merifluor DFA Kit for *Cryptosporidium/Giardia*, modified acid-fast stain for *Cryptosporidium* spp., or Wheatley's trichrome stain for *Giardia* spp. are used at CDC for routine identification of these parasites. These techniques can be used to confirm suspicious or discrepant diagnostic results.

Trichomoniasis

Trichomoniasis, an infection caused by *Trichomonas vaginalis*, is a common sexually transmitted disease. Diagnosis is made by detection of trophozoites in vaginal secretions or urethral specimens by wet mount microscopic examination, DFA staining of specimens, or culture.

Sensitivity of the assays were reported as 60% for wet mounts and 86% for DFA when compared to cultures. A kit which employs FITC- or enzyme-labeled monoclonal antibodies for use in a DFA or EIA procedure is available for detection of whole parasites in fluids. A latex agglutination test for antigen detection in vaginal swab specimens is available; the manufacturer's evaluation indicated good sensitivity and specificity.

Table 16.1.

Organism	Kit Name	Manufacturer/ Distributors	Type of Test
Cryptosporidium **spp.**	Crypto CELISA	Cellabs	EIA
	PARA-TECT™ Cryptosporidium Antigen 96	Medical Chemical Corporation	EIA
	ProSpecT Rapid	Remel	EIA
	ProSpecT	Remel	EIA
	Cryptosporidium	TechLab	EIA
	Cryptosporidium	Wampole	EIA
	Crypto CEL	Cellabs	IFA
	XPect Crypto	Remel	Rapid
Cryptosporidium spp./Giardia duodenalis	PARA-TECT™ Cryptosporidium/ Giardia DFA 75	Medical Chemical Corporation	DFA
	Merifluor	Meridian	DFA
	ProSpecT	Remel	EIA
	Crypto/Giardia CEL	Cellabs	IFA
	ColorPAC	Becton Dickinson	Rapid
	ImmunoCard STAT!	Meridian	Rapid
	XPect	Remel	Rapid
Cryptosporidium spp./Giardia duodenalis/ Entamoeba histolytica/dispar	Triage	BioSite	Rapid

Organism	Kit Name	Manufacturer/ Distributors	Type of Test
Entamoeba histolytica	Entamoeba CELISA	Cellabs	EIA
	E. histolytica	Wampole	EIA
	E. histolytica II	TechLab	EIA
Entamoeba histolytica/E. dispar	ProSpecT	Remel	EIA
Giardia duodenalis	Giardia CELISA	Cellabs	EIA
	PARA-TECT™ Giardia Antigen 96	Medical Chemical Corporation	EIA
	ProSpecT	Remel	EIA
	Giardia II	TechLab	EIA
	Giardia	Wampole	EIA
	GiardiaEIA	Antibodies, Inc.	EIA
	Giardia CEL	Cellabs	IFA
	ProSpecT	Remel	Rapid
	Simple-Read Giardia	Medical Chemical Corporation	Rapid
Wuchereria bancrofti	Filariasis CELISA	Cellabs	EIA

Chapter 17

Strep Throat Test

Strep throat is a common type of sore throat in children, but it's not very common in adults. Healthcare professionals can do a quick test to determine if a sore throat is strep throat and decide if antibiotics are needed. Proper treatment can help you feel better faster and prevent spreading it to others!

Many things can cause that unpleasant, scratchy, and sometimes painful condition known as a sore throat. Viruses, bacteria, allergens, environmental irritants (such as cigarette smoke), chronic postnasal drip and fungi can all cause a sore throat. While many sore throats will get better without treatment, some throat infections—including strep throat—may need antibiotic treatment.

How You Get Strep Throat

Strep throat is an infection in the throat and tonsils caused by group A Streptococcus bacteria (called "group A strep"). Group A strep bacteria can also live in a person's nose and throat without causing illness. The bacteria are spread through contact with droplets after an infected person coughs or sneezes. If you touch your mouth, nose, or eyes after touching something that has these droplets on it, you may become ill. If you drink from the same glass or eat from the same plate as the sick person, you could also become ill. It is also possible to get strep throat from contact with sores from group A strep skin infections.

Text in this chapter is excerpted from "Is It Strep Throat?" Centers for Disease Control and Prevention (CDC), October 20, 2014.

Common Symptoms of Strep Throat

The most common symptoms of strep throat include:

- Sore throat, usually starts quickly and can cause severe pain when swallowing

- A fever (101°F or above)

- Red and swollen tonsils, sometimes with white patches or streaks of pus

- Tiny red spots (petechiae) on the area at the back of the roof of the mouth (the soft or hard palate)

- Headache, nausea, or vomiting

- Swollen lymph nodes in the neck

- Body aches or rash

A Simple Test Gives Fast Results

Healthcare professionals can test for strep by swabbing the throat to quickly see if group A strep bacteria are causing a sore throat. **A strep test is needed to tell if you have strep throat; just looking at your throat is not enough to make a diagnosis.** If the test is positive, your healthcare professional can prescribe antibiotics. If the strep test is negative, but your clinician still strongly suspects you have this infection, then they can take a throat culture swab to test for the bacteria.

Antibiotics Get You Well Fast

The strep test results will help your healthcare professional decide if you need antibiotics, which can:

- Decrease the length of time you're sick

- Reduce your symptoms

- Help prevent the spread of infection to friends and family members

- Prevent more serious complications, such as tonsil and sinus infections, and acute rheumatic fever (a rare inflammatory disease that can affect the heart, joints, skin, and brain)

You should start feeling better in just a day or two after starting antibiotics. Call your healthcare professional if you don't feel better after taking antibiotics for 48 hours. People with strep throat should stay home from work, school, or daycare until they have taken antibiotics for at least 24 hours so they don't spread the infection to others.

Be sure to finish the entire prescription, even when you start feeling better, unless your healthcare professional tells you to stop taking the medicine. When you stop taking antibiotics early, you risk getting an infection later that is resistant to antibiotic treatment.

More Prevention Tips

The best way to keep from getting strep throat is to wash your hands often and avoid sharing eating utensils, like forks or cups. It is especially important for anyone with a sore throat to wash their hands often and cover their mouth when coughing and sneezing. There is no vaccine to prevent strep throat.

Part Four

Imaging Tests and Risks

Chapter 18

Medical X-Ray Imaging

Overview of Medical X-Ray Imaging

What Are Medical X-rays?

X-rays are a form of electromagnetic radiation, similar to visible light. Unlike light, however, X-rays have higher energy and can pass through most objects, including the body. Medical X-rays are used to generate images of tissues and structures inside the body. If X-rays travelling through the body also pass through an X-ray detector on the other side of the patient, an image will be formed that represents the "shadows" formed by the objects inside the body. One type of X-ray detector is photographic film, but there are many other types of detectors that are used to produce digital images. The X-ray images that result from this process are called radiographs.

How Do Medical X-rays work?

To create a radiograph, a patient is positioned so that the part of the body being imaged is located between an X-ray source and an X-ray detector. When the machine is turned on, X-rays travel through the body and are absorbed in different amounts by different tissues, depending on the radiological density of the tissues they pass through. Radiological density is determined by both the density and the atomic

---

Text in this chapter is excerpted from "X-rays," National Institute of Biomedical Imaging and Bioengineering (NIBIB), July 2013.

number of the materials being imaged. For example, structures such as bone contain calcium, which has a higher atomic number than most tissues. Because of this property, bones readily absorb X-rays and, thus, produce high contrast on the X-ray detector. As a result, bony structures appear whiter than other tissues against the black background of a radiograph. Conversely, X-rays travel more easily through less radiologically dense tissues such as fat and muscle, as well as through air-filled cavities such as the lungs. These structures are displayed in shades of gray on a radiograph.

When Are Medical X-rays used?

Listed below are examples of examinations and procedures that use X-ray technology to either diagnose or treat disease:

Diagnostic

X-ray radiography: Detects bone fractures, certain tumors and other abnormal masses, pneumonia, some types of injuries, calcifications, foreign objects, dental problems, etc.

Mammography: A radiograph of the breast that is used for cancer detection and diagnosis. Tumors tend to appear as regular or irregular-shaped masses that are somewhat brighter than the background on the radiograph (i.e., whiter on a black background or blacker on a white background). Mammograms can also detect tiny bits of calcium, called microcalcifications, which show up as very bright specks on a mammogram. While usually benign, microcalcifications may occasionally indicate the presence of a specific type of cancer

CT (computed tomography): Combines traditional X-ray technology with computer processing to generate a series of crosssectional images of the body that can later be combined to form a three-dimensional X-ray image. CT images are more detailed than plain radiographs and give doctors the ability to view structures within the body from many different angles.

Fluoroscopy: Uses X-rays and and a fluorescent screen to obtain real-time images of movement within the body or to view diagnostic processes, such as following the path of an injected or swallowed contrast agent. For example, fluoroscopy is used to view the movement of the beating heart, and, with the aid of radiographic contrast agents, to view blood flow to the heart muscle as well as through blood vessels and organs. This technology is also used with a radiographic contrast agent to guide an internally threaded catheter during cardiac angioplasty, which is a minimally invasive procedure for opening clogged arteries that supply blood to the heart.

Therapeutic

Radiation therapy in cancer treatment: X-rays and other types of high-energy radiation can be used to destroy cancerous tumors and cells by damaging their DNA. The radiation dose used for treating cancer is much higher than the radiation dose used for diagnostic imaging. Therapeutic radiation can come from a machine outside of the body or from a radioactive material that is placed in the body, inside or near tumor cells, or injected into the blood stream.

Chapter 19

Risks of Medical Imaging

Chapter Contents

Section 19.1

Overview on Risks of Medical Imaging

Text in this section is excerpted from "Medical X-ray Imaging," U.S.
Food and Drug Administration (FDA), February 10, 2015.

As in many aspects of medicine, there are both benefits and risks
associated with the use of computed tomography (CT). The main risks
are those associated with

1. abnormal test results, for a benign or incidental finding, lead-
    ing to unneeded, possibly invasive, follow-up tests that may
    present additional risks and

2. the increased possibility of cancer induction from X-ray radia-
    tion exposure.

The probability for absorbed X-rays to induce cancer or heritable
mutations leading to genetically associated diseases in offspring is
thought to be very small for radiation doses of the magnitude that are
associated with CT procedures. Such estimates of cancer and genetically
heritable risk from X-ray exposure have a broad range of statistical
uncertainty, and there is some scientific controversy regarding the effects
from very low doses and dose rates as discussed below. Under some rare
circumstances of prolonged, high-dose exposure, X-rays can cause other
adverse health effects, such as skin erythema (reddening), skin tissue
injury, and birth defects following in-utero exposure. But at the exposure
levels associated with most medical imaging procedures, including most
CT procedures, these other adverse effects would not occur.

Because of the rapidly growing use of pediatric CT and the potential for increased radiation exposure to children undergoing these
scans, special considerations should be applied when using pediatric CT. Doses from a single pediatric CT scan can range from about
5 mSv to 60 mSv. Among children who have undergone CT scans,
approximately one-third have had at least three scans. The National
Cancer Institute and The Society for Pediatric Radiology developed
a brochure, Radiation Risks and Pediatric Computed Tomography: A
Guide for Health Care Providers, and the FDA issued a Public Health
Notification, Reducing Radiation Risk from Computed Tomography for

Pediatric and Small Adult Patients, that discuss the value of CT and the importance of minimizing the radiation dose, especially in children.

Risk Estimates

In the field of radiation protection, it is commonly assumed that the risk for adverse health effects from cancer is proportional to the amount of radiation dose absorbed and the amount of dose depends on the type of X-ray examination. A CT examination with an effective dose of 10 millisieverts (abbreviated mSv; 1 mSv = 1 mGy in the case of X-rays.) may be associated with an increase in the possibility of fatal cancer of approximately 1 chance in 2000. This increase in the possibility of a fatal cancer from radiation can be compared to the natural incidence of fatal cancer in the U.S. population, about 1 chance in 5. In other words, for any one person the risk of radiation-induced cancer is much smaller than the natural risk of cancer. Nevertheless, this small increase in radiation-associated cancer risk for an individual can become a public health concern if large numbers of the population undergo increased numbers of CT screening procedures of uncertain benefit.

It must be noted that there is uncertainty regarding the risk estimates for low levels of radiation exposure as commonly experienced in diagnostic radiology procedures. There are some that question whether there is adequate evidence for a risk of cancer induction at low doses. However, this position has not been adopted by most authoritative bodies in the radiation protection and medical arenas.

Radiation Dose

The effective doses from diagnostic CT procedures are typically estimated to be in the range of 1 to 10 mSv. This range is not much less than the lowest doses of 5 to 20 mSv received by some of the Japanese survivors of the atomic bombs. These survivors, who are estimated to have experienced doses only slightly larger than those encountered in CT, have demonstrated a small but increased radiation-related excess relative risk for cancer mortality.

Radiation dose from CT procedures varies from patient to patient. A particular radiation dose will depend on the size of the body part examined, the type of procedure, and the type of CT equipment and its operation. Typical values cited for radiation dose should be considered as estimates that cannot be precisely associated with any individual patient, examination, or type of CT system. The actual dose from a procedure could be two or three times larger or smaller than the estimates. Facilities performing "screening" procedures may adjust the radiation dose used to levels less (by factors such as 1/2 to 1/5 for so called "low dose CT scans") than those typically used for diagnostic CT procedures. However, no comprehensive data is available to permit estimation of the extent of this practice and reducing the dose can have an adverse impact on the image quality produced. Such reduced image quality may be acceptable in certain imaging applications.

The quantity most relevant for assessing the risk of cancer detriment from a CT procedure is the "effective dose." Effective dose is evaluated in units of millisieverts (abbreviated mSv; 1 mSv = 1 mGy in the case of X-rays.) Using the concept of effective dose allows comparison of the risk estimates associated with partial or whole-body radiation exposures. This quantity also incorporates the different radiation sensitivities of the various organs in the body.

Estimates of the effective dose from a diagnostic CT procedure can vary by a factor of 10 or more depending on the type of CT procedure, patient size and the CT system and its operating technique. A list of representative diagnostic procedures and associated doses are given in the table.

Table 19.1. Radiation Dose Comparison

Diagnostic Procedure	Typical Effective Dose (mSv)[1]	Number of Chest X-rays (PA film) for Equivalent Effective Dose[2]	Time Period for Equivalent Effective Dose from Natural Background Radiation[3]
Chest X-ray (PA film)	0.02	1	2.4 days
Skull X-ray	0.1	5	12 days
Lumbar spine	1.5	75	182 days
I.V. urogram	3	150	1.0 year
Upper G.I. exam	6	300	2.0 years
Barium enema	8	400	2.7 years
CT head	2	100<	243 days
CT abdomen	8	400	2.7 years

[1] *Average effective dose in millisieverts (mSv) as compiled by Fred A. Mettler, Jr., et al., "Effective Doses in Radiology and Diagnostic Nuclear Medicine: A Catalog," Radiology Vol. 248, No. 1, pp. 254-263, July 2008.*

[2] *Based on the assumption of an average "effective dose" from chest X-ray (PA film) of 0.02 mSv.*

[3] *Based on the assumption of an average "effective dose" from natural background radiation of 3 mSv per year in the United States*

Section 19.2

FAQs on Radiation and Risks

Text in this section is excerpted from "Radfacts," U.S. Environmental
Protection Agency (EPA), June 29, 2015.

What is radiation?

Radiation is a form of energy. The radiation of concern here is called
ionizing radiation. Atoms release radiation as they change from unstable, energized forms to more stable forms.

What is a radionuclide?

All matter is composed of elements, and elements that are radioactive are generally referred to as radionuclides. Each element can
take many different forms (called isotopes). Some of these isotopes
are unstable and emit radiation; these unstable isotopes are known as
radioisotopes or radionuclides. Stable isotopes do not undergo radioactive decay and therefore do not emit radiation.

What are the types of radiation?

Alpha particles can travel only a few inches in the air and lose their
energy almost as soon as they collide with anything. They are easily
shielded by a sheet of paper or the outer layer of a person's skin. Alpha
particles are hazardous only when they are inhaled or swallowed.

Beta particles can travel in the air for a distance of a few feet. Beta
particles can pass through a sheet of paper but can be stopped by a
sheet of aluminum foil or glass. Beta particles can damage skin, but
are most hazardous when swallowed or inhaled.

Gamma rays are waves of pure energy and are similar to X-rays.
They travel at the speed of light through air or open spaces. Concrete,
lead, or steel must be used to block gamma rays. Gamma rays can
present an extreme external hazard.

Neutrons are small particles that have no electrical charge. They
can travel long distances in air and are released during nuclear fission.

Water or concrete offer the best shielding against neutrons. Like gamma rays, neutrons can present an extreme external hazard.

What terms are used for radiation measurements?

Radiation is measured in different ways. Measurements used in the United States include the following (the internationally used equivalent unit of measurement follows in parenthesis):

Rad (radiation absorbed dose) measures the amount of energy actually absorbed by a material, such as human tissue (Gray=100 rads).

Roentgen is a measure of exposure; it describes the amount of radiation energy, in the form of gamma or X-rays, in the air.

(Roentgen equivalent man) measures the biological damage of radiation. It takes into account both the amount, or dose, of radiation and the biological effect of the type of radiation in question. A millirem is one one-thousandth of a rem (Sievert=100 rems).

Curie is a unit of radioactivity. One curie refers to the amount of any radionuclide that undergoes 37 billion atomic transformations a second. A nanocurie is one one-billionth of a curie (37 Becquerel = 1 nanocurie).

What levels of radiation are people exposed to in everyday life?

To put an emergency situation in perspective, it helps to be aware of the radiation levels people encounter in everyday life. Individual exposures vary, but humans are exposed routinely to radiation from both natural sources, such as cosmic rays from the sun and indoor radon, and from manufactured sources, such as televisions and medical X-rays. Even the human body contains natural radioactive elements.

Because individual human exposures to radiation are usually small, the millirem (one one-thousandth of a rem) is generally used to express the doses humans receive. The following table shows average radiation doses from several common sources of human exposure.

Table 19.2. Radiation Source and Dosage

Radiation Source	Dose (millirems)
Chest X-ray	10
Mammogram	30
Cosmic rays	31 (annually)
Human body	39 (annually)
Household radon	200 (annually)
Cross-country airplane flight	5

Are there any legal limits for radiation exposure?

Another way to help put a radiological emergency into perspective is to be aware of the radiation exposure limits for people who work with and around radioactive materials full time, as shown in the following table:

Table 19.3. Legal Limits for Radiation Exposure

Worker Category	Legal Limit
18-year old male	5 rem/year
Pregnant woman	500 millirem (mrem) during pregnancy

What are radiation's effects on humans?

Radiation effects fall into two broad categories: deterministic and stochastic. At the cellular level, high doses of ionizing radiation can result in severe dysfunction, even death, of cells. At the organ level, if a sufficient number of cells are so affected, the function of the organ is impaired. Such effects are called "deterministic." Deterministic effects have definite threshold doses, which means that the effect is not seen until the absorbed dose is greater than a certain level. Once above that threshold level, the severity of the effect increases with dose. Also, deterministic effects are usually manifested soon after exposure. Examples of such effects include radiation skin burning, blood count effects, and cataracts.

In contrast, stochastic effects are caused by more subtle radiation-induced cellular changes (usually DNA mutations) that are random in nature and have no threshold dose. The probability of such effects increases with dose, but the severity does not. Cancer is the only observed clinical manifestation of radiation-induced stochastic effects. Not only is the severity independent of dose, but also, there is a substantial delay between the time of exposure and the appearance of the cancer, ranging from several years for leukemia to decades for solid tumors. Cancer can result from some DNA changes in the somatic cells of the body, but radiation can also damage the germ cells (ova and sperm) to produce hereditary effects. These are also classified as stochastic; however, clinical manifestations of such effects have not been observed in humans at a statistically significant level.

The nature and extent of damage caused by ionizing radiation depend on a number of factors, including the amount of exposure, the frequency of exposure, and the penetrating power of the radiation to which an individual is exposed. Rapid exposure to very large doses of ionizing radiation is rare but can cause death within a few days or months. The sensitivity of the exposed cells also influences the extent of damage. For example, rapidly growing tissues, such as developing embryos, are particularly vulnerable to harm from ionizing radiation.

What are some important emergency response terms?

RadNet (formerly the Environmental Radiation Ambient Monitoring System). RadNet is the EPA-operated monitoring system used to measure radioactivity and other contaminants in the environment. There are 260 RadNet sampling stations throughout the U.S. In an emergency, the sampling stations can be used to provide information on how far contamination has spread.

Plume The airborne "cloud" of material released to the environment. The plume may contain nuclear materials and may or may not be visible.

Protective Action Any action taken to reduce or avoid a radiation dose to the public.

Protective Action Guide (PAG) A predetermined projected dose level at which specified actions should be taken to protect the public from exposure to radiation.

Section 19.3

Radiation Exposure from CT Scan and Its Effects on Children

Text in this section is excerpted from "Diagnosis and Staging," National Cancer Institute (NCI), July 16, 2013.

Is the radiation from CT harmful?

Some people may be concerned about the amount of radiation they receive during CT. CT imaging involves the use of X-rays, which are a form of ionizing radiation. Exposure to ionizing radiation is known to increase the risk of cancer. Standard X-ray procedures, such as routine chest X-rays and mammography, use relatively low levels of ionizing radiation. The radiation exposure from CT is higher than that from standard X-ray procedures, but the increase in cancer risk from one CT scan is still small. Not having the procedure can be much more risky than having it, especially if CT is being used to diagnose cancer or another serious condition in someone who has signs or symptoms of disease.

It is commonly thought that the extra risk of any one person developing a fatal cancer from a typical CT procedure is about 1 in 2,000. In contrast, the lifetime risk of dying from cancer in the U.S. population is about 1 in 5.

It is also important to note that everyone is exposed to some background level of naturally occurring ionizing radiation every day. The average person in the United States receives an estimated effective dose of about 3 millisieverts (mSv) per year from naturally occurring radioactive materials, such as radon and radiation from outer space. By comparison, the radiation exposure from one low-dose CT scan of the chest (1.5 mSv) is comparable to 6 months of natural background radiation, and a regular-dose CT scan of the chest (7 mSv) is comparable to 2 years of natural background radiation.

The widespread use of CT and other procedures that use ionizing radiation to create images of the body has raised concerns that even small increases in cancer risk could lead to large numbers of future cancers. People who have CT procedures as children may be at higher risk because children are more sensitive to radiation and have a longer life expectancy than adults. Women are at a somewhat higher risk than men of developing cancer after receiving the same radiation exposures at the same ages.

People considering CT should talk with their doctors about whether the procedure is necessary for them and about its risks and benefits. Some organizations recommend that people keep a record of the imaging examinations they have received in case their doctors don't have access to all of their health records. A sample form, called My Medical Imaging , was developed by the Radiological Society of North America, the American College of Radiology, and the U.S. Food and Drug Administration. It includes questions to ask the doctor before undergoing any X-ray exam or treatment procedure.

What are the risks of CT scans for children?

Radiation exposure from CT scans affects adults and children differently. Children are considerably more sensitive to radiation than adults because of their growing bodies and the rapid pace at which the cells in their bodies divide. In addition, children have a longer life expectancy than adults, providing a larger window of opportunity for radiation-related cancers to develop.

Individuals who have had multiple CT scans before the age of 15 were found to have an increased risk of developing leukemia, brain tumors, and other cancers in the decade following their first scan. However, the lifetime risk of cancer from a single CT scan was small— about one case of cancer for every 10,000 scans performed on children.

In talking with health care providers, three key questions that the parents can ask are: why is the test needed? Will the results change the treatment decisions? Is there an alternative test that doesn't involve radiation? If the test is clinically justified, then the parents can be reassured that the benefits will outweigh the small long-term risks.

Chapter 20

Radiography

Medical radiography is a broad term that covers several types of studies that require the visualization of the internal parts of the body using X-ray techniques. For the purposes of this page radiography means a technique for generating and recording an X-ray pattern for the purpose of providing the user with a static image(s) after termination of the exposure. It is differentiated from *fluoroscopy, mammography*, and *computed tomography* which are discussed elsewhere. Radiography may also be used during the planning of radiation therapy treatment.

It is used to diagnose or treat patients by recording images of the internal structure of the body to assess the presence or absence of disease, foreign objects, and structural damage or anomaly.

During a radiographic procedure, an X-ray beam is passed through the body. A portion of the X-rays are absorbed or scattered by the internal structure and the remaining X-ray pattern is transmitted to a detector so that an image may be recorded for later evaluation. The recoding of the pattern may occur on film or through electronic means.

Uses

Radiography is used in many types of examinations and procedures where a record of a static image is desired. Some examples include:

Text in this chapter is excerpted from "Radiography," U.S. Food and Drug Administration (FDA), June 4, 2014.

- Dental examination

- Verification of correct placement of surgical markers prior to invasive procedures

- Mammography

- Orthopedic evaluations

- Spot film or static recording during fluoroscopy

- Chiropractic examinations

Risks

Radiography is a type of X-ray procedure, and it carries the same types of risks as other X-ray procedures. The radiation dose the patient receives varies depending on the individual procedure, but is generally less than that received during fluoroscopy and computed tomography procedures.

The major risks associated with radiography are the small possibilities of

- developing a radiation-induced cancer or cataracts some time later in life, and

- causing a disturbance in the growth or development of an embryo or fetus (teratogenic defect) when performed on a pregnant patient or one of childbearing age.

When an individual has a medical need, the benefit of radiography far exceeds the small cancer risk associated with the procedure. Even when radiography is medically necessary, it should use the lowest possible exposure and the minimum number of images. In most cases many of the possible risks can be reduced or eliminated with proper shielding.

Chapter 21

Contrast Radiography

Chapter Contents

Section 21.1

Coronary Angiography

Text in this section is excerpted from "Coronary Angiography,"
National Heart, Lung, and Blood Institute (NHLBI), March 2, 2012.

What Is Coronary Angiography?

Coronary angiography is a test that uses dye and special X-rays
to show the insides of your coronary arteries. The coronary arteries
supply oxygen-rich blood to your heart.

A waxy substance called plaque can build up inside the coronary
arteries. The buildup of plaque in the coronary arteries is called coronary heart disease (CHD).

Over time, plaque can harden or rupture (break open). Hardened
plaque narrows the coronary arteries and reduces the flow of oxygen-rich blood to the heart. This can cause chest pain or discomfort
called angina.

If the plaque ruptures, a blood clot can form on its surface. A large
blood clot can mostly or completely block blood flow through a coronary
artery. This is the most common cause of a heart attack. Over time,
ruptured plaque also hardens and narrows the coronary arteries.

Overview

During coronary angiography, special dye is released into the bloodstream. The dye makes the coronary arteries visible on X-ray pictures.
This helps doctors see blockages in the arteries.

A procedure called cardiac catheterization is used to get the dye
into the coronary arteries.

For this procedure, a thin, flexible tube called a catheter is put into
a blood vessel in your arm, groin (upper thigh), or neck. The tube is
threaded into your coronary arteries, and the dye is released into your
bloodstream. X-ray pictures are taken while the dye is flowing through
the coronary arteries.

Cardiologists (heart specialists) usually do cardiac catheterization
in a hospital. You're awake during the procedure, and it causes little

or no pain. However, you may feel some soreness in the blood vessel where the catheter was inserted.

Cardiac catheterization rarely causes serious complications.

Who Needs Coronary Angiography?

Your doctor may recommend coronary angiography if you have signs or symptoms of coronary heart disease (CHD). Signs and symptoms include:

- Angina. This is unexplained pain or pressure in your chest. You also may feel it in your shoulders, arms, neck, jaw, or back. The pain my even feel like indigestion. Angina may not only happen when you're active. Emotional stress also can trigger the pain associated with angina.

- Sudden cardiac arrest (SCA). This is a condition in which your heart suddenly and unexpectedly tops beating.

- Abnormal results from tests such as an EKG (electrocardiogram), exercise stress test, or other test.

Coronary angiography also might be done on an emergency basis, such as during a heart attack. If angiography shows blockages in your coronary arteries, your doctor may do a procedure called percutaneous coronary intervention, also known as angioplasty. This procedure can open blocked heart arteries and prevent further heart damage.

Coronary angiography also can help your doctor plan treatment after you've had a heart attack, especially if you have major heart damage or if you're still having chest pain.

What to Expect before Coronary Angiography

Before having coronary angiography, talk with your doctor about:

- How the test is done and how to prepare for it

- Any medicines you're taking, and whether you should stop taking them before the test

- Whether you have diseases or conditions that may require taking extra steps during or after the test to avoid complications. Examples of such conditions include diabetes and kidney disease.

Your doctor will tell you exactly which procedures will be done. For example, your doctor may recommend percutaneous coronary intervention, also known as coronary angioplasty, if the angiography shows a blocked artery.

You will have a chance to ask questions about the procedures. Also, you'll be asked to provide written informed consent to have the procedures.

It's not safe to drive after having cardiac catheterization, which is part of coronary angiography. You'll need to have someone drive you home after the procedure.

What to Expect during Coronary Angiography

During coronary angiography, you're kept on your back and awake. This allows you to follow your doctor's instructions during the test. You'll be given medicine to help you relax. The medicine might make you sleepy.

Your doctor will numb the area on the arm, groin (upper thigh), or neck where the catheter will enter your blood vessel. Then, he or she will use a needle to make a small hole in the blood vessel. The catheter will be inserted in the hole.

Next, your doctor will thread the catheter through the vessel and into the coronary arteries. Special X-ray movies are taken of the catheter as it's moved into the heart. The movies help your doctor see where to place the tip of the catheter.

Once the catheter is properly placed, your doctor will inject a special type of dye into the tube. The dye will flow through your coronary arteries, making them visible on an X-ray. This X-ray is called an angiogram.

If the angiogram reveals blocked arteries, your doctor may use percutaneous coronary intervention (PCI), commonly known as coronary angioplasty to restore blood flow to your heart.

After your doctor completes the procedure(s), he or she will remove the catheter from your body. The opening left in the blood vessel will then be closed up and bandaged.

A small sandbag or other type of weight might be placed on the bandage to apply pressure. This will help prevent major bleeding from the site.

What to Expect after Coronary Angiography

After coronary angiography, you'll be moved to a special care area in the hospital. You'll be carefully watched for several hours or overnight. During this time, you'll need to limit your movement to avoid bleeding from the site where the catheter was inserted.

While you recover in the special care area, nurses will check your heart rate and blood pressure regularly. They'll also watch for any bleeding at the catheter insertion site. You may develop a small bruise on your arm, groin (upper thigh), or neck at the catheter insertion site. That area may feel sore or tender for about a week.

Let your doctor know if you develop problems such as:

- A constant or large amount of blood at the catheter insertion site that can't be stopped with a small bandage

- Unusual pain, swelling, redness, or other signs of infection at or near the catheter insertion site

Your doctor will tell you whether you should avoid certain activities, such as heavy lifting, for a short time after the test.

What Are the Risks of Coronary Angiography?

Coronary angiography is a common medical test. It rarely causes serious problems. However, complications can include:

- Bleeding, infection, and pain at the catheter insertion site.

- Damage to blood vessels. Rarely, the catheter may scrape or poke a hole in a blood vessel as it's threaded to the heart.

- An allergic reaction to the dye that's used during the test.

Other, less common complications include:

- Arrhythmias (irregular heartbeats). These irregular heartbeats often go away on their own. However, your doctor may recommend treatment if they persist.

- Kidney damage caused by the dye that's used during the test.

- Blood clots that can trigger a stroke, heart attack, or other serious problems.

- Low blood pressure.

- A buildup of blood or fluid in the sac that surrounds the heart. This fluid can prevent the heart from beating properly.

As with any procedure involving the heart, complications can sometimes be fatal. However, this is rare with coronary angiography.

The risk of complications is higher in people who are older and in those who have certain diseases or conditions (such as chronic kidney disease and diabetes).

Section 21.2

Lower Gastrointestinal (GI) Series

Text in this section is excerpted from "Lower GI Series," National
Institute of Diabetes and Digestive and Kidney Diseases (NIDDK),
May 7, 2014.

A lower GI series, also called a barium enema, is an X-ray exam
used to help diagnose problems of the large intestine. An X-ray is a
picture created by using radiation and recorded on film or on a computer. To make the large intestine more visible on X-ray, a health
care provider will fill the person's intestine with a chalky liquid called
barium. The two types of lower GI series are

- a single-contrast lower GI series, which uses only barium during
  the test

- a double-contrast or air-contrast lower GI series, which uses a
  combination of barium and air to create a more detailed view of
  the large intestine

The health care provider and radiologist—a doctor who specializes in
medical imaging—will work together to determine which exam to perform.

What is the large intestine?

The large intestine is part of the GI tract, a series of hollow organs
joined in a long, twisting tube from the mouth to the anus—a 1-inch-
long opening through which stool leaves the body. The body digests food
using the movement of muscles in the GI tract, along with the release
of hormones and enzymes. Organs that make up the GI tract are the
mouth, esophagus, stomach, small intestine, large intestine—which
includes the appendix, cecum, colon, and rectum—and anus. The intestines are sometimes called the bowel. The last part of the GI tract—
called the lower GI tract—consists of the large intestine and anus.

The large intestine is about 5 feet long in adults and absorbs water
and any remaining nutrients from partially digested food passed from
the small intestine. The large intestine then changes waste from liquid
to a solid matter called stool. Stool passes from the colon to the rectum.

276

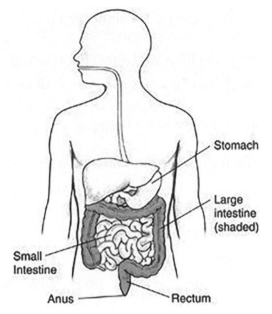

Figure 21.1. *Large intestine in the gastrointestinal tract.*

The rectum is 6 to 8 inches long in adults and is located between the last part of the colon—called the sigmoid colon—and the anus. The rectum stores stool prior to a bowel movement. During a bowel movement, stool moves from the rectum to the anus.

Why is a lower gastrointestinal series performed?

A lower GI series can help diagnose the cause of

- abdominal pain
- bleeding from the anus
- changes in bowel habits
- chronic diarrhea
- unexplained weight loss

A lower GI series can also show

- cancerous growths.
- diverticula—small pouches in the colon.
- a fistula—an abnormal passage, or tunnel, between two organs, called an internal fistula, or between an organ and the outside of

277

the body, called an external fistula. Fistulas occur most often in the areas around the rectum and anus.

- inflammation, or swelling, of the intestinal lining.

- polyps—extra pieces of tissue that grow on the lining of the intestine.

- ulcers—sores on the intestinal lining.

How does a person prepare for a lower gastrointestinal series?

A person prepares for a lower GI series by

- talking with a health care provider
- cleansing the bowel

Talking with a health care provider. People should talk with their health care provider

- about medical conditions they have
- about all prescribed and over-the-counter medications, vitamins, and supplements they take
- if they've had a colonoscopy with a biopsy or polyp removal in the last 4 weeks

Women should let their health care provider know if they may be pregnant to avoid potential risks to the developing baby. The health care provider will take special precautions to minimize exposure to radiation, or he or she may suggest a different procedure.

Cleansing the bowel. The health care provider will give written bowel prep instructions to follow at home. The health care provider orders a bowel prep so that little to no stool is present inside the person's intestine. A complete bowel prep lets the person pass stool that is clear. Stool inside the colon can prevent the X-ray from making a clear image of the intestine. Instructions may include following a clear liquid diet for 1 to 3 days before the procedure and avoiding drinks that contain red or purple dye. The instructions will provide specific direction about when to start and stop the clear liquid diet. During this diet, people may drink or eat the following:

- fat-free bouillon or broth
- gelatin in flavors such as lemon, lime, or orange

- plain coffee or tea, without cream or milk

- sports drinks in flavors such as lemon, lime, or orange

- strained fruit juice, such as apple or white grape—orange juice is not recommended

- water

The person needs to take laxatives and enemas the night before a lower GI series. A laxative is medication that loosens stool and increases bowel movements. An enema involves flushing water or laxative into the rectum using a special wash bottle. Laxatives and enemas can cause diarrhea, so the person should stay close to a bathroom during the bowel prep.

A person may take laxatives swallowed as a pill or as a powder dissolved in water. Some people will need to drink a large amount, usually a gallon, of liquid laxative over the course of the bowel prep at scheduled times. People may find this step difficult; however, it is very important to complete the prep. The images will not be clear if the prep is incomplete.

People should call their health care provider if they are having side effects that make them feel they can't finish the prep.

How is a lower gastrointestinal series performed?

An X-ray technician and a radiologist perform a lower GI series at a hospital or an outpatient center. A person does not need anesthesia. The procedure usually takes 30 to 60 minutes.

For the test,

- the person lies on a table while the radiologist inserts a flexible tube into the person's anus and fills the large intestine with barium

- the radiologist prevents leaking of barium from the anus by inflating a balloon on the end of the tube

- the technician may ask the person to change position several times to evenly coat the large intestine with the barium

- if the health care provider has ordered a double-contrast lower GI series, the radiologist will inject air through the tube to inflate the intestine

During the test, the person may have some discomfort and feel the urge to have a bowel movement.

The person will need to hold still in various positions while the radiologist and technician take X-ray images and possibly X-ray video, called fluoroscopy. The radiologist and technician will view the large intestine from different angles.

When the imaging is complete, the radiologist or technician will deflate the balloon on the tube, and most of the barium will drain through the tube. The person will expel the remaining barium into a bedpan or nearby toilet. A nurse or technician may give the person an enema to further flush out the barium.

What can a person expect after a lower gastrointestinal series?

After a lower GI series, a person can expect the following:

- abdominal cramps and bloating that may occur for a short time after the procedure

- to resume most normal activities after leaving the hospital or outpatient center

- barium in the large intestine that causes stools to be white or light colored for several days after the procedure

A person should carefully read and follow the discharge instructions, which will explain how to flush the remaining barium from the intestine. The radiologist will interpret the images and send a report of the findings to the person's health care provider.

What are the risks of a lower gastrointestinal series?

The risks of a lower GI series include

- constipation from the barium enema—the most common complication of a lower GI series.

- an allergic reaction to the barium.

- bowel obstruction—partial or complete blockage of the small or large intestine. Although rare, bowel obstruction can be a life-threatening condition that requires emergency medical treatment.

- leakage of barium into the abdomen—the area between the chest and the hips—through an undetected tear or hole in the lining of the large intestine. This complication is rare; however, it usually requires emergency surgery to repair.

Radiation exposure can cause cancer, although the level of radiation exposure that leads to cancer is unknown. Health care providers estimate the risk of cancer from this type of test to be small.

Seek Immediate Care

People who have any of the following symptoms after a lower GI series should seek immediate medical attention:

- severe abdominal pain
- bloody bowel movements or bleeding from the anus
- inability to pass gas
- fever
- severe constipation

Section 21.3

Upper Gastrointestinal (GI) Series

Text in this section is excerpted from "Upper GI Series," National Institute of Diabetes and Digestive and Kidney Diseases (NIDDK), May 7, 2014.

An upper GI series, also called a barium swallow, uses X-rays and fluoroscopy to help diagnose problems of the upper GI tract. An X-ray is a picture created by using radiation and recorded on film or on a computer. Fluoroscopy is a form of X-ray that makes it possible to see the internal organs and their motion on a video monitor. To make the upper GI tract more visible on X-ray, a health care provider will fill the person's upper GI tract with a chalky liquid called barium. The two types of upper GI series are

- a standard barium upper GI series, which uses only barium during the test

- a double-contrast upper GI series, which uses a combination of air and barium to create a more detailed view of the stomach lining

281

What is the upper gastrointestinal tract?

The upper GI tract is the first part of the GI tract, which includes a series of hollow organs joined in a long, twisting tube from the mouth to the anus—a 1-inch-long opening through which stool leaves the body. The upper GI tract includes the mouth, esophagus, stomach, duodenum, and small intestine. The duodenum is the first part of the small intestine.

The esophagus carries food and liquids from the mouth to the stomach. The muscular layers of the esophagus are normally pinched together at both the upper and lower ends by muscles called sphincters. When a person swallows, the sphincters relax to let food or drink pass from the mouth into the stomach. The muscles then close rapidly to prevent the food or drink from leaking out of the stomach back into the esophagus. This process is automatic and people are usually not aware of it, though people sometimes feel food in their esophagus when they swallow something too large, try to eat too quickly, or drink very hot or cold liquids.

The stomach slowly pumps the food and liquids into the small intestine, which absorbs needed nutrients. The body digests food using the

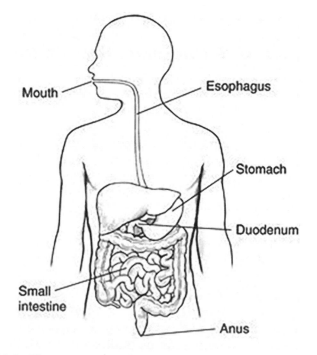

Figure 21.2. *The upper gastrointestinal tract*

movement of the muscles in the GI tract, along with the release of hormones and enzymes.

Why is an upper GI series performed?

An upper GI series can help diagnose the cause of

- abdominal pain
- nausea and vomiting
- problems swallowing
- unexplained weight loss

An upper GI series can also show

- abnormal growths.
- esophageal varices—abnormal, enlarged veins in the lower part of the esophagus.
- gastroesophageal reflux, which occurs when stomach contents flow back up into the esophagus.
- a hiatal hernia, or when the upper part of the stomach slips through the diaphragm and moves up into the chest. The diaphragm is the muscle wall that separates the stomach from the chest.
- inflammation, or swelling, of the GI tract.
- scars or strictures—abnormal narrowing of openings in the body.
- ulcers—sores on the stomach or intestinal lining.

How does a person prepare for an upper gastrointestinal series?

A person prepares for an upper GI series by

- talking with a health care provider
- clearing the upper GI tract

Talking with a health care provider. A person should talk with his or her health care provider about

- medical conditions he or she has
- all prescribed and over-the-counter medications, vitamins, and supplements he or she takes

Women should let their health care provider know if they may be pregnant to avoid potential risks to the developing baby. The health care provider will take special precautions to minimize the exposure to radiation, or he or she may suggest a different procedure.

Clearing the upper GI tract. This procedure uses X-ray images to examine the upper GI tract during the procedure. The X-ray can't show the lining of the organs clearly if food or drink is inside the upper GI tract. To ensure the upper GI tract is clear, health care providers usually advise people not to eat, drink, smoke, or chew gum during the 8 hours before the procedure.

How is an upper gastrointestinal series performed?

An X-ray technician and a radiologist—a doctor who specializes in medical imaging—perform an upper GI series at a hospital or an outpatient center. A person does not need anesthesia. The procedure usually takes about 2 hours to complete. However, if the barium moves slowly through the small intestine, the test may take up to 5 hours to complete.

For the test,

- the person stands or sits in front of an X-ray machine and drinks barium, which coats the lining of the upper GI tract

- the person lies on the X-ray table and the radiologist watches the barium move through the GI tract on the X-rays and fluoroscopy

- the technician may press on the abdomen—the area between the chest and hips—or ask the person to change positions to fully coat the upper GI tract with the barium

If a person has a double-contrast study, he or she will swallow gas-forming crystals, which activate when they mix with the barium. The gas expands the barium-coated stomach, filling it with air and exposing finer details of the upper GI tract lining. The technician will take additional X-rays.

What can a person expect after an upper gastrointestinal series?

After an upper GI series, a person can expect the following:

- bloating or nausea for a short time after the procedure

- to resume most normal activities after leaving the hospital or outpatient center

- barium in the GI tract that causes stools to be white or light colored for several days after the procedure

A person should carefully read and follow the discharge instructions, which will explain how to flush the remaining barium from the GI tract. The radiologist will interpret the images and send a report of the findings to the person's health care provider.

What are the risks of an upper gastrointestinal series?

The risks of an upper GI series include

- constipation from the barium—the most common complication of an upper GI series.

- an allergic reaction to the barium or flavoring in the barium.

- bowel obstruction—partial or complete blockage of the small or large intestine. Although rare, bowel obstruction can be a life-threatening condition that requires emergency medical treatment.

Radiation exposure can cause cancer, although the level of radiation exposure that leads to cancer is unknown. Health care providers estimate the risk of cancer from this type of test to be small.

Seek Immediate Care

People who have any of the following symptoms after an upper GI series should seek immediate medical attention:

- failure to have a bowel movement within 2 days of the procedure
- fever
- inability to pass gas
- severe abdominal pain
- severe constipation

Section 21.4

Lung Ventilation / Perfusion Scan

Text in this section is excerpted from "Lung Ventilation/Perfusion
Scan," National Institute of Diabetes and Digestive and Kidney
Diseases (NIDDK), July 25, 2014.

A lung ventilation/perfusion scan, or VQ scan, is a test that measures air and blood flow in your lungs. A VQ scan most often is used to help diagnose or rule out a pulmonary embolism (PE).

A PE is a sudden blockage in a lung artery. The blockage usually is caused by a blood clot that travels to the lung from a vein in the leg. PE is a serious condition that can cause low blood oxygen levels, damage to the lungs, or even death.

A VQ scan also can detect poor blood flow in the lungs' blood vessels and uneven air distribution, and it can provide pictures that help doctors prepare for some types of lung surgery.

Overview

A VQ scan involves two types of scans: ventilation and perfusion. The ventilation scan shows where air flows in your lungs. The perfusion scan shows where blood flows in your lungs.

Both scans use radioisotopes (a low-risk radioactive substance). For the ventilation scan, you inhale a small amount of radioisotope gas. For the perfusion scan, the radioisotopes are injected into a vein in your arm.

Radioisotopes release energy inside your body. Special scanners outside of your body use the energy to create images of air and blood flow patterns in your lungs.

Outlook

VQ scans involve little pain or risk for most people. During the perfusion scan, you may feel some discomfort when the radioisotopes are injected. You also may have a bruise at the injection site after the test.

The amount of radiation in the radioisotopes used for both tests is very small. The amount of radiation in the gas and injection together are about the same as the amount a person is naturally exposed to in 1 year.

Very rarely, the radioisotopes used in VQ scans can cause an allergic reaction. Hives or a rash may result. Medicines can relieve this reaction.

Other Names for Lung Ventilation / Perfusion Scans

Lung ventilation / perfusion scans also are called VQ scans, pulmonary ventilation/perfusion scans, and nuclear medicine tests.

Who Needs a Lung Ventilation / Perfusion Scan?

You may need a lung ventilation / perfusion (VQ) scan if you have signs or symptoms of a pulmonary embolism (PE). A PE is a sudden blockage in a lung artery. A blood clot usually causes the blockage.

Signs and symptoms of a PE include chest pain, trouble breathing, rapid breathing, coughing, and coughing up blood. An irregular heartbeat called an arrhythmia also may suggest a PE.

Some blood clots that can cause a PE travel to the lungs from veins deep in the legs. This can cause pain and swelling in the affected limb.

Doctors use VQ scans to help find out whether a PE is causing these signs and symptoms. A VQ scan alone, however, won't confirm whether you have a PE. Your doctor also will consider other factors when making a diagnosis.

Doctors also use VQ scans to detect poor blood flow in the lungs' blood vessels, air trapping or uneven air distribution, and to examine the lungs before some types of surgery.

What to Expect before a Lung Ventilation / Perfusion Scan?

A lung ventilation / perfusion (VQ) scan may be done during an emergency to help diagnose or rule out a pulmonary embolism (PE). A PE is a sudden blockage in a lung artery. This serious condition can cause low blood oxygen levels, damage to the lungs, or even death.

If your VQ scan isn't done during an emergency, your doctor will tell you how to prepare for the test. Most people don't need to take any special steps to prepare for a VQ scan.

Your doctor may ask you to wear clothing that has no metal hooks or snaps. These materials can block the scanner's view. Or, you may be asked to wear a hospital gown for the test.

Tell your doctor whether you're pregnant or may be pregnant. If possible, you should avoid radiation exposure during pregnancy, as it may harm the fetus.

You and your doctor will decide whether the benefits of a VQ scan outweigh the small risk to the fetus, or whether another test might be better.

If you're breastfeeding, ask your doctor how long you should wait after the test before you breastfeed. The radioisotopes used for VQ scans can pass through your breast milk to your baby.

You may want to prepare for the scan by pumping and saving milk for 24 to 48 hours in advance. You can bottle-feed your baby in the hours after the VQ scan.

What to Expect during a Lung Ventilation / Perfusion Scan

Lung ventilation / perfusion (VQ) scans are done at radiology clinics or hospitals.

For the test, you lie on a table for about 1 hour and have two types of scans: ventilation and perfusion. The ventilation scan shows the pattern of air flow in your lungs. The perfusion scan shows the pattern of blood flow in your lungs.

You must lie very still during the tests or the pictures may blur. If you're having trouble staying still, your doctor may give you medicine to help you relax.

Both scans use radioisotopes (a low-risk radioactive substance). This substance releases energy inside your body. Special scanners outside of your body use the energy to create images of air and blood flow in your lungs.

The radioisotopes used in VQ scans can cause an allergic reaction, including itching and hives. Medicines can relieve these symptoms.

Ventilation

For this scan, you lie on a table that moves under the arm of the scanner. You wear a breathing mask over your nose and mouth and inhale a small amount of radioisotope gas mixed with oxygen.

As you breathe, the scanner takes pictures that show air going into your lungs. You'll need to hold your breath for a few seconds at the start of each picture.

The scan is painless, and each picture takes only a few minutes. However, wearing the mask can make some people feel anxious. If this happens, your doctor may give you medicine to help you relax.

Perfusion

For this scan, a small amount of radioisotope is injected into a vein in your arm. The scanner then takes pictures of blood flow through your lungs.

The scan itself doesn't hurt, but you may feel some discomfort from the radioisotope injection.

What to Expect after a Lung Ventilation/Perfusion Scan

Most people can return to their normal activities right after a lung ventilation / perfusion (VQ) scan.

If you got medicine to help you relax during the scan, your doctor will tell you when you can return to your normal activities. The medicine may make you tired, so you'll need someone to drive you home.

You may have a bruise on your arm where the radioisotopes were injected. You'll need to drink plenty of fluids to flush the radioisotopes out of your body. Your doctor can advise you about how much fluid to drink.

If you're breastfeeding, ask your doctor how long you should wait after the test before you breastfeed. The radioisotopes used for VQ scans can pass through your breast milk to your baby.

You may want to prepare for the scan by pumping and saving milk for 24 to 48 in advance. You can bottle-feed your baby in the hours after the VQ scan.

What Does a Lung Ventilation/Perfusion Scan Show?

A lung ventilation / perfusion (VQ) scan shows how well air and blood are flowing through your lungs. Normal results show full air and blood flow to all parts of your lungs.

If air flow is normal but blood flow isn't, you may have a pulmonary embolism (PE). A PE is a sudden blockage in a lung artery. The blockage usually is caused by a blood clot that travels to the lung from a vein in the leg.

The results of the scan show whether you're at high, medium, or low risk for a PE. However, a VQ scan alone won't confirm whether you have a PE. A scan showing low blood flow in spots may reflect other lung problems, such as lung damage from COPD (chronic obstructive pulmonary disease).

Your doctor uses the VQ scan results—along with results from a physical exam, chest X-ray, and other tests—to make a diagnosis.

What Are the Risks of a Lung Ventilation/Perfusion Scan?

Lung ventilation / perfusion (VQ) scans involve little risk for most people. The radioisotopes used for both tests expose you to a small amount of radiation. The amount of radiation in the gas and injection together are about the same as the amount a person is naturally exposed to in 1 year.

Although rare, the radioisotopes may cause an allergic reaction.

Radiation

The radiation from a VQ scan leaves your body after a few days. Exposure to radiation is associated with a risk of cancer. However, it's not known whether the amount of radiation from a VQ scan increases your risk for cancer.

You and your doctor will decide whether the benefits of a VQ scan outweigh the possible risks. Your doctor also will try to avoid ordering multiple VQ scans for you over a short period.

If you're pregnant or breastfeeding, talk with your doctor about the risk of radiation to your baby. He or she will consider whether another test can be used instead.

Allergic Reaction

Very rarely, the radioisotopes used in VQ scans can cause an allergic reaction. Hives or a rash may result. Medicines can relieve this reaction.

Chapter 22

Ultrasound Imaging

Chapter Contents

Section 22.1

Overview of Ultrasound Imaging

Text in this section is excerpted from "Ultrasound Imaging," Food and Drug Administration (FDA), December 16, 2014.

Description

Ultrasound imaging (sonography) uses high-frequency sound waves to view inside the body. Because ultrasound images are captured in real-time, they can also show movement of the body's internal organs as well as blood flowing through the blood vessels. Unlike X-ray imaging, there is no ionizing radiation exposure associated with ultrasound imaging.

In an ultrasound exam, a transducer (probe) is placed directly on the skin or inside a body opening. A thin layer of gel is applied to the skin so that the ultrasound waves are transmitted from the transducer through the gel into the body.

The ultrasound image is produced based on the reflection of the waves off of the body structures. The strength (amplitude) of the sound signal and the time it takes for the wave to travel through the body provide the information necessary to produce an image.

Uses

Ultrasound imaging is a medical tool that can help a physician evaluate, diagnose and treat medical conditions. Common ultrasound imaging procedures include:

- Abdominal ultrasound (to visualize abdominal tissues and organs)

- Bone sonometry (to assess bone fragility)

- Breast ultrasound (to visualize breast tissue)

- Doppler fetal heart rate monitors (to listen to the fetal heart beat)

- Doppler ultrasound (to visualize blood flow through a blood vessel, organs, or other structures)

- Echocardiogram (to view the heart)
- Fetal ultrasound (to view the fetus in pregnancy)
- Ultrasound-guided biopsies (to collect a sample of tissue)
- Ophthalmic ultrasound (to visualize ocular structures
- Ultrasound-guided needle placement (in blood vessels or other tissues of interest)

Benefits / Risks

Ultrasound imaging has been used for over 20 years and has an excellent safety record. It is based on non-ionizing radiation, so it does not have the same risks as X-rays or other types of imaging systems that use ionizing radiation.

Although ultrasound imaging is generally considered safe when used prudently by appropriately trained health care providers, ultrasound energy has the potential to produce biological effects on the body. Ultrasound waves can heat the tissues slightly. In some cases, it can also produce small pockets of gas in body fluids or tissues (cavitation). The long-term consequences of these effects are still unknown. Because of the particular concern for effects on the fetus, organizations such as the American Institute of Ultrasound in Medicine disclaimer iconhave advocated prudent use of ultrasound imaging in pregnancy. Furthermore, the use of ultrasound solely for non-medical purposes such as obtaining fetal 'keepsake' videos has been discouraged. Keepsake images or videos are reasonable if they are produced during a medically-indicated exam, and if no additional exposure is required.

Information for Patients including Expectant Mothers

For all medical imaging procedures, the FDA recommends that patients talk to their health care provider to understand the reason for the examination, the medical information that will be obtained, the potential risks, and how the results will be used to manage the medical condition or pregnancy. Because ultrasound is not based on ionizing radiation, it is particularly useful for women of child-bearing age when CT or other imaging methods would otherwise result in exposure to radiation.

Expectant Mothers

Ultrasound is the most widely used medical imaging method for viewing the fetus during pregnancy. Routine examinations are performed to assess and monitor the health status of the fetus and mother. Ultrasound examinations provide parents with a valuable opportunity to view and hear the heartbeat of the fetus, bond with the unborn baby, and capture images to share with family and friends.

In fetal ultrasound, three-dimensional (3D) ultrasound allows the visualization of some facial features and possibly other parts such as fingers and toes of the fetus. Four-dimensional (4D) ultrasound is 3D ultrasound in motion. While ultrasound is generally considered to be safe with very low risks, the risks may increase with unnecessary prolonged exposure to ultrasound energy, or when untrained users operate the device.

Expectant mothers should also be aware of purchasing over-the-counter fetal heartbeat monitoring systems (also called doptones). These devices should only be used by trained health care providers when medically necessary. Use of these devices by untrained persons could expose the fetus to prolonged and unsafe energy levels, or could provide information that is interpreted incorrectly by the user.

Section 22.2

Carotid Ultrasound

Text in this section is excerpted from "Carotid Ultrasound," National Heart, Lung, and Blood Institute (NHLBI), February 3, 2012.

Carotid ultrasound is a painless and harmless test that uses high-frequency sound waves to create pictures of the insides of your carotid arteries.

You have two common carotid arteries, one on each side of your neck. They each divide into internal and external carotid arteries.

The internal carotid arteries supply oxygen-rich blood to your brain. The external carotid arteries supply oxygen-rich blood to your face, scalp, and neck.

Overview

Carotid ultrasound shows whether a waxy substance called plaque (plak) has built up in your carotid arteries. The buildup of plaque in the carotid arteries is called carotid artery disease.

Carotid Arteries

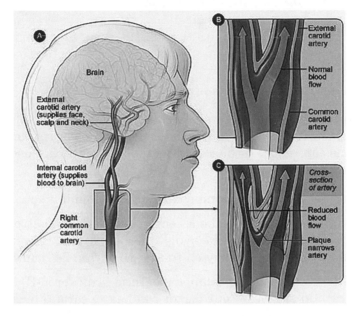

Figure 22.1. Carotid Ultrasound: *"A" shows the location of the right carotid artery in the head and neck. "B" shows the inside of a normal carotid artery that has normal blood flow. "C" shows the inside of a carotid artery that has plaque buildup and reduced blood flow.*

Over time, plaque can harden or rupture (break open). Hardened plaque narrows the carotid arteries and reduces the flow of oxygen-rich blood to the brain.

If the plaque ruptures, a blood clot can form on its surface. A clot can mostly or completely block blood flow through a carotid artery, which can cause a stroke.

A piece of plaque or a blood clot also can break away from the wall of the carotid artery. The plaque or clot can travel through the bloodstream and get stuck in one of the brain's smaller arteries. This can block blood flow in the artery and cause a stroke.

A standard carotid ultrasound shows the structure of your carotid arteries. Your carotid ultrasound test might include a Doppler ultrasound. Doppler ultrasound is a special test that shows the movement of blood through your blood vessels.

Your doctor might need results from both types of ultrasound to fully assess whether you have a blood flow problem in your carotid arteries.

Other Names for Carotid Ultrasound

- Doppler ultrasound

- Carotid duplex ultrasound

Who Needs Carotid Ultrasound?

A carotid ultrasound shows whether you have plaque buildup in your carotid arteries. Over time, plaque can harden or rupture (break open). This can reduce or block the flow of oxygen-rich blood to your brain and cause a stroke.

Your doctor may recommend a carotid ultrasound if you:

- Had a stroke or mini-stroke recently. During a mini-stroke, you may have some or all of the symptoms of a stroke. However, the symptoms usually go away on their own within 24 hours.

- Have an abnormal sound called a carotid bruit (broo-E) in one of your carotid arteries. Your doctor can hear a carotid bruit using a stethoscope. A bruit might suggest a partial blockage in your carotid artery, which could lead to a stroke.

Your doctor also may recommend a carotid ultrasound if he or she thinks you have:

- Blood clots in one of your carotid arteries

- A split between the layers of your carotid artery wall. The split can weaken the wall or reduce blood flow to your brain.

A carotid ultrasound also might be done to see whether carotid artery surgery, also called carotid endarterectomy, has restored normal blood flow through a carotid artery.

If you had a procedure called carotid stenting, your doctor might use carotid ultrasound afterward to check the position of the stent in your carotid artery. (The stent, a small mesh tube, supports the inner artery wall.)

Carotid ultrasound sometimes is used as a preventive screening test in people at increased risk of stroke, such as those who have high blood pressure and diabetes.

What to Expect before Carotid Ultrasound

Carotid ultrasound is a painless test, and typically there is little to do in advance. Your doctor will tell you how to prepare for your carotid ultrasound.

What to Expect during Carotid Ultrasound

Carotid ultrasound usually is done in a doctor's office or hospital. The test is painless and often doesn't take more than 30 minutes.

The ultrasound machine includes a computer, a screen, and a transducer. The transducer is a hand-held device that sends and receives ultrasound waves.

You will lie on your back on an exam table for the test. Your technician or doctor will put gel on your neck where your carotid arteries are located. The gel helps the ultrasound waves reach the arteries.

Your technician or doctor will put the transducer against different spots on your neck and move it back and forth. The transducer gives off ultrasound waves and detects their echoes as they bounce off the artery walls and blood cells. Ultrasound waves can't be heard by the human ear.

The computer uses the echoes to create and record pictures of the insides of the carotid arteries. These pictures usually appear in black and white. The screen displays these live images for your doctor to review.

Your carotid ultrasound test might include a Doppler ultrasound. Doppler ultrasound is a special test that shows the movement of blood through your arteries. Blood flow through the arteries usually appears in color on the ultrasound pictures.

What to Expect after Carotid Ultrasound

You usually can return to your normal activities as soon as the carotid ultrasound is over. Your doctor will likely be able to tell you the results of the carotid ultrasound when it occurs or soon afterward.

What Does a Carotid Ultrasound Show?

A carotid ultrasound can show whether plaque buildup has narrowed one or both of your carotid arteries. If so, you might be at risk of having a stroke. The risk depends on the extent of the blockage and how much it has reduced blood flow to your brain.

To lower your risk of stroke, your doctor may recommend medical or surgical treatments to reduce or remove plaque from your carotid arteries.

What Are the Risks of Carotid Ultrasound?

Carotid ultrasound has no risks because the test uses harmless sound waves. They are the same type of sound waves that doctors use to record pictures of fetuses in pregnant women.

Chapter 23

Computed Tomography (CT) Scan

Chapter Contents

Section 23.1

Overview of Computed Tomography

Text in this section is excerpted from "Computed Tomography (CT),"
U.S. Food and Drug Administration (FDA), August 7, 2014.

Description

Computed tomography (CT), sometimes called "computerized tomography" or "computed axial tomography" (CAT), is a noninvasive medical examination or procedure that uses specialized X-ray equipment to produce cross-sectional images of the body. Each cross-sectional image represents a "slice" of the person being imaged, like the slices in a loaf of bread. These cross-sectional images are used for a variety of diagnostic and therapeutic purposes.

CT scans can be performed on every region of the body for a variety of reasons (e.g., diagnostic, treatment planning, interventional, or screening). Most CT scans are performed as outpatient procedures.

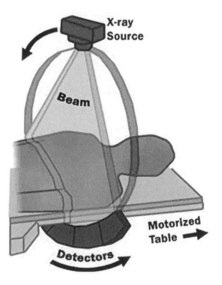

Figure 23.1. *Drawing of CT fan beam (left) and patient in a CT imaging system*

How a CT system works:

- A motorized table moves the patient through a circular opening in the CT imaging system.

- While the patient is inside the opening, an X-ray source and a detector assembly within the system rotate around the patient. A single rotation typically takes a second or less. During rotation the X-ray source produces a narrow, fan-shaped beam of X-rays that passes through a section of the patient's body.

- Detectors in rows opposite the X-ray source register the X-rays that pass through the patient's body as a snapshot in the process of creating an image. Many different "snapshots" (at many angles through the patient) are collected during one complete rotation.

- For each rotation of the X-ray source and detector assembly, the image data are sent to a computer to reconstruct all of the individual "snapshots" into one or multiple cross-sectional images (slices) of the internal organs and tissues.

CT images of internal organs, bones, soft tissue, and blood vessels provide greater clarity and more details than conventional X-ray images, such as a chest X-Ray.

Uses

CT is a valuable medical tool that can help a physician:

- Diagnose disease, trauma or abnormality

- Plan and guide interventional or therapeutic procedures

- Monitor the effectiveness of therapy (e.g., cancer treatment)

Benefits/Risks

When used appropriately, the benefits of a CT scan far exceed the risks. CT scans can provide detailed information to diagnose, plan treatment for, and evaluate many conditions in adults and children. Additionally, the detailed images provided by CT scans may eliminate the need for exploratory surgery.

Concerns about CT scans include the risks from exposure to ionizing radiation and possible reactions to the intravenous contrast agent, or dye, which may be used to improve visualization. The exposure to

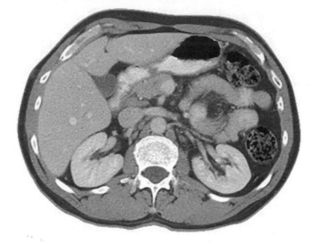

Figure 23.2. *CT image of the abdomen*

ionizing radiation may cause a small increase in a person's lifetime risk of developing cancer. Exposure to ionizing radiation is of particular concern in pediatric patients because the cancer risk per unit dose of ionizing radiation is higher for younger patients than adults, and younger patients have a longer lifetime for the effects of radiation exposure to manifest as cancer.

However, in children and adults, the risk from a medically necessary imaging exam is quite small when compared to the benefit of accurate diagnosis or intervention. It is especially important to make sure that CT scans in children are performed with appropriate exposure factors, as use of exposure settings designed for adults can result in a larger radiation dose than necessary to produce a useful image for a pediatric patient.

Information for Patients and Parents

If a physician recommends a CT scan for you or your child, the FDA encourages you to discuss the benefits and risks of the CT scan, as well as any past X-ray procedures you or your child have had, with your physician. A CT scan should always be performed if it is medically necessary and other exams using no or less radiation are unsuitable. At this time, the FDA does not see a benefit to whole-body scanning of individuals without symptoms.

Section 23.2

Full-Body Computed Tomography

Text in this section is excerpted from "Full-Body CT Scans -
What You Need to Know," Food and Drug Administration (FDA),
March 23, 2015.

Using a technology that "takes a look" at people's insides and promises early warnings of cancer, cardiac disease, and other abnormalities, clinics and medical imaging facilities nationwide are touting a new service for health-conscious people: "Whole-body CT screening." This typically involves scanning the body from the chin to below the hips with a form of X-ray imaging that produces cross-sectional images.

The technology used is called "X-ray computed tomography" (CT), sometimes referred to as "computerized axial tomography" (CAT). A number of different types of X-ray CT systems are being promoted for various types of screening. For example, "multi-slice" CT (MSCT) and "electron beam" CT (EBCT) – also called "electron beam tomography" (EBT) – are X-ray CT systems that produce images rapidly and are often promoted for screening the buildup of calcium in arteries of the heart.

CT, MSCT and EBCT all use X-rays to produce images representing "slices" of the body – like the slices of a loaf of bread. Each image slice corresponds to a wafer-thin section which can be viewed to reveal body structures in great detail.

CT is recognized as an invaluable medical tool for the diagnosis of disease, trauma, or abnormality in patients with signs or symptoms of disease. It's also used for planning, guiding, and monitoring therapy. What's new is that CT is being marketed as a preventive or proactive health care measure to healthy individuals who have no symptoms of disease.

No Proven Benefits for Healthy People

Taking preventive action, finding unsuspected disease, uncovering problems while they are treatable, these all sound great, almost too good to be true! In fact, at this time the Food and Drug Administration

303

(FDA) knows of no scientific evidence demonstrating that whole-body scanning of individuals without symptoms provides more benefit than harm to people being screened. The FDA is responsible for assuring the safety and effectiveness of such medical devices, and it prohibits manufacturers of CT systems to promote their use for whole-body screening of asymptomatic people. The FDA, however, does not regulate practitioners and they may choose to use a device for any use they deem appropriate.

Compared to most other diagnostic X-ray procedures, CT scans result in relatively high radiation exposure. The risks associated with such exposure are greatly outweighed by the benefits of diagnostic and therapeutic CT. However, for whole-body CT screening of asymptomatic people, the benefits are questionable:

- Can it effectively differentiate between healthy people and those who have a hidden disease?

- Do suspicious findings lead to additional invasive testing or treatments that produce additional risk with little benefit?

- Does a "normal" finding guarantee good health?

Many people don't realize that getting a whole body CT screening exam won't necessarily give them the "peace of mind" they are hoping for, or the information that would allow them to prevent a health problem. An abnormal finding, for example, may not be a serious one, and a normal finding may be inaccurate. CT scans, like other medical procedures, will miss some conditions, and "false" leads can prompt further, unnecessary testing.

Points to consider if you are thinking of having a whole-body screening:

- Whole-body CT screening has not been demonstrated to meet generally accepted criteria for an effective screening procedure.

- Medical professional societies have not endorsed whole-body CT scanning for individuals without symptoms.

- CT screening of high-risk individuals for specific diseases such as lung cancer or colon cancer is currently being studied.

- The radiation from a CT scan may be associated with a very small increase in the possibility of developing cancer later in a person's life.

- The FDA provides additional information regarding whole-body CT screening on its Computed Tomography (CT) Web site.

FDA's Recommendation

Before having a CT screening procedure, carefully investigate and consider the potential risks and benefits and discuss them with your physician.

Section 23.3

Chest Computed Tomography Scan

Text in this section is excerpted from "Chest CT Scan," National Heart, Lung, and Blood Institute (NHLBI), February 29, 2012.

A chest computed tomography scan, or chest CT scan, is a painless, noninvasive test. It creates precise pictures of the structures in your chest, such as your lungs. "Noninvasive" means that no surgery is done and no instruments are inserted into your body.

A chest CT scan is a type of X-ray. However, a CT scan's pictures show more detail than pictures from a standard chest X-ray.

Like other X-ray tests, chest CT scans use a form of energy called ionizing radiation. This energy helps create pictures of the inside of your chest.

Overview

Doctors use chest CT scans to:

- Show the size, shape, and position of your lungs and other structures in your chest.

- Follow up on abnormal findings from standard chest X-rays.

- Find the cause of lung symptoms, such as shortness of breath or chest pain.

- Find out whether you have a lung problem, such as a tumor, excess fluid around the lungs, or a pulmonary embolism (a blood clot in the lungs). The test also is used to check for other conditions, such as tuberculosis, emphysema, and pneumonia.

The chest CT scanning machine takes many pictures, called slices, of the lungs and the inside of the chest. A computer processes these pictures; they can be viewed on a screen or printed on film. The computer also can stack the pictures to create a very detailed, three-dimensional (3D) model of organs.

Sometimes, a substance called contrast dye is injected into a vein in your arm for the CT scan. This substance highlights areas in your chest, which helps create clearer images.

Outlook

Chest CT scans have few risks. Because the test uses radiation, there may be a slight risk of cancer. Children are more sensitive to radiation than adults because they're smaller and still growing.

The amount of radiation will vary with the type of CT scan. On average, though, the amount of radiation will not exceed the amount a person is naturally exposed to over 3 years. The benefits of a CT scan should always be weighed against the possible risks.

Rarely, people have allergic reactions to the contrast dye that's sometimes used during chest CT scans. If this happens, medicine is given to relieve the symptoms.

Types of Chest CT Scans

A CT scanner is a large, tunnel-like machine with a hole in the center. During a chest CT scan, you lie on a table as it moves small distances at a time through the hole.

An X-ray beam rotates around your body as you move through the hole. A computer takes data from the X-rays and creates a series of pictures, called slices, of the inside of your chest.

Different types of chest CT scans have different diagnostic uses.

High-Resolution Chest CT Scan

High-resolution CT (HRCT) scans provide more than one slice in a single rotation of the X-ray tube. Each slice is very thin and provides a lot of details about the organs and other structures in your chest.

Spiral Chest CT Scan

For this scan, the table moves continuously through the tunnel-like hole as the X-ray tube rotates around you. This allows the X-ray beam to follow a spiral path.

The machine's computer can process the many slices into a very detailed, three-dimensional (3D) picture of the lungs and other structures in the chest.

Other Names for Chest CT Scans

- Lung imaging test

- Computed axial tomography (CAT) scan

- Helical CT scan (another name for spiral CT scan)

Who Needs a Chest CT Scan?

Your doctor may recommend a chest CT scan if you have symptoms of lung problems, such as chest pain or trouble breathing. The scan can help find the cause of the symptoms.

A chest CT scan looks for problems such as tumors, excess fluid around the lungs, and pulmonary embolism (a blood clot in the lungs). The scan also checks for other conditions, such as tuberculosis, emphysema, and pneumonia.

Your doctor may recommend a chest CT scan if a standard chest X-ray doesn't help diagnose the problem. The chest CT scan can:

- Provide more detailed pictures of your lungs and other chest structures than a standard chest X-ray

- Find the exact location of a tumor or other problem

- Show something that isn't visible on a chest X-ray

What to Expect before a Chest CT Scan

What to Wear

Wear loose-fitting, comfortable clothing for the test. Sometimes the CT scan technician (a person specially trained to do CT scans) may ask you to wear a hospital gown.

You also may want to avoid wearing jewelry and other metal objects. You'll be asked to take off any jewelry, eyeglasses, and metal objects that might interfere with the test.

You may be asked to remove hearing aids and dentures as well. Let the technician know if you have any body piercing on your chest.

Pregnancy and Other Conditions

Tell your doctor whether you're pregnant or may be pregnant. If possible, you should avoid unnecessary radiation exposure during pregnancy. This is because of the concern that radiation may harm the fetus.

You and your doctor will decide whether the benefits of a chest CT scan outweigh the possible risks to the fetus, or whether another test might be better. If you do have the chest CT scan, the technician will take extra steps to reduce the fetus' exposure to radiation.

You also should tell your doctor whether:

- You're taking any medicines

- You have any allergies

- You've recently been ill

- You have any medical conditions (for example, heart disease, asthma, diabetes, kidney disease, or thyroid problems)

These factors or conditions may raise your risk of having a bad reaction to the test.

CT Scanner

The CT scanner is a large, tunnel-like machine with a hole in the center. You'll lie on a table that goes through the hole.

Tell your doctor if you're afraid of tight or closed spaces. He or she may give you medicine to help you relax. This medicine may make you sleepy, so you'll need to arrange for a ride home after the test.

Contrast Dye

Your doctor may inject a substance called contrast dye into a vein in your arm for the test. You may feel some discomfort when the needle is inserted. As the dye is injected, you also may feel warm and have a metallic taste in your mouth. These feelings last only a few minutes.

The contrast dye highlights areas inside your chest, which helps create clearer pictures.

Your doctor may ask you to not eat or drink for a few hours before the test, especially if contrast dye is part of the test.

Some people are allergic to the contrast dye. If you have allergic symptoms, such as itching or hives, tell the technician or doctor right away. He or she can give you medicine to relieve the symptoms.

The most common type of contrast dye used in CT scans contains iodine. Let your doctor know if you're allergic to iodine.

If you're breastfeeding, ask your doctor how long you should wait after the test before you breastfeed. The contrast dye can be passed to your baby through your breast milk.

You may want to prepare for the test by pumping and saving milk for 24 to 48 hours in advance. You can bottle-feed your baby in the hours after the CT scan.

What to Expect during a Chest CT Scan

A chest CT scan takes about 30 minutes, which includes preparation time. The actual scanning time is much shorter, only a few minutes or less.

The CT scanner is a large, tunnel-like machine that has a hole in the middle. You'll lie on a narrow table that moves through the hole.

While you're inside the scanner, an X-ray tube moves around your body. You'll hear soft buzzing, clicking, or whirring noises as the scanner takes pictures.

The CT scan technician who controls the machine will be in the next room. He or she can see you through a glass window and talk to you through a speaker.

Moving your body can cause the pictures to blur. The technician will ask you to lie still and hold your breath for short periods. This will help make the pictures as clear as possible.

The scan itself doesn't hurt, but you may feel anxious if you get nervous in tight or closed spaces. Your doctor may give you medicine to help you relax.

What to Expect after a Chest CT Scan

You usually can return to your normal routine right after a chest CT scan.

If you got medicine to help you relax during the CT scan, your doctor will tell you when you can return to your normal routine. The medicine may make you sleepy, so you'll need someone to drive you home.

If contrast dye was used during the test, you may have a bruise where the needle was inserted. Your doctor may give you special instructions, such as drinking plenty of liquids to flush out the contrast dye.

If you're breastfeeding, the contrast dye can be passed to your baby through your breast milk. Ask your doctor how long you should wait after the test before you breastfeed.

You may want to prepare for the test by pumping and saving milk for 24 to 48 hours in advance. You can bottle-feed your baby in the hours after the CT scan.

What Does a Chest CT Scan Show?

A chest CT scan provides detailed pictures of the size, shape, and position of your lungs and other structures in your chest. Doctors use this test to:

- Follow up on abnormal results from standard chest X-rays.

- Find the cause of lung symptoms, such as shortness of breath or chest pain.

- Find out whether you have a lung problem, such as a tumor, excess fluid around the lungs, or a pulmonary embolism (a blood clot in the lungs). The test also is used to check for other conditions, such as tuberculosis, emphysema, and pneumonia.

What Are the Risks of a Chest CT Scan?

Radiation

Chest CT scans use radiation. The amount of radiation will vary based on the type of CT scan. On average, though, the amount of radiation will not exceed the amount you're naturally exposed to over 3 years. The radiation from the test is gone from the body within a few days.

Children are more sensitive to radiation because they're smaller than adults and still growing.

Exposure to radiation is associated with a risk of cancer. However, it's not known whether the amount of radiation from a chest CT scan increases your risk of cancer.

You and your doctor will decide whether the benefits of the CT scan outweigh any possible risks. Your doctor also will try to avoid ordering repeated CT scans over a short period.

Allergic Reaction

The contrast dye used in some chest CT scans can cause an allergic reaction, such as hives or trouble breathing. The risk of this happening is slight. If you have an allergic reaction, your doctor can give you medicine to relieve it.

The most common contrast dye used in CT scans contains iodine. Tell your doctor if you're allergic to iodine.

Section 23.4

Computed Tomography and Its Role in Cancer Treatment

Text in this section is excerpted from "Computed Tomography (CT) Scans and Cancer," National Cancer Institute (NCI), July 16, 2013.

How is CT used in cancer?

CT is used in cancer in many different ways:

- To detect abnormal growths

- To help diagnose the presence of a tumor

- To provide information about the stage of a cancer

- To determine exactly where to perform (i.e., guide) a biopsy procedure

- To guide certain local treatments, such as cryotherapy, radiofrequency ablation, and the implantation of radioactive seeds

- To help plan external-beam radiation therapy or surgery

- To determine whether a cancer is responding to treatment

- To detect recurrence of a tumor

How is CT used in cancer screening?

Studies have shown that CT can be effective in both colorectal cancer screening (including screening for large polyps) and lung cancer screening.

Colorectal cancer

CT colonography (also known as virtual colonoscopy) can be used to screen for both large colorectal polyps and colorectal tumors. CT colonography uses the same dose of radiation that is used in standard CT of the abdomen and pelvis, which is about 10 millisieverts (mSv). (By comparison, the estimated average annual dose received from natural sources of radiation is about 3 mSv.) As with standard (optical) colonoscopy, a thorough cleansing of the colon is performed before this test. During the examination, air or carbon dioxide gas is pumped into the colon to expand it for better viewing.

The National CT Colonography Trial, an NCI-sponsored clinical trial, found that the accuracy of CT colonography is similar to that of standard colonoscopy. CT colonography is less invasive than standard colonoscopy and has a lower risk of complications. However, if polyps or other abnormal growths are found on CT colonography, a standard colonoscopy is usually performed to remove them.

Whether CT colonography can help reduce the death rate from colorectal cancer is not yet known, and most insurance companies (and Medicare) do not currently reimburse the costs of this procedure. Also, because CT colonography can produce images of organs and tissues outside the colon, it is possible that non-colorectal abnormalities may be found. Some of these "extra-colonic" findings will be serious, but many will not be, leading to unnecessary additional tests and surgeries.

Lung cancer

The NCI-sponsored National Lung Screening Trial (NLST) showed that people aged 55 to 74 years with a history of heavy smoking are 20 percent less likely to die from lung cancer if they are screened with low-dose helical CT than if they are screened with standard chest X-rays. (Previous studies had shown that screening with standard chest X-rays does not reduce the death rate from lung cancer.) The estimated amount of radiation in a low-dose helical CT procedure is 1.5 mSv.

Despite the effectiveness of low-dose helical CT for lung cancer screening in heavy smokers, the NLST identified risks as well as benefits. For example, people screened with low-dose helical CT had a higher overall rate of false-positive results (that is, findings that appeared to be abnormal even though no cancer was present), a higher rate of false-positive results that led to an invasive procedure (such as bronchoscopy or biopsy), and a higher rate of serious complications from an invasive procedure than those screened with standard X-rays.

The benefits of helical CT in screening for lung cancer may vary, depending on how similar someone is to the people who participated in the NLST. The benefits may also be greater for those with a higher lung cancer risk, and the harms may be more pronounced for those who have more medical problems (like heart or other lung disease), which could increase problems arising from biopsies and other surgery.

People who think that they have an increased risk of lung cancer and are interested in screening with low-dose helical CT should discuss the appropriateness and the benefits and risks of lung cancer screening with their doctors. They should also be aware that, because the technique is fairly new, some insurance plans do not currently cover it.

What is total, or whole-body, CT?

Total, or whole-body, CT creates pictures of nearly every area of the body—from the chin to below the hips. This procedure, which is used routinely in patients who already have cancer, can also be used in people who do not have any symptoms of disease. However, whole-body CT has not been shown to be an effective screening method for healthy people. Most abnormal findings from this procedure do not indicate a serious health problem, but the tests that must be done to follow up and rule out a problem can be expensive, inconvenient, and uncomfortable. In addition, whole-body CT can expose people to relatively large amounts of ionizing radiation—about 12 mSv, or four times the estimated average annual dose received from natural sources of radiation. Most doctors recommend against whole-body CT for people without any signs or symptoms of disease.

What is combined PET/CT?

Combined PET/CT uses two imaging methods, CT and positron emission tomography (PET), in one procedure. CT is done first to create anatomic pictures of the organs and structures in the body, and then PET is done to create colored pictures that show chemical or other functional changes in tissues.

Different types of positron-emitting (radioactive) substances can be used in PET. Depending on the substance used, different kinds of chemical or functional changes can be imaged. The most common type of PET procedure uses an imaging agent called FDG (a radioactive form of the sugar glucose), which shows the metabolic activity of tissues. Because cancerous tumors are usually more metabolically active than normal tissues, they appear different from other tissues on a PET scan. Other PET imaging agents can provide information about the level of oxygen in a particular tissue, the formation of new blood vessels, the presence of bone growth, or whether tumor cells are actively dividing and growing.

Combining CT and PET may provide a more complete picture of a tumor's location and growth or spread than either test alone. The combined procedure may improve the ability to diagnose cancer, to determine how far a tumor has spread, to plan treatment, and to monitor response to treatment. Combined PET/CT may also reduce the number of additional imaging tests and other procedures a patient needs.

Is the radiation from CT harmful?

Some people may be concerned about the amount of radiation they receive during CT. CT imaging involves the use of X-rays, which are a form of ionizing radiation. Exposure to ionizing radiation is known to increase the risk of cancer. Standard X-ray procedures, such as routine chest X-rays and mammography, use relatively low levels of ionizing radiation. The radiation exposure from CT is higher than that from standard X-ray procedures, but the increase in cancer risk from one CT scan is still small. Not having the procedure can be much more risky than having it, especially if CT is being used to diagnose cancer or another serious condition in someone who has signs or symptoms of disease.

It is commonly thought that the extra risk of any one person developing a fatal cancer from a typical CT procedure is about 1 in 2,000. In contrast, the lifetime risk of dying from cancer in the U.S. population is about 1 in 5.

It is also important to note that everyone is exposed to some background level of naturally occurring ionizing radiation every day. The average person in the United States receives an estimated effective dose of about 3 millisieverts (mSv) per year from naturally occurring radioactive materials, such as radon and radiation from outer space. By comparison, the radiation exposure from one low-dose CT scan of the chest (1.5 mSv) is comparable to 6 months of natural background radiation, and a regular-dose CT scan of the chest (7 mSv) is comparable to 2 years of natural background radiation.

The widespread use of CT and other procedures that use ionizing radiation to create images of the body has raised concerns that even small increases in cancer risk could lead to large numbers of future cancers. People who have CT procedures as children may be at higher risk because children are more sensitive to radiation and have a longer life expectancy than adults. Women are at a somewhat higher risk than men of developing cancer after receiving the same radiation exposures at the same ages.

People considering CT should talk with their doctors about whether the procedure is necessary for them and about its risks and benefits. Some organizations recommend that people keep a record of the imaging examinations they have received in case their doctors don't have access to all of their health records. A sample form, called My Medical Imaging History, was developed by the Radiological Society of North America, the American College of Radiology, and the U.S. Food and Drug Administration. It includes questions to ask the doctor before undergoing any X-ray exam or treatment procedure.

What are the risks of CT scans for children?

Radiation exposure from CT scans affects adults and children differently. Children are considerably more sensitive to radiation than adults because of their growing bodies and the rapid pace at which the cells in their bodies divide. In addition, children have a longer life expectancy than adults, providing a larger window of opportunity for radiation-related cancers to develop.

Individuals who have had multiple CT scans before the age of 15 were found to have an increased risk of developing leukemia, brain tumors, and other cancers in the decade following their first scan. However, the lifetime risk of cancer from a single CT scan was small — about one case of cancer for every 10,000 scans performed on children.

In talking with health care providers, three key questions that the parents can ask are: why is the test needed? Will the results change the treatment decisions? Is there an alternative test that doesn't involve radiation? If the test is clinically justified, then the parents can be reassured that the benefits will outweigh the small long-term risks.

What is being done to reduce the level of radiation exposure from CT?

In response to concerns about the increased risk of cancer associated with CT and other imaging procedures that use ionizing radiation, several organizations and government agencies have developed guidelines and recommendations regarding the appropriate use of these procedures.

- In 2010, the U.S. Food and Drug Administration (FDA) launched the Initiative to Reduce Unnecessary Radiation Exposure from Medical Imaging. This initiative focuses on the safe use of medical imaging devices, informed decision-making about when to use specific imaging procedures, and increasing patients' awareness of their radiation exposure. Key components of the initiative include avoiding repeat procedures, keeping doses as low as possible while maximizing image quality, and using imaging only when appropriate. The FDA also produced *Reducing Radiation from Medical X-rays*, a guide for consumers that includes information about the risks of medical X-rays, steps consumers can take to reduce radiation risks, and a table that shows the radiation dose of some common medical X-ray exams.

• The NIH Clinical Center requires that radiation dose exposures from CT and other imaging procedures be included in the electronic medical records of patients treated at the center. In addition, all imaging equipment purchased by NIH must provide data on exposure in a form that can be tracked and reported electronically. This patient protection policy is being adopted by other hospitals and imaging facilities.

• NCI's website includes a guide for health care providers, *Radiation Risks and Pediatric Computed Tomography (CT): A Guide for Health Care Providers*. The guide addresses the value of CT as a diagnostic tool in children, unique considerations for radiation exposure in children, risks to children from radiation exposure, and measures to minimize exposure.

• The American College of Radiology (ACR) has developed the *ACR Appropriateness Criteria®*, evidence-based guidelines to help providers make appropriate imaging and treatment decisions for a number of clinical conditions. These guidelines and supporting documents are available on ACR's website.

• ACR has also established the Dose Index Registry, which collects anonymized information related to dose indices for all CT exams at participating facilities. Data from the registry can be used to compare radiology facilities and to establish national benchmarks.

• CT scanner manufacturers are developing newer cameras and detector systems that can provide higher quality images at much lower radiation doses.

What is NCI doing to improve CT imaging?

Researchers funded by NCI are studying ways to improve the use of CT in cancer screening, diagnosis, and treatment. NCI also conducts and sponsors clinical trials that are testing ways to improve CT or new uses of CT imaging technology. Some of these clinical trials are run by the American College of Radiology Imaging Network (ACRIN), a clinical trials cooperative group that is funded in part by NCI. ACRIN performed the National CT Colonography Trial, which tested the use of CT for colorectal cancer screening, and participated in the NLST, which tested the use of CT for lung cancer screening in high-risk individuals.

NCI's Cancer Imaging Program (CIP), part of the Division of Cancer Treatment and Diagnosis (DCTD), funds cancer-related basic, translational, and clinical research in imaging sciences and technology. CIP supports the development of novel imaging agents for CT and other types of imaging procedures to help doctors better locate cancer cells in the body.

Where can people get more information about CT?

Additional information about CT imaging is available from the U.S. Food and Drug Administration (FDA), the federal agency that regulates food, drugs, medical devices, cosmetics, biologics, and radiation-emitting products.

Section 23.5

Virtual Colonoscopy

Text in this section is excerpted from "Virtual Colonoscopy," National Institute of Diabetes and Digestive and Kidney Diseases (NIDDK), September 25, 2013.

Virtual colonoscopy, also called computerized tomography (CT) colonography, is a procedure that uses a combination of X-rays and computer technology to create images of the rectum and entire colon. Virtual colonoscopy can show irritated and swollen tissue, ulcers, and polyps—extra pieces of tissue that grow on the lining of the intestine.

This procedure is different from colonoscopy, which uses a long, flexible, narrow tube with a light and tiny camera on one end, called a colonoscope or scope, to look inside the rectum and entire colon.

What are the rectum and colon?

The rectum and colon are part of the gastrointestinal (GI) tract, a series of hollow organs joined in a long, twisting tube from the mouth to the anus, a 1-inch-long opening through which stool leaves the body. The body digests food using the movement of muscles in the GI tract, along with the release of hormones and enzymes. Organs that make up the GI tract are the mouth, esophagus, stomach, small intestine, large intestine—which includes the appendix, cecum, colon, and rectum—and anus. The intestines are sometimes called the bowel. The last part of the GI tract—called the lower GI tract—consists of the large intestine and anus.

The large intestine is about 5 feet long in adults and absorbs water and any remaining nutrients from partially digested food passed from the small intestine. The large intestine then changes waste from liquid to a solid matter called stool. Stool passes from the colon to the rectum. The rectum is 6 to 8 inches long in adults and is located between the last part of the colon—called the sigmoid colon—and the anus. The rectum stores stool prior to a bowel movement. During a bowel movement, stool moves from the rectum to the anus.

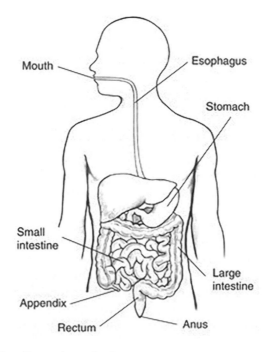

Figure 23.3. *The Gastrointestinal tract*

Why is a virtual colonoscopy performed?

A virtual colonoscopy is performed to help diagnose

- changes in bowel habits
- abdominal pain
- bleeding from the anus
- weight loss

A gastroenterologist—a doctor who specializes in digestive diseases—may also order a virtual colonoscopy as a screening test for colon cancer. Screening is testing for diseases when people have no symptoms. Screening may find a disease at an early stage, when a gastroenterologist has a better chance of curing the disease. However, while some gastroenterologists use a virtual colonoscopy to screen for colon cancer, not enough evidence exists to fully assess its effectiveness as a screening tool. Instead, the U.S. Preventive Services Task Force recommends fecal occult blood testing, sigmoidoscopy, or colonoscopy for colon cancer screening.

The American College of Gastroenterology recommends screening for colon cancer

- at age 50 for people who are not at increased risk of the disease
- at age 45 for African Americans because they have an increased risk of developing the disease

A gastroenterologist may recommend earlier screening for people with a family history of colon cancer, a personal history of inflammatory bowel disease—a long-lasting disorder that causes irritation and sores in the GI tract—or other risk factors for colon cancer.

Medicare and private insurance companies sometimes change whether and how often they pay for cancer screening tests. People should check with their insurance company to find out how often they can get a screening virtual colonoscopy that their insurance will cover.

How does a person prepare for a virtual colonoscopy?

Preparation for a virtual colonoscopy includes the following steps:

- **Talk with a gastroenterologist.** When people schedule a virtual colonoscopy, they should talk with their gastroenterologist about medical conditions they have and all prescribed and over-the-counter medications, vitamins, and supplements they take, including

- aspirin or medications that contain aspirin
- nonsteroidal anti-inflammatory drugs such as ibuprofen or naproxen
- arthritis medications
- blood thinners
- diabetes medications
- vitamins that contain iron or iron supplements

Women should let their gastroenterologist know if they are pregnant. Developing fetuses are particularly sensitive to X-rays. The X-ray technician should take special precautions to minimize exposure, or the gastroenterologist may suggest an alternative procedure, such as a colonoscopy.

- **Cleanse the bowel.** The gastroenterologist will give written bowel prep instructions to follow at home. A gastroenterologist orders a bowel prep so that little to no stool is present inside the person's intestine. A complete bowel prep lets the person pass stool that is clear. Stool inside the colon can prevent the CT scanner from taking clear images of the intestinal lining. Instructions may include following a clear liquid diet for 1 to 3 days before the procedure and avoiding drinks that contain red or purple dye. The instructions will provide specific direction about when to start and stop the clear liquid diet. People may drink or eat the following:
  - fat-free bouillon or broth
  - strained fruit juice, such as apple or white grape—orange juice is not recommended
  - water
  - plain coffee or tea, without cream or milk
  - sports drinks in flavors such as lemon, lime, or orange
  - gelatin in flavors such as lemon, lime, or orange

The person needs to take laxatives and enemas the night before a virtual colonoscopy. A laxative is medication that loosens stool and increases bowel movements. An enema involves flushing water or laxative into the rectum using a special wash bottle. Laxatives and enemas can cause diarrhea, so the person should stay close to a bathroom during the bowel prep.

Laxatives are usually swallowed in pill form or as a powder dissolved in water. Some people will need to drink a large amount, usually a gallon, of liquid laxative at scheduled times. People may find this part of the bowel prep difficult; however, it is very important to complete the prep. The images will not be clear if the prep is incomplete.

People should call the gastroenterologist if they are having side effects that are preventing them from finishing the prep.

- **Drink contrast medium.** The night before the procedure, the person will drink a liquid that contains a special dye, called contrast medium. Contrast medium is visible on X-rays and can help distinguish between stool and polyps.

How is a virtual colonoscopy performed?

A radiologist—a doctor who specializes in medical imaging—performs a virtual colonoscopy at an outpatient center or a hospital. A person does not need anesthesia.

For the test, the person will lie on a table while the radiologist inserts a thin tube through the anus and into the rectum. The tube inflates the large intestine with air for a better view. The table slides into a tunnel-shaped device where the radiologist takes the X-ray images. The radiologist may ask the person to hold his or her breath several times during the test to steady the images. The radiologist will ask the person to turn over on the side or stomach so the radiologist can take different images of the large intestine. The procedure lasts about 10 to 15 minutes.

What can a person expect after a virtual colonoscopy?

After a virtual colonoscopy, a person can expect

- cramping or bloating during the first hour after the test

- to resume regular activities immediately after the test

- to return to a normal diet

After the test, a radiologist interprets the images, evaluates the results to find any abnormalities, and sends a report to the gastroenterologist. If the radiologist finds abnormalities, a gastroenterologist may perform a colonoscopy the same day or at a later time.

Seek Help for Emergency Symptoms

People who have any of the following symptoms after a virtual colonoscopy should seek immediate medical attention:

- severe abdominal pain
- fever
- bloody bowel movements or bleeding from the anus
- dizziness
- weakness

What are the risks of virtual colonoscopy?

The risks of virtual colonoscopy include

- exposure to radiation

- perforation—a hole or tear in the lining of the colon

Radiation exposure can cause cancer. However, though the level of radiation exposure that leads to cancer is unknown, the risk from these types of tests is thought to be small. Inflating the colon with air has a small risk of perforating the intestinal lining. Perforation may need to be treated with surgery.

Virtual colonoscopy shows the entire abdomen—the area between the chest and the hips—and can show abnormalities outside of the GI tract. These findings may lead to additional testing, cost, and anxiety.

Work with a Gastroenterologist to Determine the Best Screening Method

Virtual colonoscopy has several advantages and disadvantages when compared with a colonoscopy. The advantages of virtual colonoscopy include the following:

- Virtual colonoscopy does not require the insertion of a colonoscope into the entire length of the colon.
- People do not need anesthesia. People can return to their normal activities or go home after the procedure without the help of another person.

- Virtual colonoscopy takes less time than colonoscopy.
- The radiologist can use a virtual colonoscopy to view the inside of a colon that is narrowed because of inflammation or the presence of a polyp.

The disadvantages of virtual colonoscopy include the following:

- People require bowel prep and the insertion of a tube into the rectum.
- The radiologist cannot remove tissue samples or polyps or stop bleeding if a perforation occurs.
- If a virtual colonoscopy shows a polyp or cancer, a colonoscopy may be needed to confirm or treat the abnormality; with a colonoscopy, treatment can occur at the same time as diagnosis.
- Virtual colonoscopy may not be as effective as colonoscopy at detecting certain polyps.
- Virtual colonoscopy may interfere with personal medical devices. People should tell the gastroenterologist about any implanted medical devices.
- Medicare and private insurance companies sometimes change whether and how often they pay for cancer screening tests. People should check with their insurance company to find out how often they can get a screening virtual colonoscopy that their insurance will cover.
- Virtual colonoscopy is a newer technology and not all medical facilities make this procedure available.
- Gastroenterologists do not recommend techniques that use X-ray radiation for pregnant women because the radiation may harm the fetus.

Chapter 24

Magnetic Resonance Imaging (MRI) Scan

Chapter Contents

Section 24.1

Overview of Magnetic Resonance Imaging Scan

Text in this section begins with excerpts from "MRI (Magnetic Resonance Imaging)," U.S. Food and Drug Administration (FDA), June 4, 2014; and text from "Are there risks?" is excerpted from "Magnetic Resonance Imaging (MRI)," National Institute of Biomedical Imaging and Bioengineering (NIBIB), April 1, 2013.

Description

Magnetic resonance imaging (MRI) is a medical imaging procedure that uses strong magnetic fields and radio waves to produce cross-sectional images of organs and internal structures in the body. Because the signal detected by an MRI machine varies depending on the water content and local magnetic properties of a particular area of the body, different tissues or substances can be distinguished from one another in the study image.

MRI can give different information about structures in the body than can be obtained using a standard X-ray, ultrasound, or computed tomography (CT) exam. For example, an MRI exam of a joint can provide detailed images of ligaments and cartilage, which are not visible using other study types. In some cases, a magnetically active material (called a contrast agent) is used to show internal structures or abnormalities more clearly.

In most MRI devices, an electric current is passed through coiled wires to create a temporary magnetic field around a patient's body. (In open-MRI devices, permanent magnets are used.) Radio waves are sent from and received by a transmitter/receiver in the machine, and these signals are used to produce digital images of the area of interest.

Uses

Using MRI scans, physicians can diagnose or monitor treatments for a variety of medical conditions, including:

- Abnormalities of the brain and spinal cord

- Tumors, cysts, and other abnormalities in various parts of the body
- Injuries or abnormalities of the joints
- Certain types of heart problems
- Diseases of the liver and other abdominal organs
- Causes of pelvic pain in women (e.g. fibroids, endometriosis)
- Suspected uterine abnormalities in women undergoing evaluation for infertility

Are there risks?

Although MRI does not emit the damaging ionizing radiation that is found in X-ray and CT imaging, it does employ a strong magnetic field. The magnetic field extends beyond the machine and exerts very powerful forces on objects of iron, some steels, and other magnetizable objects; it is strong enough to fling a wheelchair across the room. Patients should notify their physicians of any form of medical or implant prior to an MR scan.

When having an MRI scan, the following should be taken into consideration:

- People with implants, particularly those containing iron,---pacemakers, vagus nerve stimulators, implantable cardioverter-defibrillators, loop recorders, insulin pumps, cochlear implants, deep brain stimulators, and capsules from capsule endoscopy should not enter an MRI machine.

- Noise—loud noise commonly referred to as clicking and beeping, as well as sound intensity up to 120 decibels in certain MR scanners, may require special ear protection.

- Nerve Stimulation—a twitching sensation sometimes results from the rapidly switched fields in the MRI.

- Contrast agents—patients with severe renal failure who require dialysis may risk a rare but serious illness called nephrogenic systemic fibrosis that may be linked to the use of certain gadolinium-containing agents, such as gadodiamide and others. Although a causal link has not been established, current guidelines in the United States recommend that dialysis patients should only receive gadolinium agents when essential, and that dialysis should be performed as soon as possible after the scan to remove the agent from the body promptly.

- Pregnancy—while no effects have been demonstrated on the fetus, it is recommended that MRI scans be avoided as a precaution especially in the first trimester of pregnancy when the fetus' organs are being formed and contrast agents, if used, could enter the fetal bloodstream.

- Claustrophobia—people with even mild claustrophobia may find it difficult to tolerate long scan times inside the machine. Familiarization with the machine and process, as well as visualization techniques, sedation, and anesthesia provide patients with mechanisms to overcome their discomfort. Additional coping mechanisms include listening to music or watching a video or movie, closing or covering the eyes, and holding a panic button. The open MRI is a machine that is open on the sides rather than a tube closed at one end, so it does not fully surround the patient. It was developed to accommodate the needs of patients who are uncomfortable with the narrow tunnel and noises of the traditional MRI and for patients whose size or weight make the traditional MRI impractical. Newer open MRI technology provides high quality images for many but not all types of examinations.

Section 24.2

Cardiac MRI

Text in this section is excerpted from "Cardiac MRI," National Heart, Lung, and Blood Institute (NHLBI), February 2, 2012.

What to Expect before Cardiac MRI

You'll be asked to fill out a screening form before having cardiac MRI. The form may ask whether you've had any previous surgeries. It also may ask whether you have any metal objects or medical devices (like a cardiac pacemaker) in your body.

Some implanted medical devices, such as man-made heart valves and coronary stents, are safe around the MRI machine, but others are not. For example, the MRI machine can:

- Cause implanted cardiac pacemakers and defibrillators to malfunction.

- Damage cochlear (inner-ear) implants. Cochlear implants are small, electronic devices that help people who are deaf or who can't hear well understand speech and the sounds around them.

- Cause brain aneurysm (AN-u-rism) clips to move as a result of the MRI's strong magnetic field. This can cause severe injury.

Talk to your doctor or the MRI technician if you have concerns about any implanted devices that may interfere with the MRI.

Your doctor will let you know if you shouldn't have a cardiac MRI because of a medical device. If so, consider wearing a medical ID bracelet or necklace or carrying a medical alert card that states that you shouldn't have an MRI.

If you're pregnant, make sure your doctor knows before you have an MRI. No harmful effects of MRI during pregnancy have been reported; however, more research on the safety of MRI during pregnancy is needed.

Your doctor or technician will tell you whether you need to change into a hospital gown for the test. Don't bring hearing aids, credit cards, jewelry and watches, eyeglasses, pens, removable dental work, or anything that's magnetic near the MRI machine.

Tell your doctor if being in a fairly tight or confined space causes you anxiety or fear. If so, your doctor might give you medicine to help you relax. Your doctor may ask you to fast (not eat) for 6 hours before you take this medicine on the day of the test.

Some newer cardiac MRI machines are open on all sides. If you're fearful in tight or confined spaces, ask your doctor to help you find a facility that has an open MRI machine.

Your doctor will let you know whether you need to arrange for a ride home after the test.

What to Expect during Cardiac MRI

Cardiac MRI takes place in a hospital or medical imaging facility. A radiologist or other doctor who has special training in medical imaging oversees MRI testing.

Cardiac MRI usually takes 30 to 90 minutes, depending on how many pictures are needed. The test may take less time with some newer MRI machines.

The MRI machine will be located in a special room that prevents radio waves from disrupting the machine. It also prevents the MRI machine's strong magnetic fields from disrupting other equipment.

Traditional MRI machines look like long, narrow tunnels. Newer MRI machines (called short-bore systems) are shorter, wider, and don't completely surround you. Some newer machines are open on all sides. Your doctor will help decide which type of machine is best for you.

Cardiac MRI is painless and harmless. You'll lie on your back on a sliding table that goes inside the tunnel-like machine.

The MRI technician will control the machine from the next room. He or she will be able to see you through a glass window and talk to you through a speaker. Tell the technician if you have a hearing problem.

The MRI machine makes loud humming, tapping, and buzzing noises. Some facilities let you wear earplugs or listen to music during the test.

You will need to remain very still during the MRI. Any movement can blur the pictures. If you're unable to lie still, you may be given medicine to help you relax.

The technician might ask you to hold your breath for 10 to 15 seconds at a time while he or she takes pictures of your heart. Researchers are studying ways that will allow someone having a cardiac MRI to breathe freely during the exam, while achieving the same image quality.

A contrast agent, such as gadolinium, might be used to highlight your blood vessels or heart in the pictures. The substance usually is injected into a vein in your arm using a needle.

You may feel a cool sensation during the injection and discomfort when the needle is inserted. Gadolinium doesn't contain iodine, so it won't cause problems for people who are allergic to iodine.

Your cardiac MRI might include a stress test to detect blockages in your coronary arteries. If so, you'll get other medicines to increase the blood flow in your heart or to increase your heart rate.

What to Expect after Cardiac MRI

You'll be able to return to your normal routine once the cardiac MRI is done.

If you took medicine to help you relax during the test, your doctor will tell you when you can return to your normal routine. The medicine will make you sleepy, so you'll need someone to drive you home.

What Does Cardiac MRI Show?

The doctor supervising your scan will provide your doctor with the results of your cardiac MRI. Your doctor will discuss the findings with you.

Cardiac MRI can reveal various heart diseases and conditions, such as:

- Coronary heart disease

- Damage caused by a heart attack

- Heart failure

- Heart valve problems

- Congenital heart defects (heart defects present at birth)

- Pericarditis (a condition in which the membrane, or sac, around your heart is inflamed)

- Cardiac tumors

Cardiac MRI is a fast, accurate tool that can help diagnose a heart attack. The test does this by detecting areas of the heart that don't move normally, have poor blood supply, or are scarred.

Cardiac MRI also can show whether any of the coronary arteries are blocked. A blockage prevents your heart muscle from getting enough oxygen-rich blood, which can lead to a heart attack.

Currently, coronary angiography is the most common procedure for looking at blockages in the coronary arteries. Coronary angiography is an invasive procedure that uses X-rays and iodine-based dye.

Researchers have found that cardiac MRI can sometimes replace coronary angiography, avoiding the need to use X-ray radiation and iodine-based dye. This use of MRI is called MR angiography (MRA).

Echocardiography (echo) is the main test for diagnosing heart valve disease. However, your doctor also might recommend cardiac MRI to assess the severity of valve disease.

A cardiac MRI can confirm information about valve defects or provide more detailed information about heart valve disease.

This information can help your doctor plan your treatment. An MRI also might be done before heart valve surgery to help your surgeon plan for the surgery.

Researchers are finding new ways to use cardiac MRI. In the future, cardiac MRI may replace X-rays as the main way to guide invasive procedures such as cardiac catheterization.

Also, improvements in cardiac MRI will likely lead to better methods for detecting heart disease in the future.

What Are the Risks of Cardiac MRI?

The magnetic fields and radio waves used in cardiac MRI have no side effects. This method of taking pictures of organs and tissues doesn't carry a risk of causing cancer or birth defects.

Serious reactions to the contrast agent used during some MRI tests are very rare. However, side effects are possible and include the following:

- Headache

- Nausea (feeling sick to your stomach)

- Dizziness

- Changes in taste

- Allergic reactions

Rarely, the contrast agent can harm people who have severe kidney or liver disease. The substance may cause a disease called nephrogenic systemic fibrosis.

If your cardiac MRI includes a stress test, more medicines will be used during the test. These medicines may have other side effects that aren't expected during a regular MRI scan, such as:

- Arrhythmias, or irregular heartbeats

- Chest pain

- Shortness of breath

- Palpitations (feelings that your heart is skipping a beat, fluttering, or beating too hard or fast)

Chapter 25

Nuclear Heart Scan

A nuclear heart scan is a test that provides important information about the health of your heart.

For this test, a safe, radioactive substance called a tracer is injected into your bloodstream through a vein. The tracer travels to your heart and releases energy. Special cameras outside of your body detect the energy and use it to create pictures of your heart.

Nuclear heart scans are used for three main purposes:

1. To check how blood is flowing to the heart muscle. If part of the heart muscle isn't getting blood, it may be a sign of coronary heart disease (CHD). CHD can lead to chest pain called angina, a heart attack, and other heart problems. When a nuclear heart scan is done for this purpose, it's called myocardial perfusion scanning.

2. To look for damaged heart muscle. Damage might be the result of a previous heart attack, injury, infection, or medicine. When a nuclear heart scan is done for this purpose, it's called myocardial viability testing.

3. To see how well your heart pumps blood to your body. When a nuclear heart scan is done for this purpose, it's called ventricular function scanning.

Text in this chapter is excerpted from "Nuclear Heart Scan," National Heart, Lung, and Blood Institute (NHLBI), March 9, 2012.

Usually, two sets of pictures are taken during a nuclear heart scan. The first set is taken right after a stress test, while your heart is beating fast.

During a stress test, you exercise to make your heart work hard and beat fast. If you can't exercise, you might be given medicine to increase your heart rate. This is called a pharmacological (FAR-ma-ko-LOJ-ih-kal) stress test.

The second set of pictures is taken later, while your heart is at rest and beating at a normal rate.

Types of Nuclear Heart Scans

The two main types of nuclear heart scans are single photon emission computed tomography (SPECT) and cardiac positron emission tomography (PET).

Single Photon Emission Computed Tomography

Doctors use SPECT to help diagnose coronary heart disease (CHD). Combining SPECT with a stress test can show problems with blood flow to the heart. Sometimes doctors can detect these problems only when the heart is working hard and beating fast.

Doctors also use SPECT to look for areas of damaged or dead heart muscle tissue. These areas might be the result of a previous heart attack or other cause.

SPECT also can show how well the heart's lower left chamber (left ventricle) pumps blood to the body. Weak pumping ability might be the result of a heart attack, heart failure, and other causes.

Tracers commonly used during SPECT include thallium-201, technetium-99m sestamibi (Cardiolite®), and technetium-99m tetrofosmin (Myoview™).

Positron Emission Tomography

Doctors can use PET for the same purposes as SPECT—to diagnose CHD, check for damaged or dead heart muscle tissue, and check the heart's pumping strength.

Compared with SPECT, PET takes a clearer picture through thick layers of tissue (such as abdominal or breast tissue). PET also is better at showing whether CHD is affecting more than one of your heart's blood vessels.

Right now, however, there's no clear advantage of using one scan over the other in all situations. Research into advances in both SPECT and PET is ongoing.

PET uses different tracers than SPECT.

Other Names for a Nuclear Heart Scan

- Nuclear stress test
- SPECT scan
- PET scan
- Radionuclide scan

What to Expect before a Nuclear Heart Scan

A nuclear heart scan can take a lot of time. Most scans take between 2–5 hours, especially if your doctor needs two sets of pictures.

Discuss with your doctor how a nuclear heart scan is done. Talk with him or her about your overall health, including health problems such as asthma, COPD (chronic obstructive pulmonary disease), diabetes, and kidney disease.

If you have lung disease or diabetes, your doctor will give you special instructions before the nuclear heart scan.

If you're having a stress test as part of your nuclear heart scan, wear comfortable walking shoes and loose-fitting clothes for the test. You may be asked to wear a hospital gown during the test.

Let your doctor know about any medicines you take, including prescription and over-the-counter medicines, vitamins, minerals, and other supplements. Some medicines and supplements can interfere with the medicines that might be used during the stress test to raise your heart rate.

What to Expect during a Nuclear Heart Scan

Many nuclear medicine centers are located in hospitals. A doctor who has special training in nuclear heart scans—a cardiologist or radiologist—will oversee the test.

Cardiologists are doctors who specialize in diagnosing and treating heart problems. Radiologists are doctors who have special training in medical imaging techniques.

Before the test begins, the doctor or a technician will use a needle to insert an intravenous (IV) line into a vein in your arm. Through this IV line, he or she will put radioactive tracer into your bloodstream at the right time.

You also will have EKG (electrocardiogram) patches attached to your body to check your heart rate during the test. (An EKG is a simple test that detects and records the heart's electrical activity.)

During the Stress Test

If you're having an exercise stress test as part of your nuclear scan, you'll walk on a treadmill or pedal a stationary bike. During this time, you'll be attached to EKG and blood pressure monitors.

Your doctor will ask you to exercise until you're too tired to continue, short of breath, or having chest or leg pain. You can expect that your heart will beat faster, you'll breathe faster, your blood pressure will increase, and you'll sweat.

Tell your doctor if you have any chest, arm, or jaw pain or discomfort. Also, report any dizziness, light-headedness, or other unusual symptoms.

If you're unable to exercise, your doctor may give you medicine to increase your heart rate. This is called a pharmacological stress test. The medicine might make you feel anxious, sick, dizzy, or shaky for a short time. If the side effects are severe, your doctor may give you other medicine to relieve the symptoms.

Before the exercise or pharmacological stress test ends, the tracer is injected through the IV line.

During the Nuclear Heart Scan

The nuclear heart scan will start shortly after the stress test. You'll lie very still on a padded table.

The nuclear heart scan camera, called a gamma camera, is enclosed in metal housing. The camera can be put in several positions around your body as you lie on the padded table.

For some nuclear heart scans, the metal housing is shaped like a doughnut (with a hole in the middle). You lie on a table that slowly moves through the hole. A computer nearby or in another room collects pictures of your heart.

Usually, two sets of pictures are taken. One will be taken right after the stress test and the other will be taken after a period of rest. The pictures might be taken all in 1 day or over 2 days. Each set of pictures takes about 15–30 minutes.

Some people find it hard to stay in one position during the test. Others may feel anxious while lying in the doughnut-shaped scanner. The table may feel hard, and the room may feel chilly because of the air conditioning needed to maintain the machines.

Let your doctor or technician know how you're feeling during the test so he or she can respond as needed.

What to Expect after a Nuclear Heart Scan

Your doctor may ask you to return to the nuclear medicine center on a second day for more pictures. Outpatients will be allowed to go home after the scan or leave the nuclear medicine center between the two scans.

Most people can go back to their daily routines after a nuclear heart scan. The radioactivity will naturally leave your body in your urine or stool. It's helpful to drink plenty of fluids after the test, as your doctor advises.

The cardiologist or radiologist will read and interpret the results of your test. He or she will report the results to your doctor, who will contact you to discuss them. Or, the cardiologist or radiologist may contact you directly to discuss the results.

What Does a Nuclear Heart Scan Show?

The results from a nuclear heart scan can help doctors:

- Diagnose heart conditions, such as coronary heart disease (CHD), and decide the best course of treatment.

- Manage certain heart diseases, such as CHD and heart failure, and predict short-term or long-term survival.

- Determine your risk for a heart attack.

- Decide whether other heart tests or procedures will help you. Examples of these tests and procedures include coronary angiography and cardiac catheterization.

- Decide whether procedures that increase blood flow to the coronary arteries will help you. Examples of these procedures include percutaneous coronary intervention, also known as coronary angioplasty, and coronary artery bypass grafting (CABG).

- Monitor procedures or surgeries that have been done, such as CABG or a heart transplant.

What Are the Risks of a Nuclear Heart Scan?

The radioactive tracer used during nuclear heart scanning exposes the body to a very small amount of radiation. No long-term effects have been reported from these doses.

Radiation dose might be a concern for people who need multiple scans. However, advances in hardware and software may greatly reduce the radiation dose people receive.

Some people are allergic to the radioactive tracer, but this is rare.

If you have coronary heart disease, you may have chest pain during the stress test while you're exercising or taking medicine to raise your heart rate. Medicine can relieve this symptom.

If you're pregnant, tell your doctor or technician before the scan. It might be postponed until after the pregnancy.

Chapter 26

Coronary Calcium Scan

A coronary calcium scan is a test that looks for specks of calcium in the walls of the coronary (heart) arteries. These specks of calcium are called calcifications.

Calcifications in the coronary arteries are an early sign of coronary heart disease (CHD). CHD is a disease in which a waxy substance called plaque builds up in the coronary arteries.

Over time, plaque can harden or rupture (break open). Hardened plaque narrows the coronary arteries and reduces the flow of oxygen-rich blood to the heart. This can cause chest pain or discomfort called angina.

If the plaque ruptures, a blood clot can form on its surface. A large blood clot can mostly or completely block blood flow through a coronary artery. This is the most common cause of a heart attack. Over time, ruptured plaque also hardens and narrows the coronary arteries.

CHD also can lead to heart failure and arrhythmias. Heart failure is a condition in which your heart can't pump enough blood to meet your body's needs. Arrhythmias are problems with the rate or rhythm of your heartbeat.

Text in this chapter is excerpted from "Coronary Calcium Scan," National Heart, Lung, and Blood Institute (NHLBI), March 30, 2012.

Overview

Two machines can show calcium in the coronary arteries—electron beam computed tomography (EBCT) and multidetector computed tomography (MDCT).

Both use X-rays to create detailed pictures of your heart. Your doctor will study the pictures to see whether you're at risk for future heart problems.

A coronary calcium scan is a fairly simple test. You'll lie quietly in the scanner machine for about 10 minutes while it takes pictures of your heart. The pictures will show whether you have calcifications in your coronary arteries.

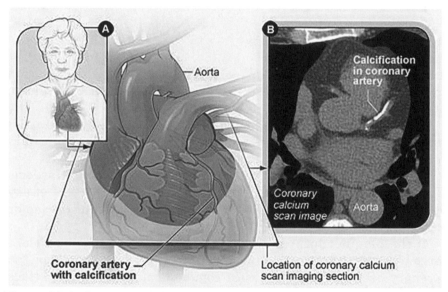

Figure 26.1. *Coronary Calcium Scan: "A" shows the position of the heart in the body and the location and angle of the coronary calcium scan image. "B" is a coronary calcium scan image showing calcifications in a coronary artery.*

Because calcifications are an early sign of CHD, a coronary calcium scan can show whether you're at risk for a heart attack or other heart problems before other signs and symptoms occur.

Outlook

A coronary calcium scan is most useful for people who are at moderate risk for heart attacks. You or your doctor can calculate your 10-year risk using the Risk Assessment Tool from the National Cholesterol Education Program.

People who are at moderate risk have a 10–20 percent chance of having a heart attack within the next 10 years. The coronary calcium scan may help doctors decide who within this group needs treatment.

Other Names for a Coronary Calcium Scan

- Calcium scan test

- Cardiac CT for calcium scoring

Some people refer to coronary calcium scans by the name of the machine used to take pictures of the heart:

- Electron beam computed tomography (EBCT) or electron beam tomography (EBT)

- Multidetector computed tomography (MDCT)

What To Expect Before a Coronary Calcium Scan

You don't need to take any special steps before having a coronary calcium scan. However, your doctor may ask you to avoid caffeine and smoking for 4 hours before the test.

For the scan, you'll remove your clothes above the waist and wear a hospital gown. You also will remove any jewelry from around your neck or chest.

What To Expect During a Coronary Calcium Scan

A coronary calcium scan is done in a hospital or outpatient office. The X-ray machine that's used for the scan is called a computed tomography (CT) scanner.

The technician who runs the scanner will clean areas of your chest and apply sticky patches with sensors called electrodes. The patches are connected to an EKG (electrocardiogram) machine.

The EKG will record your heart's electrical activity during the scan. This makes it possible to take pictures of your heart when it's relaxed between beats.

The CT scanner is a large machine that has a hollow, circular tube in the center. You'll lie on your back on a sliding table. The table can move up and down, and it goes inside the tunnel-like machine.

The table will slowly slide into the opening in the machine. Inside the scanner, an X-ray tube will move around your body to take pictures of your heart. The technician will control the CT scanner from the next room. He or she will be able to see you through a glass window and talk to you through a speaker.

The technician will ask you to lie still and hold your breath for short periods while each picture is taken. You may be given medicine to slow your heart rate. This helps the machine take clearer pictures of your heart. The medicine will be given by mouth or injected into a vein.

The coronary calcium scan will take about 10–15 minutes, although the actual scanning will take only a few seconds. During the test, the machine will make clicking and whirring sounds as it takes pictures. The scan causes no discomfort, but the exam room might be chilly to keep the machine working properly.

If you get nervous in enclosed or tight spaces, you might receive medicine to help you stay calm. Your head will remain outside the opening in the machine during the test.

What to Expect after a Coronary Calcium Scan

You'll be able to return to your normal activities after the coronary calcium scan is done. Your doctor will discuss the results of the test with you.

What Does a Coronary Calcium Scan Show?

After a coronary calcium scan, you'll get a calcium score called an Agatston score. The score is based on the amount of calcium found in your coronary (heart) arteries. You may get an Agatston score for each major artery and a total score.

The test is negative if no calcifications are found in your arteries. This means your chance of having a heart attack in the next 2–5 years is low.

The test is positive if calcifications are found in your arteries. Calcifications are a sign of atherosclerosis and coronary heart disease (CHD). (Atherosclerosis is a condition in which plaque builds up in the arteries.) The higher your Agatston score is, the more severe the atherosclerosis.

An Agatston score of 0 is normal. In general, the higher your score, the more likely you are to have CHD. If your score is high, your doctor may recommend more tests.

What Are the Risks of a Coronary Calcium Scan?

Coronary calcium scans have very few risks. The test isn't invasive, which means that no surgery is done and no instruments are inserted into your body.

Unlike some CT scans, coronary calcium scans don't require an injection of contrast dye to make your heart or arteries visible on X-ray images.

Coronary calcium scans involve radiation, although the amount used is considered small. Electron beam computed tomography (EBCT) uses less radiation than multidetector computed tomography (MDCT).

In either case, the amount of radiation is about equal to the amount of radiation you're naturally exposed to in a single year.

Chapter 27

Mammography

A mammogram is an X-ray picture of the breast. Mammograms can be used to check for breast cancer in women who have no signs or symptoms of the disease. This type of mammogram is called a screening mammogram. Screening mammograms usually involve two X-ray pictures, or images, of each breast. The X-ray images make it possible to detect tumors that cannot be felt. Screening mammograms can also find microcalcifications (tiny deposits of calcium) that sometimes indicate the presence of breast cancer.

Mammograms can also be used to check for breast cancer after a lump or other sign or symptom of the disease has been found. This type of mammogram is called a diagnostic mammogram. Besides a lump, signs of breast cancer can include breast pain, thickening of the skin of the breast, nipple discharge, or a change in breast size or shape; however, these signs may also be signs of benign conditions. A diagnostic mammogram can also be used to evaluate changes found during a screening mammogram or to view breast tissue when it is difficult to obtain a screening mammogram because of special circumstances, such as the presence of breast implants.

How are screening and diagnostic mammograms different?

Diagnostic mammography takes longer than screening mammography because more X-rays are needed to obtain views of the breast from

Text in this chapter is excerpted from "Mammograms," National Cancer Institute (NCI), March 25, 2014.

several angles. The technician may magnify a suspicious area to produce a detailed picture that can help the doctor make an accurate diagnosis.

What are the benefits of screening mammograms?

Early detection of breast cancer with screening mammography means that treatment can be started earlier in the course of the disease, possibly before it has spread. Results from randomized clinical trials and other studies show that screening mammography can help reduce the number of deaths from breast cancer among women ages 40 to 74, especially for those over age 50. However, studies to date have not shown a benefit from regular screening mammography in women under age 40 or from baseline screening mammograms (mammograms used for comparison) taken before age 40.

What are some of the potential limitations of screening mammograms?

False-positive results. False-positive results occur when radiologists decide mammograms are abnormal but no cancer is actually present. All abnormal mammograms should be followed up with additional testing (diagnostic mammograms, ultrasound, and/or biopsy) to determine whether cancer is present.

False-positive results are more common for younger women, women who have had previous breast biopsies, women with a family history of breast cancer, and women who are taking estrogen (for example, menopausal hormone therapy).

False-positive mammogram results can lead to anxiety and other forms of psychological distress in affected women. The additional testing required to rule out cancer can also be costly and time consuming and can cause physical discomfort.

Overdiagnosis and overtreatment. Screening mammograms can find cancers and cases of ductal carcinoma in situ (DCIS, a noninvasive tumor in which abnormal cells that may become cancerous build up in the lining of breast ducts) that need to be treated. However, they can also find cancers and cases of DCIS that will never cause symptoms or threaten a woman's life, leading to "overdiagnosis" of breast cancer. Treatment of these latter cancers and cases of DCIS is not needed and leads to "overtreatment." Overtreatment exposes women unnecessarily to the adverse effects associated with cancer therapy.

Because doctors often cannot distinguish cancers and cases of DCIS that need to be treated from those that do not, they are all treated.

False-negative results. False-negative results occur when mammograms appear normal even though breast cancer is present. Overall, screening mammograms miss about 20 percent of breast cancers that are present at the time of screening.

The main cause of false-negative results is high breast density. Breasts contain both dense tissue (i.e., glandular tissue and connective tissue, together known as fibroglandular tissue) and fatty tissue. Fatty tissue appears dark on a mammogram, whereas fibroglandular tissue appears as white areas. Because fibroglandular tissue and tumors have similar density, tumors can be harder to detect in women with denser breasts.

False-negative results occur more often among younger women than among older women because younger women are more likely to have dense breasts. As a woman ages, her breasts usually become more fatty, and false-negative results become less likely. False-negative results can lead to delays in treatment and a false sense of security for affected women.

Some of the cancers missed by screening mammograms can be detected by clinical breast exams (physical exams of the breast done by a health care provider).

Finding cancer early does not always reduce a woman's chance of dying from breast cancer. Even though mammograms can detect malignant tumors that cannot be felt, treating a small tumor does not always mean that the woman will not die from the cancer. A fast-growing or aggressive cancer may have already spread to other parts of the body before it is detected. Women with such tumors live a longer period of time knowing that they likely have a fatal disease.

In addition, screening mammograms may not help prolong the life of a woman who is suffering from other, more life-threatening health conditions.

Radiation exposure. Mammograms require very small doses of radiation. The risk of harm from this radiation exposure is extremely low, but repeated X-rays have the potential to cause cancer. The benefits of mammography, however, nearly always outweigh the potential harm from the radiation exposure. Nevertheless, women should talk with their health care providers about the need for each X-ray. In addition, they should always let their health care provider and the X-ray technician know if there is any possibility that they are pregnant, because radiation can harm a growing fetus.

Where can I find current recommendations for screening mammography?

Many organizations and professional societies, including the United States Preventive Services Task Force (which is convened by the Agency for Healthcare Research and Quality, a federal agency), have developed guidelines for mammography screening. All recommend that women should talk with their doctor about the benefits and harms of mammography, when to start screening, and how often to be screened.

Although NCI does not issue guidelines for cancer screening, it conducts and facilitates basic and translational research that informs standard clinical practice and medical decision making that other organizations may use to develop their guidelines.

What is the best method of detecting breast cancer as early as possible?

Getting a high-quality screening mammogram and having a clinical breast exam on a regular basis are the most effective ways to detect breast cancer early.

Checking one's own breasts for lumps or other unusual changes is called a breast self-exam, or BSE. This type of exam cannot replace regular screening mammograms or clinical breast exams. In clinical trials, BSE alone was not found to help reduce the number of deaths from breast cancer.

Although regular BSE is not specifically recommended for breast cancer screening, many women choose to examine their own breasts. Women who do so should remember that breast changes can occur because of pregnancy, aging, or menopause; during menstrual cycles; or when taking birth control pills or other hormones. It is normal for breasts to feel a little lumpy and uneven. Also, it is common for breasts to be swollen and tender right before or during a menstrual period. If a woman notices any unusual changes in her breasts, she should contact her health care provider.

How much does a mammogram cost?

For most women with private insurance, the cost of screening mammograms is covered without copayments or deductibles, but women should contact their mammography facility or health insurance company for confirmation of the cost and coverage.

Medicare pays for annual screening mammograms for all female Medicare beneficiaries who are age 40 or older. Medicare will also pay for one baseline mammogram for female beneficiaries between the ages of 35 and 39. There is no deductible requirement for this benefit.

How can uninsured or low-income women obtain a free or low-cost screening mammogram?

Some state and local health programs and employers provide mammograms free or at low cost. For example, the Centers for Disease Control and Prevention (CDC) coordinates the National Breast and Cervical Cancer Early Detection Program. This program provides screening services, including clinical breast exams and mammograms, to low-income, uninsured women throughout the United States and in several U.S. territories. Contact information for local programs is available on the CDC website or by calling 1–800–CDC–INFO (1–800–232–4636). Information about free or low-cost mammography screening programs is also available from NCI's Cancer Information Service at 1–800–4–CANCER (1–800–422–6237) and from local hospitals, health departments, women's centers, or other community groups.

Where can women get high-quality mammograms?

Women can get high-quality mammograms in breast clinics, hospital radiology departments, mobile vans, private radiology offices, and doctors' offices.

The Mammography Quality Standards Act (MQSA) is a Federal law that requires mammography facilities across the nation to meet uniform quality standards. Under the law, all mammography facilities must: 1) be accredited by an FDA-approved accreditation body; 2) be certified by the FDA, or an agency of a state that has been approved by the FDA, as meeting the standards; 3) undergo an annual MQSA inspection; and 4) prominently display the certificate issued by the agency.

Women can ask their doctors or staff at a local mammography facility about FDA certification before making an appointment. Women should look for the MQSA certificate at the mammography facility and check its expiration date. MQSA regulations also require that mammography facilities give patients an casy-to-read report of their mammogram results.

What should women with breast implants do about screening mammograms?

Women with breast implants should continue to have mammograms. (A woman who had an implant following a mastectomy should ask her doctor whether a mammogram of the reconstructed breast is necessary.) It is important to let the mammography facility know about breast implants when scheduling a mammogram. The technician and radiologist must be experienced in performing mammography on women who have breast implants. Implants can hide some breast tissue, making it more difficult for the radiologist to detect an abnormality on the mammogram. If the technician performing the procedure is aware that a woman has breast implants, steps can be taken to make sure that as much breast tissue as possible can be seen on the mammogram. A special technique called implant displacement views may be used.

What is digital mammography? How is it different from conventional (film) mammography?

Digital and conventional mammography both use X-rays to produce an image of the breast; however, in conventional mammography, the image is stored directly on film, whereas, in digital mammography, an electronic image of the breast is stored as a computer file. This digital information can be enhanced, magnified, or manipulated for further evaluation more easily than information stored on film.

Because digital mammography allows a radiologist to adjust, store, and retrieve digital images electronically, digital mammography may offer the following advantages over conventional mammography:

- Health care providers can share image files electronically, making long-distance consultations between radiologists and breast surgeons easier.

- Subtle differences between normal and abnormal tissues may be more easily noted.

- Fewer follow-up procedures may be needed.

- Fewer repeat images may be needed, reducing the exposure to radiation.

To date, there is no evidence that digital mammography helps to reduce a woman's risk of dying from breast cancer compared with film mammography. Results from a large NCI-sponsored clinical trial that compared digital mammography with film mammography found no difference between digital and film mammograms in detecting breast cancer in the general population of women in the trial; however, digital mammography appeared to be more accurate than conventional film mammography in younger women with dense breasts. A subsequent analysis of women aged 40 through 79 who were undergoing screening in U.S. community-based imaging facilities also found that digital and film mammography had similar accuracy in most women. Digital screening had higher sensitivity in women with dense breasts.

Some health care providers recommend that women who have a very high risk of breast cancer, such as those with a known mutation in either the *BRCA1* or *BRCA2* gene or extremely dense breasts, have digital mammograms instead of conventional mammograms; however, no studies have shown that digital mammograms are superior to conventional mammograms in reducing the risk of death for these women.

Digital mammography can be done only in facilities that are certified to practice conventional mammography and have received FDA approval to offer digital mammography. The procedure for having a mammogram with a digital system is the same as with conventional mammography.

What is 3D mammography?

Three-dimensional (3D) mammography, also known as breast tomosynthesis, is a type of digital mammography in which X-ray machines are used to take pictures of thin slices of the breast from different angles and computer software is used to reconstruct an image. This process is similar to how a computed tomography (CT) scanner produces images of structures inside of the body. 3D mammography uses very low dose X-rays, but, because it is generally performed at the same time as standard two-dimensional (2D) digital mammography, the radiation dose is slightly higher than that of standard mammography. The accuracy of 3D mammography has not been compared with that of 2D mammography in randomized studies. Therefore, researchers do not know whether 3D mammography is better or worse than standard mammography at avoiding false-positive results and identifying early cancers.

What other technologies are being developed for breast cancer screening?

NCI is supporting the development of several new technologies to detect breast tumors. This research ranges from methods being developed in research labs to those that are being studied in clinical trials. Efforts to improve conventional mammography include digital mammography, magnetic resonance imaging (MRI), positron emission tomography (PET) scanning, and diffuse optical tomography, which uses light instead of X-rays to create pictures of the breast.

Chapter 28

Pediatric X-Ray Imaging

Description

Medical imaging has led to improvements in the diagnosis and treatment of numerous medical conditions in children and adults.

There are many types – or modalities – of medical imaging procedures that are used on children, each of which uses different technologies and techniques. Computed tomography (CT), fluoroscopy, and radiography (conventional X-ray) all use ionizing radiation to generate images of the body. Ionizing radiation is a form of radiation that has enough energy to potentially cause damage to DNA and may elevate a person's lifetime risk of developing cancer.

CT, radiography, and fluoroscopy all work on the same basic principle: an X-ray beam is passed through the body where a portion of the X-rays are either absorbed or scattered by the internal structures, and the remaining X-ray pattern is transmitted to a detector for recording or further processing by a computer. These exams differ in their purpose:

- Radiography – a single image is recorded for later evaluation.

- Fluoroscopy – a continuous X-ray image is displayed on a monitor, allowing for real-time monitoring of a procedure or passage of a contrast agent, or "dye" through the body. Fluoroscopy can result in relatively high radiation doses, especially for

Text in this chapter is excerpted from "Pediatric X-ray Imaging," Food and Drug Administration (FDA), June 5, 2014.

interventional procedures (such as placing catheters, or other devices inside the body) which require fluoroscopy be administered for a long period of time.

- CT – many X-ray images are recorded as the detector moves around the patient's body. A computer reconstructs all the individual images into cross-sectional images or "slices" of internal organs and tissues. A CT exam involves a higher radiation dose than conventional radiography because the CT image is reconstructed from many individual X-ray projections.

Benefits / Risks

X-ray imaging exams are recognized as a valuable medical tool for a wide variety of examinations and procedures including:

- noninvasive and painless diagnosis of disease and monitoring of therapy;

- support of medical and surgical treatment planning; and

- interventional procedures such as placing catheters, stents, or other devices inside the body, or removing blood clots or other blockages.

The individual risk from a necessary imaging exam is generally quite small when compared to the benefit of helping with accurate diagnosis or intervention. Risks from X-ray imaging include risks from exposure to ionizing radiation and possible reactions to the intravenous contrast agent, or "dye" that is sometimes used to improve visualization.

Types of radiation risks include:

- tissue effects such as cataracts, skin reddening, and hair loss, which occur at relatively high levels of radiation exposure and are very rare in children; and

- a small increase in the possibility that a person exposed to X-rays will develop cancer later in life. Radiation-induced cancer risks depend on the radiation dose, the patient's age at exposure, the sex of the patient (women are more radiosensitive than men), and the organ irradiated.

While the benefit of a clinically appropriate X-ray imaging exam generally far outweighs the risk, efforts should be made to minimize this risk by reducing unnecessary exposure to ionizing radiation.

Ionizing radiation exposure to pediatric patients from medical imaging procedures is of particular concern because pediatric patients:

- are more radiosensitive than adults (i.e., the cancer risk per unit dose of ionizing radiation is higher);

- have a longer expected lifetime for any effects of radiation exposure to manifest as cancer; and

- use of equipment and exposure settings designed for adults may result in excessive radiation exposure if used on smaller patients.

The medical community has emphasized dose reduction in CT because of the relatively high doses of CT exams and their increased use, as reported in the National Council on Radiation Protection and Measurements (NCRP) Report No. 160. However, the increased radiosensitivity of pediatric patients compared to adults makes it important to adjust equipment settings to optimize radiation exposure to pediatric patients for all types of X-ray imaging exams.

If there is a medical need for a particular imaging procedure and other exams using no or less radiation are unsuitable, then the benefits exceed the risks, and radiation risk considerations should not influence the physician's decision to perform the study or the patient's decision to have the procedure. However, "As Low as Reasonably Achievable" (ALARA) principles should always be followed when choosing equipment settings to minimize radiation exposure to the pediatric patient.

Information for Patients and Parents

The FDA recommends that medical imaging exams should be performed only after careful consideration of the patient's health needs. They should be performed only when the child's physician judges them to be necessary to answer a clinical question or to guide treatment of a disease. The clinical benefit of a medically appropriate X-ray imaging exam will outweigh the small radiation risk. However, efforts should be made to help minimize this risk.

The FDA recommends that parents:

- Keep track of their child's medical-imaging histories as part of a discussion with the referring physician when a new exam is recommended

- Ask the referring physician about the benefits and risks of imaging procedures, such as:

- How will the exam improve my child's health care?

- Are there alternative exams that do not use ionizing radiation and are equally as useful?

- Ask the imaging facility:

  - What safeguards are in place to mitigate the risks to my child? For example, does the facility use reduced radiation techniques for children?

  - Are there any additional steps that may be necessary to perform the imaging study (e.g., administration of a contrast agent, sedation, or advanced preparation)?

Chapter 29

Fluoroscopy

Description

Fluoroscopy is a type of medical imaging that shows a continuous X-ray image on a monitor, much like an X-ray movie. During a fluoroscopy procedure, an X-ray beam is passed through the body. The image is transmitted to a monitor so the movement of a body part or of an instrument or contrast agent ("X-ray dye") through the body can be seen in detail.

Benefits / Risks

Fluoroscopy is used in a wide variety of examinations and procedures to diagnose or treat patients. Some examples are:

- Barium X-rays and enemas (to view the gastrointestinal tract)
- Catheter insertion and manipulation (to direct the movement of a catheter through blood vessels, bile ducts or the urinary system)
- Placement of devices within the body, such as stents (to open narrowed or blocked blood vessels)
- Angiograms (to visualize blood vessels and organs)

Text in this chapter is excerpted from "Fluoroscopy," U.S. Food and Drug Administration (FDA), June 17, 2014.

- Orthopedic surgery (to guide joint replacements and treatment of fractures)

Fluoroscopy carries some risks, as do other X-ray procedures. The radiation dose the patient receives varies depending on the individual procedure. Fluoroscopy can result in relatively high radiation doses, especially for complex interventional procedures (such as placing stents or other devices inside the body) which require fluoroscopy be administered for a long period of time. Radiation-related risks associated with fluoroscopy include:

- radiation-induced injuries to the skin and underlying tissues ("burns"), which occur shortly after the exposure, and

- radiation-induced cancers, which may occur some time later in life.

The probability that a person will experience these effects from a fluoroscopic procedure is statistically very small. Therefore, if the procedure is medically needed, the radiation risks are outweighed by the benefit to the patient. In fact, the radiation risk is usually far less than other risks not associated with radiation, such as anesthesia or sedation, or risks from the treatment itself. To minimize the radiation risk, fluoroscopy should always be performed with the lowest acceptable exposure for the shortest time necessary.

Information for Patients

Fluoroscopy procedures are performed to help diagnose disease, or to guide physicians during certain treatment procedures. Some fluoroscopy procedures may be performed as outpatient procedures while the patient is awake – for example, upper gastrointestinal series to examine the esophagus, stomach and small intestine, or a barium enema to examine the colon.

Other procedures are performed as same-day hospital procedures or sometimes as inpatient procedures, typically while the patient is sedated – for example, cardiac catheterization to examine the heart and the coronary arteries that supply blood to the heart muscle. Still other fluoroscopy procedures may be performed under general anesthesia during surgery – for example to help align and fix fractured bones.

The clinical benefit of a medically appropriate X-ray imaging exam outweighs the small radiation risk. The FDA encourages patients and parents of pediatric patients to engage in a discussion with their health care provider about the benefits and risks of fluoroscopy procedures.

Extensive information is available on fluoroscopy, diseases and conditions where fluoroscopy is used for diagnosis or treatment, and on the risks and benefits of fluoroscopy. In addition to the patient information links on the Medical X-ray Imaging webpage, more specific information on procedures conducted using fluoroscopy is provided below:

- Patient Information on interventional radiology procedures from the Society of Interventional Radiology

- Information on heart disease and cardiology procedures, including cardiac catheterization and coronary artery stenting can be found at the Society for Cardiovascular Angiography and Interventions

- The Heart Rhythm Society's Patient Information addresses heart disease, abnormal heart rhythms and treatment of abnormal heart rhythms

- The Society of Vascular Surgery's Vascular Conditions, Tests, Treatments contain information on diagnosis and treatment of abnormalities of blood vessels

Part Five

Catheterization, Endoscopic, and Electrical Tests and Assessments

Chapter 30

Cardiac Catheterization

Cardiac catheterization is a medical procedure used to diagnose and treat some heart conditions.

A long, thin, flexible tube called a catheter is put into a blood vessel in your arm, groin (upper thigh), or neck and threaded to your heart. Through the catheter, your doctor can do diagnostic tests and treatments on your heart.

For example, your doctor may put a special type of dye in the catheter. The dye will flow through your bloodstream to your heart. Then, your doctor will take X-ray pictures of your heart. The dye will make your coronary (heart) arteries visible on the pictures. This test is called coronary angiography.

The dye can show whether a waxy substance called plaque has built up inside your coronary arteries. Plaque can narrow or block the arteries and restrict blood flow to your heart.

The buildup of plaque in the coronary arteries is called coronary heart disease (CHD) or coronary artery disease.

Doctors also can use ultrasound during cardiac catheterization to see blockages in the coronary arteries. Ultrasound uses sound waves to create detailed pictures of the heart's blood vessels.

Doctors may take samples of blood and heart muscle during cardiac catheterization or do minor heart surgery.

Text in this chapter is excerpted from "Cardiac Catheterization," National Heart, Lung, and Blood Institute (NHLBI), January 30, 2012.

Cardiologists (heart specialists) usually do cardiac catheterization in a hospital. You're awake during the procedure, and it causes little or no pain. However, you may feel some soreness in the blood vessel where the catheter was inserted.

Cardiac catheterization rarely causes serious complications.

Who Needs Cardiac Catheterization?

Doctors may recommend cardiac catheterization for various reasons. The most common reason is to evaluate chest pain.

Chest pain might be a symptom of coronary heart disease (CHD). Cardiac catheterization can show whether plaque is narrowing or blocking your coronary arteries.

Doctors also can treat CHD during cardiac catheterization using a procedure called percutaneous coronary intervention (PCI), also known as coronary angioplasty.

During PCI, a catheter with a balloon at its tip is threaded to the blocked coronary artery. Once in place, the balloon is inflated, pushing the plaque against the artery wall. This creates a wider path for blood to flow to the heart.

Sometimes a stent is placed in the artery during PCI. A stent is a small mesh tube that supports the inner artery wall.

Most people who have heart attacks have narrow or blocked coronary arteries. Thus, cardiac catheterization might be used as an emergency procedure to treat a heart attack. When used with PCI, the procedure allows your doctor to open up blocked arteries and prevent further heart damage.

Cardiac catheterization also can help your doctor figure out the best treatment plan for you if:

- You recently recovered from a heart attack, but are having chest pain

- You had a heart attack that caused major heart damage

- You had an EKG (electrocardiogram), stress test, or other test with results that suggested heart disease

Cardiac catheterization also might be used if your doctor thinks you have a heart defect or if you're about to have heart surgery. The procedure shows the overall shape of your heart and the four large spaces (heart chambers) inside it. This inside view of the heart will show certain heart defects and help your doctor plan your heart surgery.

Sometimes doctors use cardiac catheterization to see how well the heart valves work. Valves control blood flow in your heart. They open and shut to allow blood to flow between your heart chambers and into your arteries.

Your doctor can use cardiac catheterization to measure blood flow and oxygen levels in different parts of your heart. He or she also can check how well a man-made heart valve is working and how well your heart is pumping blood.

If your doctor thinks you have a heart infection or tumor, he or she may take samples of your heart muscle through the catheter. With the help of cardiac catheterization, doctors can even do minor heart surgery, such as repair certain heart defects.

What to Expect before Cardiac Catheterization

Before having cardiac catheterization, discuss with your doctor:

- How to prepare for the procedure

- Any medicines you're taking, and whether you should stop taking them before the procedure

- Whether you have any conditions (such as diabetes or kidney disease) that may require taking extra steps during or after the procedure to avoid problems

Your doctor will let you know whether you need to arrange for a ride home after the procedure.

What to Expect during Cardiac Catheterization

Cardiac catheterization is done in a hospital. During the procedure, you'll be kept on your back and awake. This allows you to follow your doctor's instructions during the procedure. You'll be given medicine to help you relax, which might make you sleepy.

Your doctor will numb the area on the arm, groin (upper thigh), or neck where the catheter will enter your blood vessel. Then, a needle will be used to make a small hole in the blood vessel. Your doctor will put a tapered tube called a sheath through the hole.

Next, your doctor will put a thin, flexible guide wire through the sheath and into your blood vessel. He or she will thread the wire through your blood vessel to your heart.

Your doctor will use the guide wire to correctly place the catheter. He or she will put the catheter through the sheath and slide it over the guide wire and into the coronary arteries.

Special X-ray movies will be taken of the guide wire and the catheter as they're moved into the heart. The movies will help your doctor see where to put the tip of the catheter.

When the catheter reaches the right spot, your doctor will use it to do tests or treatments on your heart. For example, your doctor may perform a percutaneous coronary intervention (PCI), also known as coronary angioplasty, and stenting.

During the procedure, your doctor may put a special type of dye in the catheter. The dye will flow through your bloodstream to your heart. Then, your doctor will take X-ray pictures of your heart. The dye will make your coronary (heart) arteries visible on the pictures. This test is called coronary angiography.

Coronary angiography can show how well the heart's lower chambers, called the ventricles, are pumping blood.

When the catheter is inside your heart, your doctor may use it to take blood and tissue samples or do minor heart surgery.

To get a more detailed view of a blocked coronary artery, your doctor may do intracoronary ultrasound. For this test, your doctor will thread a tiny ultrasound device through the catheter and into the artery. This device gives off sound waves that bounce off the artery wall (and its blockage). The sound waves create a picture of the inside of the artery.

If the angiogram or intracoronary ultrasound shows blockages in the coronary arteries, your doctor may use PCI to treat the blocked arteries.

After your doctor does all of the needed tests or treatments, he or she will pull back the catheter and take it out along with the sheath. The opening left in the blood vessel will be closed up and bandaged.

A small weight might be put on top of the bandage for a few hours to apply more pressure. This will help prevent major bleeding from the site.

What to Expect after Cardiac Catheterization

After cardiac catheterization, you will be moved to a special care area. You will rest there for several hours or overnight. During that time, you'll have to limit your movement to avoid bleeding from the site where the catheter was inserted.

While you recover in this area, nurses will check your heart rate and blood pressure regularly. They also will check for bleeding from the catheter insertion site.

A small bruise might form at the catheter insertion site, and the area may feel sore or tender for about a week. Let your doctor know if you have problems such as:

- A constant or large amount of bleeding at the insertion site that can't be stopped with a small bandage

- Unusual pain, swelling, redness, or other signs of infection at or near the insertion site

Talk to your doctor about whether you should avoid certain activities, such as heavy lifting, for a short time after the procedure.

What Are the Risks of Cardiac Catheterization?

Cardiac catheterization is a common medical procedure. It rarely causes serious problems. However, complications can include:

- Bleeding, infection, and pain at the catheter insertion site.

- Damage to blood vessels. Rarely, the catheter may scrape or poke a hole in a blood vessel as it's threaded to the heart.

- An allergic reaction to the dye that's used during coronary angiography.

Other, less common complications include:

- Arrhythmias (irregular heartbeats). These irregular heartbeats often go away on their own. However, your doctor may recommend treatment if they persist.

- Kidney damage caused by the dye used during coronary angiography.

- Blood clots that can trigger a stroke, heart attack, or other serious problems.

- Low blood pressure.

- A buildup of blood or fluid in the sac that surrounds the heart. This fluid can prevent the heart from beating properly.

As with any procedure involving the heart, complications sometimes can be fatal. However, this is rare with cardiac catheterization.

The risks of cardiac catheterization are higher in people who are older and in those who have certain diseases or conditions (such as chronic kidney disease and diabetes).

Chapter 31

Endoscopic Procedures

Chapter Contents

Section 31.1

Bronchoscopy

Text in this section is excerpted from "What Is Bronchoscopy?,"
National Heart, Lung, and Blood Institute (NHLBI),
February 8, 2012.

What Is Bronchoscopy?

Bronchoscopy is a procedure used to look inside the lungs' airways, called the bronchi and bronchioles. The airways carry air from the trachea, or windpipe, to the lungs.

During the procedure, your doctor passes a thin, flexible tube called a bronchoscope through your nose (or sometimes your mouth), down your throat, and into your airways. If you have a breathing tube, the bronchoscope can be passed through the tube to your airways.

The bronchoscope has a light and small camera that allow your doctor to see your windpipe and airways and take pictures. You'll be given medicine to make you relaxed and sleepy during the procedure.

If there's a lot of bleeding in your lungs or a large object stuck in your throat, your doctor may use a bronchoscope with a rigid tube. The rigid tube, which is passed through the mouth, is wider. This allows your doctor to see inside it more easily, treat bleeding, and remove stuck objects.

A rigid bronchoscopy usually is done in a hospital operating room using general anesthesia. The term "anesthesia" refers to a loss of feeling and awareness. General anesthesia temporarily puts you to sleep.

Overview

Bronchoscopy usually is done to find the cause of a lung problem. Your doctor may take samples of mucus or tissue from your lungs during the procedure to test in a lab.

Bronchoscopy may show a tumor, signs of an infection, excess mucus in the airways, the site of bleeding, or something blocking the airway, like a piece of food.

Sometimes bronchoscopy is used to treat lung problems. It may be done to insert a stent in an airway. An airway stent is a small tube that holds the airway open. It's used when a tumor or other condition blocks an airway.

In children, the procedure most often is used to remove something blocking an airway. In some cases, it's used to find out what's causing a cough that has lasted for at least a few weeks.

Outlook

Bronchoscopy usually is a safe procedure. You may be hoarse and have a sore throat after the procedure. There's a slight risk of minor bleeding or developing a fever or pneumonia.

A rare, but more serious risk is a pneumothorax, or collapsed lung. In this condition, air collects in the space around the lungs, which causes one or both lungs to collapse. Usually, this problem is easily treated.

Scientists are studying new methods of bronchoscopy, including virtual bronchoscopy. This is a type of computed tomography, or CT, scan. A CT scan uses special X-rays to take clear, detailed pictures of the inside of your body.

During the scan, you lie on a table that slides through the center of a tunnel-shaped X-ray machine. X-ray tubes in the scanner rotate around you and take pictures of your lungs.

Virtual bronchoscopy still isn't widely used.

Who Needs Bronchoscopy?

The most common reason why your doctor may decide to do a bronchoscopy is if you have an abnormal chest X-ray or chest computed tomography (CT) scan. These tests may show a tumor, a pneumothorax (collapsed lung), or signs of an infection.

A chest X-ray takes a picture of your heart and lungs. A chest CT scan uses special X-rays to take pictures of the inside of your body.

Other reasons for bronchoscopy include if you're coughing up blood or if you have a cough that has lasted more than a few weeks.

The procedure also can be done to remove something that's stuck in an airway (like a piece of food), to place medicine in a lung to treat a lung problem, or to insert a stent (small tube) in an airway to hold it open when a tumor or other condition causes a blockage.

Bronchoscopy also can be used to check for swelling in the upper airways and vocal cords of people who were burned around the throat area or who inhaled smoke from a fire.

371

In children, the procedure most often is used to remove something blocking an airway. In some cases, it's used to find out what's causing a cough that has lasted for at least a few weeks.

What to Expect before Bronchoscopy

Your doctor will do the bronchoscopy in a special clinic or in a hospital. To prepare for the procedure, tell your doctor:

- What medicines you're taking, including prescription and over-the-counter medicines. It's helpful to give your doctor a list of the medicines you take.

- About any previous bleeding problems.

- About any allergies to medicines or latex.

The medicine you'll get before the procedure will make you sleepy, so you should arrange for a ride home from the clinic or hospital.

Avoid eating or drinking for 4 to 8 hours before the procedure. Your doctor will let you know the right amount of time.

What to Expect during Bronchoscopy

Your doctor will do the bronchoscopy in an exam room at a special clinic or in a hospital. The bronchoscopy itself usually lasts about 30 minutes. But the entire procedure, including preparation and recovery time, takes about 4 hours.

Your doctor will give you medicine through an intravenous (IV) line in your bloodstream or by mouth to make you sleepy and relaxed.

Your doctor also will squirt or spray a liquid medicine into your nose and throat to make them numb. This helps prevent coughing and gagging when the bronchoscope (long, thin tube) is inserted.

Then, your doctor will insert the bronchoscope through your nose or mouth and into your airways. As the tube enters your mouth, you may gag a little. Once it enters your throat, that feeling will go away.

Your doctor will look at your vocal cords and airways through the bronchoscope (which has a light and a small camera).

During the procedure, your doctor may take a sample of lung fluid or tissue for further testing. Samples can be taken using:

- Bronchoalveolar lavage. For this method, your doctor passes a small amount of salt water (a saline solution) through the bronchoscope and into part of your lung. He or she then suctions the salt water back out. The fluid picks up cells and bacteria from the airway, which your doctor can study.

- Transbronchial lung biopsy. For this method, your doctor inserts forceps into the bronchoscope and takes a small sample of tissue from inside the lung.

- Transbronchial needle aspiration. For this method, your doctor inserts a needle into the bronchoscope and removes cells from the lymph nodes in your lungs. These nodes are small, bean-shaped masses. They trap bacteria and cancer cells and help fight infection.

You may feel short of breath during bronchoscopy, but enough air is getting to your lungs. Your doctor will check your oxygen level. If the level drops, you'll be given oxygen.

If you have a lot of bleeding in your lungs or a large object stuck in your throat, your doctor may use a bronchoscope with a rigid tube. The rigid tube, which is passed through the mouth, is wider. This allows your doctor to see inside it more easily, treat bleeding, and remove stuck objects.

A rigid bronchoscopy usually is done in a hospital operating room using general anesthesia. The term "anesthesia" refers to a loss of feeling and awareness. General anesthesia temporarily puts you to sleep.

After the procedure is done, your doctor will remove the bronchoscope.

What to Expect after Bronchoscopy

After bronchoscopy, you'll need to stay at the clinic or hospital for up to a few hours. If your doctor uses a bronchoscope with a rigid tube, the recovery time is longer. While you're at the clinic or hospital:

- You may have a chest X-ray if your doctor took a sample of lung tissue. This test will check for a pneumothorax and bleeding. A pneumothorax is a condition in which air or gas collects in the space around the lungs. This can cause one or both lungs to collapse. Usually, this condition is easily treated.

- A nurse will check your breathing and blood pressure.

- You can't eat or drink until the numbness in your throat wears off. This takes 1 to 2 hours.

After recovery, you'll need to have someone take you home. You'll be too sleepy to drive.

If samples of tissue or fluid were taken during the procedure, they'll be tested in a lab. Talk to your doctor about when you'll get the lab results.

Recovery and Recuperation

Your doctor will let you know when you can return to your normal activities, such as driving, working, and physical activity. For the first few days, you may have a sore throat, cough, and hoarseness. Call your doctor right away if you:

- Develop a fever

- Have chest pain

- Have trouble breathing

- Cough up more than a few tablespoons of blood

What Does Bronchoscopy Show?

Bronchoscopy may show a tumor, signs of an infection, excess mucus in the airways, the site of bleeding, or something blocking your airway.

Your doctor will use the procedure results to decide how to treat any lung problems that were found. Other tests may be needed.

What Are the Risks of Bronchoscopy?

Bronchoscopy usually is a safe procedure. However, there's a small risk for problems, such as:

- A drop in your oxygen level during the procedure. Your doctor will give you oxygen if this happens.

- Minor bleeding and developing a fever or pneumonia.

A rare, but more serious side effect is a pneumothorax. A pneumothorax is a condition in which air or gas collects in the space around the lungs. This can cause one or both lungs to collapse.

Usually, this condition is easily treated or may go away on its own. If it interferes with breathing, a tube may need to be placed in the space around the lungs to remove the air.

A chest X-ray may be done after bronchoscopy to check for problems.

Section 31.2

Capsule Endoscopy

Text in this section is excerpted from "What is a Capsule Endoscopy?" National Heart, Lung, and Blood Institute (NHLBI), March 22, 2014.

What is a Capsule Endoscopy?

Capsule endoscopy, often referred to as the "pill camera," is one way to look at the entire small intestine. The capsule, which is the size of a large pill, is swallowed. The pill travels through the intestine taking two pictures per second. A recorder worn on a belt holds the pictures. A doctor will review the pictures on a computer. You will pass the capsule in the stool.

Why Do I Need The Test?

You may need the test if you have symptoms, such as blood in your bowel movements (BMs). Symptoms may also include chronic (long-term) stomach pain and diarrhea (liquid BMs). The pictures may show if you have growths, swelling, and bleeding areas in your small bowel. The pictures from this test may show signs of Crohn's or Celiac disease. The test may help you and your doctor learn the cause of your symptoms. Learning what is causing your symptoms may allow you to receive needed treatment and prevent further problems.

What Do I Need To Do For The Test?

The Day before the Test

1. You may have a regular breakfast and a regular lunch. After lunch, you will start a clear liquid diet. You may have clear liquids until 10:00 pm the night before your capsule endoscopy. **(Nothing to eat or drink after 10:00 pm!)**

2. You may take your necessary medications with a sip of water the morning of your test at least 2 hours before your scheduled appointment time.

3. Do not smoke 24 hours before the test.

Stop taking Carafate, Maalox, Mylanta, Pepto Bismol, and other similar medications 24 hours prior to the test.

Table 31.1. Clear Liquid Diet

TEA – no cream	BOUILLION CUBES
COFFEE – no cream	SPRITE
JELL-O – not red	7-UP
GINGERALE	POPSICLES – not red
GATORADE – not red	LIFESAVERS – not red
CRYSTAL LIGHT DRINKS – not red	APPLE JUICE
CRANBERRY JUICE – natural juice	KOOL-AID – not red

Stop all iron supplements 5 days before your test

The Day of Your Capsule Endoscopy

1. At the Endoscopy Center, you will be checked in and asked to give your informed consent.

Small sensors will be taped on your abdomen and connected to a recorder. The recorder will be attached to a belt that you will wear around your waist. After that, you will be instructed to swallow the capsule (which is called the PillCam SB2 capsule).

After Swallowing the PillCam SB Capsule

1. After swallowing the PillCam SB capsule, do not eat or drink for 4 hours. After 4 hours, you may have a light snack, such as chicken noodle soup or Jell-O (non-red). After the test is done, you may return to your normal diet. These instructions apply unless your doctor tells you differently.

2. Do not lift, stoop, or bend over during the testing. Also avoid strenuous activity that may make you sweat.

3. While you are wearing the DataRecorder, you will need to check (about every 30 minutes) that the light on the top of the DataRecorder is blinking twice per second. If it stops blinking at this rate, record the time and call our office. You should also record the time and nature of any event such as eating, drinking, activity, and unusual sensations.

4. After swallowing the PillCam SB2, and until it is passed, you should not be near any source of powerful electromagnetic fields, such as one created near an MRI device or amateur (ham) radio. Occasionally, some images may be lost due to radio interference. On rare occasions, this may result in the need to repeat the SB Capsule Endoscopy testing.

5. The Capsule Endoscopy lasts approximately 8 hours.

Do not disconnect the equipment or remove the belt at any time during this period. Since the DataRecorder is actually a small computer, it should be treated with utmost care and protection. Avoid sudden movement and banging of the DataRecorder.

Section 31.3

Colonoscopy

Text in this section is excerpted from "Colonoscopy," National Institute of Diabetes and Digestive and Kidney Diseases (NIDDK), November 13, 2014.

Colonoscopy is a procedure in which a trained specialist uses a long, flexible, narrow tube with a light and tiny camera on one end, called a colonoscope or scope, to look inside your rectum and colon. Colonoscopy can show irritated and swollen tissue, ulcers, polyps, and cancer.

How is virtual colonoscopy different from colonoscopy?

Virtual colonoscopy and colonoscopy are different in several ways. Virtual colonoscopy is an X-ray test, takes less time, and doesn't require a doctor to insert a colonoscope into the entire length of your colon. However, virtual colonoscopy may not be as effective as colonoscopy at detecting certain polyps. Also, doctors cannot treat problems during virtual colonoscopy, while they can treat some problems during colonoscopy. Your health insurance coverage for virtual colonoscopy and colonoscopy may also be different.

377

Why do doctors use colonoscopy?

A colonoscopy can help a doctor find the cause of unexplained symptoms, such as

- changes in your bowel activity

- pain in your abdomen

- bleeding from your anus

- unexplained weight loss

Doctors also use colonoscopy as a screening tool for colon polyps and cancer. Screening is testing for diseases when you have no symptoms. Screening may find diseases at an early stage, when a doctor has a better chance of curing the disease.

Screening for Colon and Rectal Cancer

Your doctor will recommend screening for colon and rectal cancer at age 50 if you don't have health problems or other factors that make you more likely to develop colon cancer.

Risk factors for colorectal cancer include

- someone in your family has had polyps or cancer of the colon or rectum

- a personal history of inflammatory bowel disease, such as ulcerative colitis and Crohn's disease

- other factors, such as if you weigh too much or smoke cigarettes

If you are at higher risk for colorectal cancer, your doctor may recommend screening at a younger age, and you may need to be tested more often.

If you are older than 75, talk with your doctor about whether you should be screened.

Government health insurance plans, such as Medicare, and private health insurance plans sometimes change whether and how often they pay for cancer screening tests. Check with your insurance plan to find out how often your insurance will cover a screening colonoscopy.

How do I prepare for a colonoscopy?

To prepare for a colonoscopy, you will need to talk with your doctor, arrange for a ride home, clean out your bowel, and change your diet.

Talk with your doctor

You should talk with your doctor about any medical conditions you have and all prescribed and over-the-counter medicines, vitamins, and supplements you take, including:

- aspirin or medicines that contain aspirin
- nonsteroidal anti-inflammatory drugs such as ibuprofen or naproxen
- arthritis medicines
- blood thinners
- diabetes medicines
- vitamins that contain iron or iron supplements

Arrange for a ride home

For safety reasons, you can't drive for 24 hours after the procedure, as the sedatives or anesthesia used during the procedure needs time to wear off. You will need to make plans for getting a ride home after the procedure.

Clean out your bowel and change your diet

A health care professional will give you written bowel prep instructions to follow at home before the procedure. A health care professional orders a bowel prep so that little to no stool is present in your intestine. A complete bowel prep lets you pass stool that is clear. Stool inside your colon can prevent your doctor from clearly seeing the lining of your intestine.

You may need to follow a clear liquid diet for 1 to 3 days before the procedure and avoid drinks that contain red or purple dye. The instructions will provide specific direction about when to start and stop the clear liquid diet. In most cases, you may drink or eat the following:

- fat-free bouillon or broth
- strained fruit juice, such as apple or white grape—doctors recommend avoiding orange juice
- water
- plain coffee or tea, without cream or milk
- sports drinks in flavors such as lemon, lime, or orange
- gelatin in flavors such as lemon, lime, or orange

Your doctor will tell you before the procedure when you should have nothing by mouth.

A health care professional will ask you to follow the directions for a bowel prep before the procedure. The bowel prep will cause diarrhea, so you should stay close to a bathroom.

Different bowel preps may contain different combinations of laxatives, pills that you swallow or powders that you dissolve in water and other clear liquids, and enemas. Some people will need to drink a large amount, often a gallon, of liquid laxative over a scheduled amount of time—most often the night before the procedure. You may find this part of the bowel prep difficult; however, completing the prep is very important. Your doctor will not be able to see your colon clearly if the prep is incomplete.

Call a health care professional if you have side effects that prevent you from finishing the prep.

How do doctors perform a colonoscopy?

A trained specialist performs a colonoscopy in a hospital or an outpatient center.

A health care professional will place an intravenous (IV) needle in a vein in your arm to give you sedatives, anesthesia, or pain medicine so you can relax during the procedure. The health care staff will monitor your vital signs and keep you as comfortable as possible.

For the procedure, you'll be asked to lie on a table while the doctor inserts a colonoscope into your anus and slowly guides it through your rectum and into your colon. The scope pumps air into your large intestine to give the doctor a better view. The camera sends a video image of the intestinal lining to a monitor, allowing the doctor to examine your intestinal tissues. The doctor may move you several times on the table to adjust the scope for better viewing. Once the scope has reached the opening to your small intestine, the doctor slowly withdraws it and examines the lining of your large intestine again.

During the procedure, the doctor may remove polyps and send them to a lab for testing. Colon polyps are common in adults and are harmless in most cases. However, most colon cancer begins as a polyp, so removing polyps early is an effective way to prevent cancer.

The doctor may also perform a biopsy. You won't feel the biopsy. Colonoscopy typically takes 30 to 60 minutes.

What should I expect after a colonoscopy?

After a colonoscopy, you can expect the following:

- You'll stay at the hospital or outpatient center for 1 to 2 hours after the procedure.

- You may have abdominal cramping or bloating during the first hour after the procedure.

- The sedatives or anesthesia takes time to wear off completely.

- You should expect a full recovery by the next day, and you should be able to go back to your normal diet.

- After the procedure, you—or a friend or family member—will receive instructions on how to care for yourself after the procedure. You should follow all instructions.

- A friend or family member will need to drive you home after the procedure.

If the doctor removed polyps or performed a biopsy, you may have light bleeding from your anus. This bleeding is normal. Some results from a colonoscopy are available right after the procedure. After the sedatives or anesthesia has worn off, the doctor will share results with you or, if you choose, with your friend or family member. A pathologist will examine the biopsy tissue. Biopsy results take a few days or longer to come back.

What are the risks of colonoscopy?

The risks of colonoscopy include

- bleeding

- perforation of the colon

- abnormal reaction to the sedative, including respiratory or cardiac problems

- abdominal pain

- death, although this risk is rare

Bleeding and perforation are the most common complications from colonoscopy. Most cases of bleeding occur in patients who have polyps removed. The doctor can treat bleeding that occurs during the colonoscopy right away. However, you may have delayed bleeding up to 2 weeks after the procedure. The doctor diagnoses and treats delayed bleeding with a repeat colonoscopy. The doctor may need to treat perforation with surgery.

A study of screening colonoscopies found roughly two serious complications for every 1,000 procedures.

Seek Care Right Away

If you have any of the following symptoms after a colonoscopy, seek medical care right away:

- severe abdominal pain

- fever

- continued bloody bowel movements or continued bleeding from the anus

- dizziness

- weakness

Section 31.4

Cystoscopy and Ureteroscopy

Text in this section is excerpted from "Cystoscopy and Ureteroscopy," National Institute of Diabetes and Digestive and Kidney Diseases (NIDDK), June 30, 2015.

Cystoscopy and ureteroscopy are common procedures performed by a urologist to look inside the urinary tract. A urologist is a doctor who specializes in urinary tract problems.

Cystoscopy. Cystoscopy uses a cystoscope to look inside the urethra and bladder. A cystoscope is a long, thin optical instrument with an eyepiece at one end, a rigid or flexible tube in the middle, and a tiny lens and light at the other end of the tube. By looking through the cystoscope, the urologist can see detailed images of the lining of the urethra and bladder. The urethra and bladder are part of the urinary tract.

Ureteroscopy. Ureteroscopy uses a ureteroscope to look inside the ureters and kidneys. Like a cystoscope, a ureteroscope has an eyepiece at one end, a rigid or flexible tube in the middle, and a tiny lens and light at the other end of the tube. However, a ureteroscope is longer and thinner than a cystoscope so the urologist can see detailed images of the lining of the ureters and kidneys. The ureters and kidneys are also part of the urinary tract.

What is the urinary tract and how does it work?

The urinary tract is the body's drainage system for removing urine, which is composed of wastes and extra fluid. In order for normal urination to occur, all body parts in the urinary tract need to work together in the correct order.

Kidneys. The kidneys are two bean-shaped organs, each about the size of a fist. They are located just below the rib cage, one on each side of the spine. Every day, the kidneys filter about 120 to 150 quarts of blood to produce about 1 to 2 quarts of urine. The kidneys work around the clock; a person does not control what they do.

Ureters. Ureters are the thin tubes of muscle—one on each side of the bladder—that carry urine from each of the kidneys to the bladder.

Bladder. The bladder, located in the pelvis between the pelvic bones, is a hollow, muscular, balloon-shaped organ that expands as it fills with urine. Although a person does not control kidney function, a person does control when the bladder empties. Bladder emptying is known as urination. The bladder stores urine until the person finds an appropriate time and place to urinate. A normal bladder acts like a reservoir and can hold 1.5 to 2 cups of urine. How often a person needs to urinate depends on how quickly the kidneys produce the urine that fills the bladder. The muscles of the bladder wall remain relaxed while the bladder fills with urine. As the bladder fills to capacity, signals sent to the brain tell a person to find a toilet soon. During urination, the bladder empties through the urethra, located at the bottom of the bladder.

Three sets of muscles work together like a dam, keeping urine in the bladder.

The first set is the muscles of the urethra itself. The area where the urethra joins the bladder is the bladder neck. The bladder neck, composed of the second set of muscles known as the internal sphincter, helps urine stay in the bladder. The third set of muscles is the pelvic floor muscles, also referred to as the external sphincter, which surround and support the urethra.

To urinate, the brain signals the muscular bladder wall to tighten, squeezing urine out of the bladder. At the same time, the brain signals the sphincters to relax. As the sphincters relax, urine exits the bladder through the urethra.

Why is a cystoscopy or ureteroscopy performed?

A urologist performs a cystoscopy or ureteroscopy to find the cause of, and sometimes treat, urinary tract problems.

Cystoscopy. A urologist performs a cystoscopy to find the cause of urinary tract problems such as

- frequent urinary tract infections (UTIs)

- hematuria—blood in the urine

- frequency—urination eight or more times a day

- urinary urgency—the inability to delay urination

- urinary retention—the inability to empty the bladder completely

- urinary incontinence—the accidental loss of urine

- pain or burning before, during, or after urination

- trouble starting urination, completing urination, or both

- abnormal cells, such as cancer cells, found in a urine sample

During a cystoscopy, a urologist can see

- stones—solid pieces of material in the bladder that may have formed in the kidneys or in the bladder when substances that are normally in the urine become highly concentrated.

- abnormal tissue, polyps, tumors, or cancer in the urethra or bladder.

- stricture, a narrowing of the urethra. Stricture can be a sign of an enlarged prostate in men or of scar tissue in the urethra.

During a cystoscopy, a urologist can treat problems such as bleeding in the bladder and blockage in the urethra. A urologist may also use a cystoscopy to

- remove a stone in the bladder or urethra.
- remove or treat abnormal tissue, polyps, and some types of tumors.
- take small pieces of urethral or bladder tissue for examination with a microscope—a procedure called a biopsy.
- inject material into the wall of the urethra to treat urinary leakage.
- inject medication into the bladder to treat urinary leakage.
- obtain urine samples from the ureters.
- perform retrograde pyelography—an X-ray procedure in which a urologist injects a special dye, called contrast medium, into a ureter to the kidney to create images of urinary flow. The test can show causes of obstruction, such as kidney stones and tumors.
- remove a stent that was placed in the ureter after a ureteroscopy with biopsy or stone removal. A stent is a small, soft tube.

Ureteroscopy. In addition to the causes of urinary tract problems he or she can find with a cystoscope, a urologist performs a ureteroscopy to find the cause of urine blockage in a ureter or to evaluate other abnormalities inside the ureters or kidneys.

During a ureteroscopy, a urologist can see

- a stone in a ureter or kidney
- abnormal tissue, polyps, tumors, or cancer in a ureter or in the lining of a kidney

During a ureteroscopy, a urologist can treat problems such as urine blockage in a ureter. The urologist can also

- remove a stone from a ureter or kidney
- remove or treat abnormal tissue, polyps, and some types of tumors
- perform a biopsy of a ureter or kidney

After a ureteroscopy, the urologist may need to place a stent in a ureter to drain urine from the kidney to the bladder while swelling in the ureter goes away. The stent, which is completely inside the body, may cause some discomfort in the kidney or bladder area. The discomfort is generally mild. The stent may be left in the ureter for a few days to a week or more. The urologist may need to perform a cystoscopy to remove the stent in the ureter.

How does a patient prepare for a cystoscopy or ureteroscopy?

In many cases, a patient does not need special preparations for a cystoscopy. A health care provider may ask the patient to drink plenty of liquids before the procedure, as well as urinate immediately before the procedure.

The patient may need to give a urine sample to test for a UTI. If the patient has a UTI, the urologist may treat the infection with antibiotics before performing a cystoscopy or ureteroscopy. A health care provider will provide instructions before the cystoscopy or ureteroscopy. These instructions may include

- when to stop certain medications, such as blood thinners
- when to stop eating and drinking
- when to empty the bladder before the procedure
- arranging for a ride home after the procedure

The urologist will ask about the patient's medical history, current prescription and over-the-counter medications, and allergies to medications, including anesthetics. The urologist will talk about which anesthetic is best for the procedure and explain what the patient can expect after the procedure.

How is a cystoscopy or ureteroscopy performed?

A urologist performs a cystoscopy or ureteroscopy during an office visit or in an outpatient center or a hospital. For some patients, the urologist will apply an anesthetic gel around the urethral opening or inject a local anesthetic into the urethra. Some patients may require sedation or general anesthesia. The urologist often gives patients sedatives and general anesthesia for a

- ureteroscopy
- cystoscopy with biopsy
- cystoscopy to inject material into the wall of the urethra
- cystoscopy to inject medication into the bladder

For sedation and general anesthesia, a nurse or technician places an intravenous (IV) needle in a vein in the arm or hand to give the medication. Sedation helps the patient relax and be comfortable. General anesthesia puts the patient into a deep sleep during the procedure. The medical staff will monitor the patient's vital signs and try to make him or her as comfortable as possible. During both procedures, a woman will lie on her back with the knees up and spread apart. During a cystoscopy, a man can lie on his back or be in a sitting position.

After the anesthetic has taken effect, the urologist gently inserts the tip of the cystoscope or ureteroscope into the urethra and slowly glides it through the urethra and into the bladder. A sterile liquid—water or salt water, called saline—flows through the cystoscope or ureteroscope to slowly fill the bladder and stretch it so the urologist has a better view of the bladder wall. As the bladder fills with liquid, the patient may feel some discomfort and the urge to urinate. The urologist may remove some of the liquid from the bladder during the procedure. As soon as the procedure is over, the urologist may remove the liquid from the bladder or the patient may empty the bladder.

For a cystoscopy, the urologist examines the lining of the urethra as he or she passes the cystoscope into the bladder. The urologist then examines the lining of the bladder. The urologist can insert small instruments through the cystoscope to treat problems in the urethra and bladder or perform a biopsy.

For a ureteroscopy, the urologist passes the ureteroscope through the bladder and into a ureter. The urologist then examines the lining of the ureter. He or she may pass the ureteroscope all the way up into the kidney. The urologist can insert small instruments through the ureteroscope to treat problems in the ureter or kidney or perform a biopsy.

When a urologist performs a cystoscopy or a ureteroscopy to make a diagnosis, both procedures—including preparation—take 15 to 30 minutes. The time may be longer if the urologist removes a stone in the bladder or a ureter or if he or she performs a biopsy.

What can a patient expect after a cystoscopy or ureteroscopy?

After a cystoscopy or ureteroscopy, a patient may

- have a mild burning feeling when urinating
- see small amounts of blood in the urine
- have mild discomfort in the bladder area or kidney area when urinating
- need to urinate more frequently or urgently

These problems should not last more than 24 hours. The patient should tell a health care provider right away if bleeding or pain is severe or if problems last more than a day.

The health care provider may recommend that the patient

- drink 16 ounces of water each hour for 2 hours after the procedure

- take a warm bath to relieve the burning feeling

- hold a warm, damp washcloth over the urethral opening to relieve discomfort

- take an over-the-counter pain reliever

The health care provider may prescribe an antibiotic to take for 1 or 2 days to prevent an infection. A patient should report any signs of infection—including severe pain, chills, or fever—right away to the health care provider.

Most patients go home the same day as the procedure. Recovery depends on the type of anesthesia. A patient who receives only a local anesthetic can go home immediately. A patient who receives general anesthesia may have to wait 1 to 4 hours before going home. A health care provider usually asks the patient to urinate before leaving. In some cases, the patient may need to stay overnight in the hospital. A health care provider will provide discharge instructions for rest, driving, and physical activities after the procedure.

What are the risks of cystoscopy and ureteroscopy?

The risks of cystoscopy and ureteroscopy include

- UTIs

- abnormal bleeding

- abdominal pain

- a burning feeling or pain during urination

- injury to the urethra, bladder, or ureters

- urethral narrowing due to scar tissue formation

- the inability to urinate due to swelling of surrounding tissues

- complications from anesthesia

Section 31.5

Upper Gastrointestinal (GI) Endoscopy

Text in this section is excerpted from "Upper GI Endoscopy,"
National Institute of Diabetes and Digestive and Kidney Diseases
(NIDDK), November 13, 2014.

What is upper gastrointestinal (GI) endoscopy?

Upper GI endoscopy is a procedure in which a doctor uses an endoscope—a long, flexible tube with a camera—to see the lining of your upper GI tract. A gastroenterologist, surgeon, or other trained health care provider performs the procedure, most often while you receive light sedation. Your doctor may also call the procedure an EGD or esophagogastroduodenoscopy.

Why do doctors use upper GI endoscopy?

Upper GI endoscopy can help find the cause of unexplained symptoms, such as

- persistent heartburn

- bleeding

- nausea and vomiting

- pain

- problems swallowing

- unexplained weight loss

Upper GI endoscopy can also find the cause of abnormal lab tests, such as

- anemia

- nutritional deficiencies

Upper GI endoscopy can identify many different diseases

- anemia

- gastroesophageal reflux disease
- ulcers
- cancer
- inflammation, or swelling
- precancerous abnormalities
- celiac disease

During upper GI endoscopy, a doctor obtains biopsies by passing an instrument through the endoscope to obtain a small piece of tissue. Biopsies are needed to diagnose conditions such as

- cancer
- celiac disease
- gastritis

Doctors also use upper GI endoscopy to

- treat conditions such as bleeding ulcers
- dilate strictures with a small balloon passed through the endoscope
- remove objects, including food, that may be stuck in the upper GI tract

How do I prepare for an upper GI endoscopy?

Talk with your doctor

You should talk with your doctor about medical conditions you have and all prescribed and over-the-counter medicines, vitamins, and supplements you take, including

- aspirin or medicines that contain aspirin
- arthritis medicines
- nonsteroidal anti-inflammatory drugs such as ibuprofen and naproxen
- blood thinners
- blood pressure medicines
- diabetes medicines

Arrange for a ride home

For safety reasons, you can't drive for 24 hours after the procedure, as the sedatives used during the procedure need time to wear off. You will need to make plans for getting a ride home after the procedure.

Do not eat or drink before the procedure

The doctor needs to examine the lining of your upper GI tract during the procedure. If food or drink is in your upper GI tract when you have the procedure, the doctor will not be able to see this lining clearly. To make sure your upper GI tract is clear, the doctor will most often advise you not to eat, drink, smoke, or chew gum during the 8 hours before the procedure.

How do doctors perform an upper GI endoscopy?

A doctor performs an upper GI endoscopy in a hospital or an outpatient center. An intravenous (IV) needle will be placed in your arm to provide a sedative. Sedatives help you stay relaxed and comfortable during the procedure. In some cases, the procedure can be performed without sedation. You will be given a liquid anesthetic to gargle or spray anesthetic on the back of your throat. The anesthetic numbs your throat and calms the gag reflex. The health care staff will monitor your vital signs and keep you as comfortable as possible.

You'll be asked to lie on your side on an exam table. The doctor will carefully feed the endoscope down your esophagus and into your stomach and duodenum. A small camera mounted on the endoscope will send a video image to a monitor, allowing close examination of the lining of your upper GI tract. The endoscope pumps air into your stomach and duodenum, making them easier to see.

During the upper GI endoscopy, the doctor may

- perform a biopsy of tissue in your upper GI tract. You won't feel the biopsy.

- stop any bleeding.

- perform other specialized procedures, such as dilating strictures.

The procedure most often takes between 15 and 30 minutes. The endoscope does not interfere with your breathing, and many people fall asleep during the procedure.

What should I expect from an upper GI endoscopy?

After an upper GI endoscopy, you can expect the following:

- to stay at the hospital or outpatient center for 1 to 2 hours after the procedure so the sedative can wear off

- bloating or nausea for a short time after the procedure

- a sore throat for 1 to 2 days to go back to your normal diet once your swallowing has returned to normal

- to rest at home for the remainder of the day

Following the procedure, you—or a friend or family member who is with you if you're still groggy—will receive instructions on how to care for yourself following the procedure. You should follow all instructions.

Some results from an upper GI endoscopy are available right away after the procedure. After the sedative has worn off, the doctor will share these results with you or, if you choose, with your friend or family member. A pathologist will examine the biopsy tissue to help confirm a diagnosis. Biopsy results take a few days or longer to come back.

What are the risks of an upper GI endoscopy?

The risks of an upper GI endoscopy include

- bleeding from the site where the doctor took the biopsy or removed a polyp

- perforation in the lining of your upper GI tract

- an abnormal reaction to the sedative, including respiratory or cardiac problems

Bleeding and perforation are more common in endoscopies used for treatment rather than testing. Bleeding caused by the procedure often stops without treatment. Research has shown that serious complications occur in one out of every 1,000 upper GI endoscopies. A doctor may need to perform surgery to treat some complications. A doctor can treat an abnormal reaction to a sedative with medicines or IV fluids during or after the procedure.

Seek Care Right Away

If you have any of the following symptoms after an upper GI endoscopy, seek medical care right away:

- chest pain

- problems breathing

- problems swallowing or throat pain that gets worse

- vomiting—particularly if your vomit is bloody or looks like coffee grounds

- pain in your abdomen that gets worse

- bloody or black, tar-colored stool

- fever

Section 31.6

Endoscopic Retrograde Cholangiopancreatography (ERCP)

Text in this section is excerpted from "ERCP (Endoscopic Retrograde Cholangiopancreatography)," National Institute of Diabetes and Digestive and Kidney Diseases (NIDDK), June 29, 2012.

Endoscopic retrograde cholangiopancreatography (ERCP) is a procedure that combines upper gastrointestinal (GI) endoscopy and X-rays to treat problems of the bile and pancreatic ducts. ERCP is also used to diagnose problems, but the availability of non-invasive tests such as magnetic resonance cholangiography has allowed ERCP to be used primarily for cases in which it is expected that treatment will be delivered during the procedure.

What are the bile and pancreatic ducts?

Ducts are tube-like structures in the body that carry fluids. The bile ducts carry bile, a liquid the liver makes to help break down food. A group of small bile ducts—called the biliary tree—in the liver empties bile into the larger common bile duct. Between meals, the common bile duct closes and bile collects in the gallbladder—a pear-shaped sac next to the liver.

The pancreatic ducts carry pancreatic juice, a liquid the pancreas makes to help break down food. A group of small pancreatic ducts in the pancreas empties into the main pancreatic duct.

The common bile duct and the main pancreatic duct join before emptying their contents into the duodenum through the papillary orifice at the end of the duodenal papilla—a small, nipple-like structure that extends into the duodenum.

When is ERCP used?

ERCP is used when it is suspected a person's bile or pancreatic ducts may be narrowed or blocked due to

- tumors
- gallstones that form in the gallbladder and become stuck in the ducts
- inflammation due to trauma or illness, such as pancreatitis—inflammation of the pancreas
- infection
- valves in the ducts, called sphincters, that won't open properly
- scarring of the ducts, called sclerosis
- pseudocysts—accumulations of fluid and tissue debris

How does a person prepare for ERCP?

The health care provider usually provides written instructions about how to prepare for ERCP.

The upper GI tract must be empty. Generally, no eating or drinking is allowed 8 hours before ERCP. Smoking and chewing gum are also prohibited during this time.

Patients should tell their health care provider about all health conditions they have, especially heart and lung problems, diabetes, and allergies. Patients should also tell their health care provider about all medications they take. Patients may be asked to temporarily stop taking medications that affect blood clotting or interact with sedatives, which are usually given during ERCP to help patients relax and stay comfortable.

Medications and vitamins that may be restricted before and after ERCP include

- nonsteroidal anti-inflammatory drugs, such as aspirin, ibuprofen (Advil), and naproxen (Aleve)
- blood thinners
- high blood pressure medication
- diabetes medications
- antidepressants
- dietary supplements

Driving is not permitted for 12 to 24 hours after ERCP to allow the sedatives time to completely wear off. Before the appointment, patients should make plans for a ride home.

How is ERCP performed?

ERCP is conducted at a hospital or outpatient center by a doctor and assistants who have specialized training in this procedure. Patients receive a local anesthetic that is gargled or sprayed on the back of the throat. The anesthetic numbs the throat and calms the gag reflex.

An intravenous needle is inserted into a vein in the arm if sedatives will be given. Doctors and other medical staff monitor vital signs while patients are sedated.

During ERCP, patients lie on their back or side on an X-ray table. The doctor inserts an endoscope down the esophagus, through the stomach, and into the duodenum. Video is transmitted from a small camera attached to the endoscope to a computer screen within the doctor's view. Air is pumped through the endoscope to inflate the stomach and duodenum, making them easier for the doctor to examine.

When the doctor locates the duodenal papilla, a blunt tube called a catheter is slid through the endoscope and guided through the papillary opening. Once the catheter is inside the papilla, the doctor injects a dye into the ducts. The dye, also called contrast medium, allows the ducts to be seen on X-rays. X rays are then taken to see the ducts and to look for narrowed areas or blockages.

Procedures to treat narrowed areas or blockages can be performed during ERCP. To see the ducts during treatment procedures, the doctor uses X-ray video, also called fluoroscopy. Special tools guided through the endoscope and into the ducts allow the doctor to open blocked ducts, break up or remove gallstones, remove tumors in the ducts, or insert stents. Stents are plastic or expandable metal tubes that are left in narrowed ducts to restore the flow of bile or pancreatic juice. A kind of biopsy called brush cytology allows the doctor to remove cells from inside the ducts using a brush that fits through the endoscope. The collected cells are later examined with a microscope for signs of infection or cancer.

Occasionally, ERCP is done after gallbladder surgery, if a surgical bile leak is suspected, to find and stop the leak with a temporary stent.

What does recovery from ERCP involve?

After ERCP, patients are moved to a recovery room where they wait for about an hour for the sedatives to wear off. Patients may not remember conversations with health care staff, as the sedatives reduce memory of events during and after the procedure. During this time, patients may feel bloated or nauseous. Patients may also have a sore throat, which can last a day or two.

Patients can go home after the sedatives wear off. Patients will likely feel tired and should plan to rest for the remainder of the day.

Some ERCP results are available immediately after the procedure. Biopsy results are usually ready in a few days.

Eating, Diet, and Nutrition

Unless otherwise directed, patients may immediately resume their normal diet and medications after having an ERCP. The health care provider can answer any specific questions about eating, diet, and nutrition.

What are the risks associated with ERCP?

Significant risks associated with ERCP include

- infection
- pancreatitis
- allergic reaction to sedatives
- excessive bleeding, called hemorrhage
- puncture of the GI tract or ducts
- tissue damage from radiation exposure
- death, in rare circumstances

When ERCP is performed by an experienced doctor, complications occur in about 6 to 10 percent of patients and these often require hospitalization. Patients who experience any of the following symptoms after ERCP should contact their health care provider immediately:

- swallowing difficulties

- throat, chest, or abdominal pain that worsens

- vomiting

- bloody or dark stool

- fever

Section 31.7

Flexible Sigmoidoscopy

Text in this section is excerpted from "Flexible Sigmoidoscopy,"
National Institute of Diabetes and Digestive and Kidney Diseases
(NIDDK), May 7, 2014.

Flexible sigmoidoscopy is a test that uses a flexible, narrow tube with a light and tiny camera on one end, called a sigmoidoscope or scope, to look inside the rectum and the lower, or sigmoid, colon. Flexible sigmoidoscopy can show irritated or swollen tissue, ulcers, and polyps—extra pieces of tissue that grow on the inner lining of the intestine. A health care provider performs the procedure during an office visit or at a hospital or an outpatient center.

What are the rectum and sigmoid colon?

The rectum and sigmoid colon are parts of the gastrointestinal (GI) tract, a series of hollow organs joined in a long, twisting tube from the mouth to the anus—the 1-inch opening through which stool leaves the body. Organs that make up the GI tract are the mouth, esophagus, stomach, small intestine, large intestine, and anus. The last part of the GI tract—called the lower GI tract—consists of the large intestine and anus.

Organs that make up the GI tract are the mouth, esophagus, stomach, small intestine, large intestine, and anus.

The large intestine is about 5 feet long and includes the appendix, cecum, colon, rectum, and anus. The large intestine changes waste from liquid to a solid matter called stool. Stool passes from the colon to the rectum. The rectum stores stool prior to a bowel movement.

The colon has four main parts:

- ascending colon

- transverse colon

- descending colon

- sigmoid colon

The sigmoid colon is the last section of the colon. The rectum is 6 to 8 inches long in adults and is located between the sigmoid colon and the anus. During a bowel movement, stool moves from the rectum to the anus and out of the body.

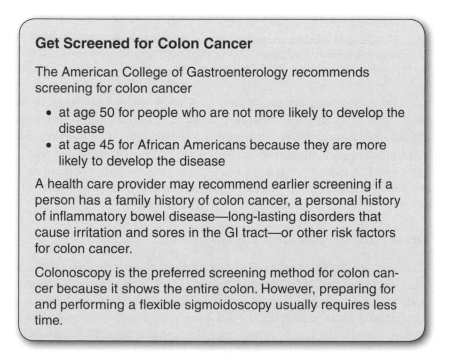

Get Screened for Colon Cancer

The American College of Gastroenterology recommends screening for colon cancer

- at age 50 for people who are not more likely to develop the disease
- at age 45 for African Americans because they are more likely to develop the disease

A health care provider may recommend earlier screening if a person has a family history of colon cancer, a personal history of inflammatory bowel disease—long-lasting disorders that cause irritation and sores in the GI tract—or other risk factors for colon cancer.

Colonoscopy is the preferred screening method for colon cancer because it shows the entire colon. However, preparing for and performing a flexible sigmoidoscopy usually requires less time.

Medicare and private insurance companies sometimes change whether and how often they pay for cancer screening tests. People should check with their insurance company to find out how often their coverage will allow a screening flexible sigmoidoscopy.

Why is a flexible sigmoidoscopy performed?

A health care provider performs a flexible sigmoidoscopy to help diagnose

- changes in bowel habits
- abdominal pain
- bleeding from the anus
- weight loss

A health care provider may also perform a flexible sigmoidoscopy as a screening test for colon cancer. Screening is testing for a disease when a person has no symptoms. Screening may find diseases at an early stage, when there may be a better chance of curing the disease.

How does a person prepare for a flexible sigmoidoscopy?

A person prepares for a flexible sigmoidoscopy by

- **talking with a health care provider.** A person should talk with his or her health care provider about medical conditions he or she has and all prescribed and over-the-counter medications, vitamins, and supplements he or she takes, including
- arthritis medications
- aspirin or medications that contain aspirin
- blood thinners
- diabetes medications
- nonsteroidal anti-inflammatory drugs such as ibuprofen or naproxen
- vitamins that contain iron or iron supplements
- **cleansing the bowel.** The health care provider will give written bowel prep instructions to follow at home. A health care

399

provider orders a bowel prep so that little to no stool is present inside the person's intestine. A complete bowel prep lets the person pass stool that is clear. Stool inside the colon can prevent the health care provider from clearly seeing the lining of the intestine. Instructions may include following a clear liquid diet for 1 to 3 days before the procedure and avoiding drinks that contain red or purple dye. The instructions will provide specific direction about when to start and stop the clear liquid diet. During this diet, people may drink or eat the following:

- fat-free bouillon or broth

- gelatin in flavors such as lemon, lime, or orange

- plain coffee or tea, without cream or milk

- sports drinks in flavors such as lemon, lime, or orange

- strained fruit juice, such as apple or white grape—orange juice is not recommended

- water

The person needs to take laxatives and enemas the night before and several hours before a flexible sigmoidoscopy. A laxative is medication that loosens stool and increases bowel movements. An enema involves flushing water or laxative into the rectum using a special wash bottle. Laxatives and enemas can cause diarrhea, so the person should stay close to a bathroom during the bowel prep.

Laxatives are usually swallowed in pill form or as a powder dissolved in water. Some people will need to drink a large amount, usually a gallon, of liquid laxative over the course of the bowel prep at scheduled times. People may find this part of the prep difficult; however, it is important to complete the prep. The health care provider will not be able to see the sigmoid colon clearly if the prep is incomplete.

People should call the health care provider if they are having side effects that make them feel they can't finish the prep.

How is a flexible sigmoidoscopy performed?

A health care provider performs a flexible sigmoidoscopy during an office visit or at a hospital or an outpatient center. A person usually does not need anesthesia, and the procedure takes about 20 minutes.

For the test, the person will lie on a table while the health care provider inserts a sigmoidoscope into the anus and slowly guides it through the rectum and into the sigmoid colon. The scope inflates the large intestine with air to give the health care provider a better view. The camera sends a video image of the intestinal lining to a computer screen, allowing the health care provider to examine the tissues lining the sigmoid colon and rectum. The health care provider may ask the person to move several times so he or she can adjust the scope for better viewing. Once the scope has reached the transverse colon, the health care provider withdraws it slowly while examining the lining of the colon again.

For the test, the person will lie on a table while the health care provider inserts a sigmoidoscope into the anus and slowly guides it through the rectum and into the sigmoid colon.

The health care provider can remove polyps during flexible sigmoidoscopy and send them to a lab for testing. Polyps are common in adults and are usually harmless. However, most colon cancer begins as a polyp, so removing polyps early is an effective way to prevent cancer.

The health care provider may also perform a biopsy, a procedure that involves taking a small piece of intestinal lining for examination with a microscope. The person will not feel the biopsy. A pathologist—a doctor who specializes in diagnosing diseases—will examine the tissue.

The health care provider may pass tiny tools through the scope to remove polyps and take a sample for biopsy. If bleeding occurs, the health care provider can usually stop it with an electrical probe or special medications passed through the scope. If the health care provider finds polyps or other abnormal tissues, he or she may suggest examining the rest of the colon with a colonoscopy.

What can a person expect after a flexible sigmoidoscopy?

After a flexible sigmoidoscopy, a person can expect

- abdominal cramps or bloating during the first hour after the test.

- resume regular activities immediately after the test.

- to return to a normal diet.

- a member of the health care team to review the discharge instructions with the person and provide a written copy. The person should follow all instructions given.

Some results from a flexible sigmoidoscopy are available immediately after the procedure, and the health care provider will share results with the person. Biopsy results take a few days to come back.

What are the risks of flexible sigmoidoscopy?

The risks of flexible sigmoidoscopy include

- bleeding.

- perforation—a hole or tear in the lining of the colon.

- severe abdominal pain.

- diverticulitis—a condition that occurs when small pouches in the colon, called diverticula, become irritated, swollen, and infected.

- cardiovascular events, such as a heart attack, low blood pressure, or the heart skipping beats or beating too fast or too slow.

- death, although this risk is rare.

Bleeding and perforation are the most common complications from flexible sigmoidoscopy. Most cases of bleeding occur in people who have polyps removed. The health care provider can treat bleeding that occurs during the flexible sigmoidoscopy right away. However, a person may have delayed bleeding up to 2 weeks after the test. The health care provider diagnoses delayed bleeding with a colonoscopy or repeat flexible sigmoidoscopy and treats it with an electrical probe or special medication. A person may need surgery to treat perforation.

Seek Immediate Care

People who have any of the following symptoms after a flexible sigmoidoscopy should seek immediate care.

- severe abdominal pain
- fever
- continued bloody bowel movements or continued bleeding from the anus
- dizziness
- weakness

Chapter 32

Transesophageal Echocardiography (TEE)

What Is Transesophageal Echocardiography?

Transesophageal echocardiography (TEE) is a test that uses sound waves to create high-quality moving pictures of the heart and its blood vessels.

TEE is a type of echocardiography (echo). Echo shows the size and shape of the heart and how well the heart chambers and valves are working.

Echo can pinpoint areas of heart muscle that aren't contracting well because of poor blood flow or injury from a previous heart attack.

Echo also can detect possible blood clots inside the heart, fluid buildup in the pericardium (the sac around the heart), and problems with the aorta. The aorta is the main artery that carries oxygen-rich blood from your heart to your body.

Overview

During echo, a device called a transducer is used to send sound waves (called ultrasound) to the heart. As the ultrasound waves bounce off the structures of the heart, a computer in the echo machine converts them into pictures on a screen.

Text in this chapter is excerpted from "Transesophageal Echocardiography," National Heart, Lung, and Blood Institute (NHLBI), March 12, 2012.

TEE involves a flexible tube (probe) with a transducer at its tip. Your doctor will guide the probe down your throat and into your esophagus (the passage leading from your mouth to your stomach). This approach allows your doctor to get more detailed pictures of your heart because the esophagus is directly behind the heart.

TEE can help doctors diagnose heart and blood vessel diseases and conditions in adults and children. Doctors also may use TEE to guide cardiac catheterization (KATH-eh-ter-ih-ZA-shun), help prepare for surgery, or assess a patient's status during or after surgery.

Doctors may use TEE in addition to transthoracic (tranz-thor-AS-ik) echo (TTE), the most common type of echo. If TTE pictures don't give doctors enough information, they may recommend TEE to get more detailed pictures.

Outlook

TEE has a low risk of complications in both adults and children. Even newborns can have TEE.

Types of Transesophageal Echocardiography

Standard transesophageal echocardiography (TEE) pictures are two-dimensional (2D). It's also possible to get three-dimensional (3D) pictures from TEE. These pictures provide even more details about the structure and function of the heart and its blood vessels.

Doctors can use 3D TEE to help diagnose heart problems, such as congenital heart disease and heart valve disease. Doctors also may use this technology to assist with heart surgery.

Who Needs Transesophageal Echocardiography?

Doctors may recommend transesophageal echocardiography (TEE) to help diagnose a heart or blood vessel disease or condition. TEE can be used for adults and children.

Doctors also may use TEE to guide cardiac catheterization, help prepare for surgery, or assess a patient's status during or after surgery.

Transesophageal Echocardiography as a Diagnostic Tool

TEE helps doctors detect problems with the structure and function of the heart and its blood vessels.

In general, transthoracic echo (TTE) is the first echo test used to diagnose heart and blood vessel problems. However, you might have

TEE if your doctor needs more information or more detailed pictures than TTE can provide.

For TTE, the transducer (the device that sends the sound waves) is placed on the chest, outside of the body. This means the sound waves may not always have a clear path to the heart and blood vessels. For example, obesity, scarring from previous heart surgery, or certain lung problems (such as a collapsed lung) may block the sound waves.

For TEE, the transducer is at the tip of a flexible tube (probe). Your doctor will guide the probe down your throat and into your esophagus (the passage leading from your mouth to your stomach).

This approach allows your doctor to get more detailed pictures of your heart because the esophagus is directly behind the heart.

Doctors may use TEE to help diagnose:

- Coronary heart disease

- Congenital heart disease

- Heart attack

- Aortic aneurysm

- Endocarditis

- Cardiomyopathy

- Heart valve disease

- Injury to the heart or aorta (the main artery that carries oxygen-rich blood from your heart to your body)

TEE also can show blood clots that may have caused a stroke or that may affect treatment for atrial fibrillation, a type of arrhythmia.

Transesophageal Echocardiography and Cardiac Catheterization

Cardiac catheterization is a medical procedure used to diagnose and/or treat certain heart conditions. During this procedure, a long, thin, flexible tube called a catheter is put into a blood vessel in your arm, groin (upper thigh), or neck and threaded to your heart.

Doctors may use TEE to help guide the catheter while they're doing the procedure.

Through the catheter, doctors can do tests and treatments on your heart. For example, cardiac catheterization might be used to repair holes in the heart, heart valve disease, and abnormal heart rhythms.

Transesophageal Echocardiography and Surgery

Doctors may use TEE to prepare for a patient's surgery and identify possible risks. For example, they may use TEE to look for possible sources of blood clots in the heart or aorta. Blood clots can cause a stroke during surgery.

TEE might be used in the operating room after a patient receives medicine to make him or her sleep during the surgery. The test can show the heart's structure and function and help guide the surgery.

TEE also helps doctors assess a patient's status during surgery. For example, TEE can help check for blood flow and blood pressure problems.

At the end of surgery, TEE might be used again to check how well the surgery worked. For example, TEE can show whether heart valves are working well. TEE also can show how well the heart is pumping.

People having surgery that isn't related to the heart also may have TEE to check their heart function if they have known heart disease or a critical illness.

What to Expect before Transesophageal Echocardiography

Transesophageal echocardiography (TEE) most often is done in a hospital. You usually will need to fast (not eat or drink) for several hours prior to the test. Your doctor will let you know exactly how long you should fast.

You should let your doctor know whether you're taking any blood-thinning medicines, have trouble swallowing, or are allergic to any medicines. If you have dentures or oral prostheses, you'll need to remove them before the test.

You may be given medicine to help you relax during TEE. If so, you'll have to arrange for a ride home after the test because the medicine can make you sleepy.

Talk with your doctor about whether you need to take any special steps before having TEE. Your doctor can tell you whether you need to change how you take your regular medicines on the day of the test or whether you need to make other changes.

What to Expect during Transesophageal Echocardiography

During transesophageal echocardiography (TEE), your doctor or your child's doctor will use a probe with a transducer at its tip. The transducer sends sound waves (ultrasound) to the heart. Probes come in many sizes; smaller probes are used for children and newborns.

The back of your mouth will be numbed with gel or spray before the probe is put down your throat. You may feel some discomfort as the probe is guided into your esophagus (the passage leading from your mouth to your stomach).

Adults having TEE may get medicine to help them relax during the test. The medicine will be injected into a vein.

Children always receive medicine to help them relax or sleep if they're having TEE. This helps them remain still so the doctor can safely insert the probe and take good pictures of the heart and blood vessels.

Your doctor will insert the probe into your mouth or nose. He or she will then gently guide it down your throat into your esophagus. Your esophagus lies directly behind your heart. During this process, your doctor will take care to protect your teeth and mouth from injury.

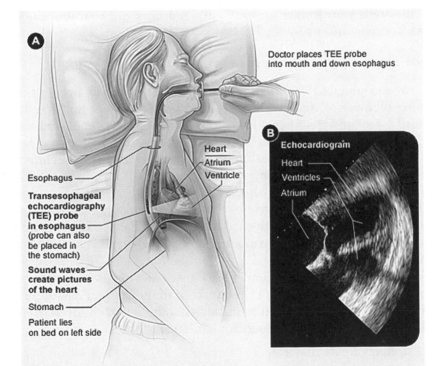

Figure 32.1. Transesophageal Echocardiography: *"A" shows a transesophageal echocardiography probe in the esophagus, which is located behind the heart. Sound waves from the probe create high-quality pictures of the heart. "B" shows an echocardiogram of the heart's lower and upper chambers (ventricles and atrium, respectively).*

Your blood pressure, blood oxygen level, and other vital signs will be checked during the test. You may be given oxygen through a tube in your nose.

TEE takes less than an hour. However, if you received medicine to help you relax, you might be watched for a few hours after the test for side effects from the medicine.

What to Expect after Transesophageal Echocardiography

After having transesophageal echocardiography (TEE), your or your child's blood pressure, blood oxygen level, and other vital signs will continue to be closely watched. You can likely go home a few hours after having the test.

After the TEE, you may have a sore throat for a few hours. You shouldn't eat or drink for 30–60 minutes after having TEE. Most people can return to their normal activities within about 24 hours of the test.

Talk with your doctor or your child's doctor to learn more about what to expect after having TEE.

What Does Transesophageal Echocardiography Show?

Transesophageal echocardiography (TEE) provides high-quality moving pictures of your heart and blood vessels. These pictures help doctors detect and treat heart and blood vessel diseases and conditions.

TEE creates pictures from inside the esophagus (the passage leading from the mouth to the stomach) or, sometimes, from inside the stomach. Because the esophagus lies directly behind the heart, TEE provides closeup pictures of the heart.

TEE also offers different views and may provide more detailed pictures than transthoracic echocardiography (TTE), the most common type of echo. (For TTE, the transducer is placed on the chest, outside of the body.)

Your doctor may recommend TEE if he or she needs more information than TTE can provide. TEE can help diagnose and assess heart and blood vessel diseases and conditions in adults and children. Examples of these diseases and conditions include:

- Coronary heart disease
- Congenital heart disease
- Heart attack
- Aortic aneurysm
- Endocarditis

- Cardiomyopathy

- Heart valve disease

- Injury to the heart or aorta (the main artery that carries oxygen-rich blood from your heart to your body)

TEE also can show blood clots that may have caused a stroke or that may affect treatment for atrial fibrillation, a type of arrhythmia.

Doctors also may use TEE during cardiac catheterization. TEE can help doctors guide the catheter (thin, flexible tube) through the blood vessels. TEE also can help doctors prepare for surgery or assess a patient's status during or after surgery.

What Are the Risks of Transesophageal Echocardiography?

Transesophageal echocardiography (TEE) has a very low risk of serious complications in both adults and children. To reduce your risk, your health care team will carefully check your heart rate and other vital signs during and after the test.

Some risks are associated with the medicine that might be used to help you relax during TEE. You may have a bad reaction to the medicine, problems breathing, or nausea (feeling sick to your stomach). Usually, these problems go away without treatment.

Your throat also might be sore for a few hours after the test. Although rare, the probe used during TEE can damage the esophagus (the passage leading from your mouth to your stomach).

Chapter 33

Electrocardiograms (EKG) and Holter and Event Monitors

Electrocardiogram (EKG)

Doctors use a test called an EKG (electrocardiogram) to help diagnose heart block. This test detects and records the heart's electrical activity. An EKG records the strength and timing of electrical signals as they pass through the heart.

The data are recorded on a graph so your doctor can study your heart's electrical activity. Different parts of the graph show each step of an electrical signal's journey through the heart.

Each electrical signal begins in a group of cells called the sinus node or sinoatrial (SA) node. The SA node is located in the right atrium, which is the upper right chamber of the heart. (Your heart has two upper chambers and two lower chambers.)

In a healthy adult heart at rest, the SA node sends an electrical signal to begin a new heartbeat 60 to 100 times a minute.

From the SA node, the signal travels through the right and left atria. This causes the atria to contract, which helps move blood into

Text in this chapter is excerpted from "Holter and Event Monitors," National Heart, Lung, and Blood Institute (NHLBI), March 16, 2012; and text from "Heart Block," National Heart, Lung, and Blood Institute (NHLBI), July 9, 2012.

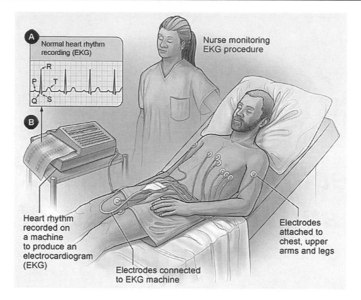

Figure 33.1. *Electrocardiogram: The image shows the standard setup for an EKG. In "A," a normal heart rhythm recording shows the electrical pattern of a regular heartbeat. In "B," a patient lies in a bed with EKG electrodes attached to his chest, upper arms, and legs. A nurse monitors the painless procedure.*

the heart's lower chambers, the ventricles. The electrical signal moving through the atria is recorded as the P wave on the EKG.

The electrical signal passes between the atria and ventricles through a group of cells called the atrioventricular (AV) node. The signal slows down as it passes through the AV node. This slowing allows the ventricles enough time to finish filling with blood. On the EKG, this part of the process is the flat line between the end of the P wave and the beginning of the Q wave.

The electrical signal then leaves the AV node and travels along a pathway called the bundle of His. From there, the signal travels into the right and left bundle branches. The signal spreads quickly across your heart's ventricles, causing them to contract and pump blood to your lungs and the rest of your body. This process is recorded as the QRS waves on the EKG.

The ventricles then recover their normal electrical state (shown as the T wave on the EKG). The muscle stops contracting to allow the heart to refill with blood. This entire process continues over and over with each new heartbeat.

What Are Holter and Event Monitors?

Holter and event monitors are medical devices that record the heart's electrical activity. Doctors most often use these monitors to diagnose arrhythmias.

Arrhythmias are problems with the rate or rhythm of the heartbeat. During an arrhythmia, the heart can beat too fast, too slow, or with an irregular rhythm.

Holter and event monitors also are used to detect silent myocardial ischemia. In this condition, not enough oxygen-rich blood reaches the heart muscle. "Silent" means that no symptoms occur.

The monitors also can check whether treatments for an arrhythmia or silent myocardial ischemia are working.

This chapter focuses on using Holter and event monitors to diagnose problems with the heart's rate or rhythm.

Overview

Holter and event monitors are similar to an EKG (electrocardiogram). An EKG is a simple test that detects and records the heart's electrical activity. It's a common test for diagnosing heart rhythm problems.

However, a standard EKG only records the heartbeat for a few seconds. It won't detect heart rhythm problems that don't occur during the test.

Holter and event monitors are small, portable devices. You can wear one while you do your normal daily activities. This allows the monitor to record your heart for a longer time than an EKG.

Some people have heart rhythm problems that occur only during certain activities, such as sleeping or physical exertion. Using a Holter or event monitor increases the chance of recording these problems.

Although similar, Holter and event monitors aren't the same. A Holter monitor records your heart's electrical activity the entire time you're wearing it. An event monitor records your heart's electrical activity only at certain times while you're wearing it.

Types of Holter and Event Monitors

Holter Monitors

Holter monitors sometimes are called continuous EKGs. This is because Holter monitors record your heart rhythm continuously for 24 to 48 hours.

A Holter monitor is about the size of a large deck of cards. You can clip it to a belt or carry it in a pocket. Wires connect the device to sensors (called electrodes) that are stuck to your chest using sticky patches. These sensors detect your heart's electrical signals, and the monitor records your heart rhythm.

Wireless Holter Monitors

Wireless Holter monitors have a longer recording time than standard Holter monitors. Wireless monitors record your heart's electrical activity for a preset amount of time.

These monitors use wireless cellular technology to send the recorded data to your doctor's office or a company that checks the data. The device sends the data automatically at certain times. Wireless monitors still have wires that connect the device to the sensors on your chest.

You can use a wireless Holter monitor for days or even weeks, until signs or symptoms of a heart rhythm problem occur. These monitors usually are used to detect heart rhythm problems that don't occur often.

Although wireless Holter monitors work for longer periods, they have a down side. You must remember to write down the time of symptoms so your doctor can match it to the heart rhythm recording. Also, the batteries in the wireless monitor must be changed every 1–2 days.

Event Monitors

Event monitors are similar to Holter monitors. You wear one while you do your normal daily activities. Most event monitors have wires that connect the device to sensors. The sensors are stuck to your chest using sticky patches.

Unlike Holter monitors, event monitors don't continuously record your heart's electrical activity. They only record during symptoms. For many event monitors, you need to start the device when you feel symptoms. Some event monitors start automatically if they detect abnormal heart rhythms.

Event monitors tend to be smaller than Holter monitors because they don't need to store as much data.

Different types of event monitors work in slightly different ways. Your doctor will explain how to use the monitor before you start wearing it.

Postevent Recorders

Postevent recorders are among the smallest event monitors. You can wear a postevent recorder like a wristwatch or carry it in your pocket. The pocket version is about the size of a thick credit card. These monitors don't have wires that connect the device to chest sensors.

To start the recorder when you feel a symptom, you hold it to your chest. To start the wristwatch version, you touch a button on the side of the watch.

A postevent recorder only records what happens after you start it. It may miss a heart rhythm problem that occurs before and during the onset of symptoms. Also, it might be hard to start the monitor when a symptom is in progress.

In some cases, the missing data could have helped your doctor diagnose the heart rhythm problem.

Presymptom Memory Loop Recorders

Presymptom memory loop recorders are the size of a small cell phone. They're also called continuous loop event recorders.

You can clip this event monitor to your belt or carry it in your pocket. Wires connect the device to sensors on your chest.

These recorders are always recording and erasing data. When you feel a symptom, you push a button on the device. The normal erase process stops. The recording will show a few minutes of data from before, during, and after the symptom. This may make it possible for your doctor to see very brief changes in your heart rhythm.

Autodetect Recorders

Autodetect recorders are about the size of the palm of your hand. Wires connect the device to sensors on your chest.

You don't need to start an autodetect recorder during symptoms. These recorders detect abnormal heart rhythms and automatically record and send the data to your doctor's office.

Implantable Loop Recorders

You may need an implantable loop recorder if other event monitors can't provide enough data. Implantable loop recorders are about the size of a pack of gum. This type of event monitor is inserted under the skin on your chest. No wires or chest sensors are used.

Your doctor can program the device to record when you start it during symptoms or automatically if it detects an abnormal heart rhythm. Devices may differ, so your doctor will tell you how to use your recorder. Sometimes a special card is held close to the recorder to start it.

Other Names for Holter and Event Monitors

- Ambulatory EKG or ECG. (The terms "EKG" and "ECG" both stand for electrocardiogram.)

- Continuous EKG or ECG.

- EKG event monitors.

- Episodic monitors.

- Mobile cardiac outpatient telemetry systems. This is another name for autodetect recorders.

- Thirty-day event recorders.

- Transtelephonic event monitors. These monitors require the patient to send the collected data by telephone to a doctor's office or a company that checks the data.

Who Needs a Holter or Event Monitor?

Your doctor may recommend a Holter or event monitor if he or she thinks you have an arrhythmia. An arrhythmia is a problem with the rate or rhythm of the heartbeat.

Holter and event monitors most often are used to detect arrhythmias in people who have:

- Issues with fainting or feeling dizzy. A monitor might be used if causes other than a heart rhythm problem have been ruled out.

- Palpitations that recur with no known cause. Palpitations are feelings that your heart is skipping a beat, fluttering, or beating too hard or fast. You may have these feelings in your chest, throat, or neck.

People who are being treated for heart rhythm problems also may need to use Holter or event monitors. The monitors can show how well their treatments are working.

Heart rhythm problems may occur only during certain activities, such sleeping or physical exertion. Holter and event monitors record your heart rhythm while you do your normal daily routine. This allows your doctor to see how your heart responds to various activities.

What to Expect before Using a Holter or Event Monitor

Your doctor will do a physical exam before giving you a Holter or event monitor. He or she may:

- Check your pulse to find out how fast your heart is beating (your heart rate) and whether your heart rhythm is steady or irregular.

- Measure your blood pressure.

- Check for swelling in your legs or feet. Swelling could be a sign of an enlarged heart or heart failure, which may cause an arrhythmia. An arrhythmia is a problem with the rate or rhythm of the heartbeat.

- Look for signs of other diseases that might cause heart rhythm problems, such as thyroid disease.

You may have an EKG (electrocardiogram) test before your doctor sends you home with a Holter or event monitor.

An EKG is a simple test that records your heart's electrical activity for a few seconds. The test shows how fast your heart is beating and its rhythm (steady or irregular). An EKG also records the strength and timing of electrical signals as they pass through your heart.

A standard EKG won't detect heart rhythm problems that don't happen during the test. For this reason, your doctor may give you a Holter or event monitor. These monitors are portable. You can wear one while doing your normal daily activities. This increases the chance of recording symptoms that only occur once in a while.

Your doctor will explain how to wear and use the Holter or event monitor. Usually, you'll leave the office wearing it.

Each type of monitor is slightly different, but most have sensors (called electrodes) that attach to the skin on your chest using sticky patches. The sensors need good contact with your skin. Poor contact can cause poor results.

Oil, too much sweat, and hair can keep the patches from sticking to your skin. You may need to shave the area on your chest where your doctor will attach the patches. If you have to replace the patches, you'll need to clean the area with a special prep pad that the doctor will provide.

You may need to use a small amount of special paste or gel to help the patches stick to your skin. Some patches come with paste or gel on them.

What to Expect while Using a Holter or Event Monitor

Your experience while using a Holter or event monitor depends on the type of monitor you have. However, most monitors have some factors in common.

Recording the Heart's Electrical Activity

All monitors record the heart's electrical activity. Thus, maintaining a clear signal between the sensors (electrodes) and the recording device is important.

In most cases, the sensors are attached to your chest using sticky patches. Wires connect the sensors to the monitor. You usually can clip the monitor to your belt or carry it in your pocket. (Postevent recorders and implantable loop recorders don't have chest sensors.)

A good stick between the patches and your skin helps provide a clear signal. Poor contact leads to a poor recording that's hard for your doctor to read.

Oil, too much sweat, and hair can keep the patches from sticking to your skin. You may need to shave the area where your doctor will attach the patches. If you have to replace the patches, you'll need to clean the area with a special prep pad that your doctor will provide.

You may need to use a small amount of special paste or gel to help the patches stick to your skin. Some patches come with paste or gel on them.

Too much movement can pull the patches away from your skin or create "noise" on the EKG (electrocardiogram) strip. An EKG strip is a graph showing the pattern of the heartbeat. Noise looks like a lot of jagged lines; it makes it hard for your doctor to see the real rhythm of your heart.

When you have a symptom, stop what you're doing. This will ensure that the recording shows your heart's activity rather than your movement.

Your doctor will tell you whether you need to adjust your activity level during the testing period. If you exercise, choose a cool location to avoid sweating too much. This will help the patches stay sticky.

Other everyday items also can disrupt the signal between the sensors and the monitor. These items include magnets; metal detectors; microwave ovens; and electric blankets, toothbrushes, and razors. Avoid using these items. Also avoid areas with high voltage.

Cell phones and MP3 players (such as iPods) may interfere with the signal between the sensors and the monitor if they're too close to the monitor. When using any electronic device, try to keep it at least 6 inches away from the monitor.

Keeping a Diary

While using a Holter or event monitor, your doctor will advise you to keep a diary of your symptoms and activities. Write down what type of symptoms you're having, when they occur, and what you were doing at the time.

The most common symptoms of heart rhythm problems include:

- Fainting or feeling dizzy.
- Palpitations. These are feelings that your heart is skipping a beat, fluttering, or beating too hard or fast. You may have these feelings in your chest, throat, or neck.

Make sure to note the time that symptoms occur, because your doctor will match the data with the information in your diary. This allows your doctor to see whether certain activities trigger changes in your heart rate and rhythm.

Also, include details in your diary about when you take any medicine or if you feel stress at certain times during the testing period.

What to Expect with Specific Monitors

Holter Monitors

Holter monitors are about the size of a large deck of cards. You'll wear one for 24 to 48 hours. You can't get your monitor wet, so you won't be able to bathe or shower. You can take a sponge bath if needed.

When the testing period is done, you'll return the device to your doctor's office. The results will be stored on the device.

The recording period for a standard Holter monitor might be too short to capture a heart rhythm problem. If this is the case, your doctor may recommend a wireless Holter monitor.

Wireless Holter Monitors

Wireless Holter monitors can record for a longer time than standard Holter monitors. You can use a wireless Holter monitor for days or even weeks, until signs or symptoms of a heart rhythm problem occur.

Wireless monitors record for a preset amount of time. Then they automatically send data to your doctor's office or a company that checks the data.

These monitors use wireless cellular technology to send data. However, they still have wires that connect the device to the sensors stuck to your chest.

The batteries in the wireless monitor must be changed every 1–2 days. You'll need to detach the sensors to shower or bathe and then reattach them.

Event Monitors

Event monitors are slightly smaller than Holter monitors. They can be worn for weeks or until symptoms occur. Most event monitors are worn like Holter monitors—clipped to a belt or carried in a pocket.

When you have symptoms, you simply push a button on your monitor to start recording. Some event monitors start automatically if they detect abnormal heart rhythms.

Postevent Recorders

Postevent recorders can be worn like a wristwatch or carried in a pocket. The pocket version is about the size of a thick credit card. These recorders don't have wires that connect the device to chest sensors.

To start the recorder when you feel a symptom, you hold it to your chest. To start the wristwatch version, you touch a button on the side of the watch.

You send the stored data to your doctor's office using a telephone. Your doctor will explain how to use the monitor before you leave his or her office.

Autodetect Recorders

Autodetect recorders are about the size of the palm of your hand. Wires connect the device to sensors on your chest.

You don't need to start an autodetect recorder. This type of monitor automatically starts recording if it detects abnormal heart rhythms. It then sends the data to your doctor's office.

Implantable Loop Recorders

Implantable loop recorders are about the size of a pack of gum. This type of event monitor is inserted under the skin on your chest. Your doctor will discuss the procedure with you. No chest sensors are used with implantable loop recorders.

Your doctor can program the device to record when you start it during symptoms or automatically if it detects an abnormal heart rhythm. Devices may differ, so your doctor will tell you how to use your recorder. Sometimes a special card is held close to the device to start it.

What to Expect after Using a Holter or Event Monitor

After you're finished using a Holter or event monitor, you'll return it to your doctor's office or the place where you picked it up.

If you were using an implantable loop recorder, your doctor will need to remove it from your chest. He or she will discuss the procedure with you.

Your doctor will tell you when to expect the results. Once your doctor has reviewed the recordings, he or she will discuss the results with you.

What Does a Holter or Event Monitor Show?

A Holter or event monitor may show what's causing symptoms of an arrhythmia. An arrhythmia is a problem with the rate or rhythm of the heartbeat.

A Holter or event monitor also can show whether a heart rhythm problem is harmless or requires treatment. The monitor might alert your doctor to medical conditions that can result in heart failure, stroke, or sudden cardiac arrest.

If the symptoms of a heart rhythm problem occur often, a Holter or event monitor has a good chance of recording them. You may not have symptoms while using a monitor. Even so, your doctor can learn more about your heart rhythm from the test results.

Sometimes Holter and event monitors can't help doctors diagnose heart rhythm problems. If this happens, talk with your doctor about other steps you can take.

One option might be to try a different type of monitor. Wireless Holter monitors and implantable loop recorders have longer recording periods. This may allow your doctor to get the data he or she needs to make a diagnosis.

What Are the Risks of Using a Holter or Event Monitor?

The sticky patches used to attach the sensors (electrodes) to your chest have a small risk of skin irritation. You also may have an allergic reaction to the paste or gel that's sometimes used to attach the patches. The irritation will go away once the patches are removed.

If you're using an implantable loop recorder, you may get an infection or have pain where the device is placed under the skin. Your doctor can prescribe medicine to treat these problems.

Part Six

Screening and Assessments for Specific Conditions and Diseases

Chapter 34

Allergy Testing

Chapter Contents

Section 34.1

Testing for Environmental Allergies

Text in this section is excerpted from "Environmental Allergies,"
National Institute of Allergy and Infectious Diseases (NIAID),
April 22, 2015.

Environmental Allergies

An allergic reaction is a specific response of the body's immune system to a normally harmless substance called an allergen. A variety of environmental allergens, such as pollen and animal dander, can trigger allergic reactions in the nose (allergic rhinitis, or hay fever) and in the lung (asthma). Not all reasons for susceptibility to environmental allergies are understood, although a family history of allergies is an important risk factor. NIAID supports and conducts research aimed at understanding how allergic rhinitis and asthma develop and identifying new strategies to diagnose, treat, and prevent environmental allergies.

Understanding Environmental Allergies

Causes of Environmental Allergies

Both genetic and environmental factors can contribute to the development of allergies. Allergic rhinitis (hay fever) and asthma are triggered by exposure to airborne allergens. Sources of allergens include pollens, pet dander, house dust mites, molds, cockroaches, and rodents.

Pollen

Each spring, summer, and fall, plants release tiny pollen grains to fertilize other plants of the same species.

People with allergic rhinitis or asthma aggravated by pollen have symptoms only for the period or season when the pollen grains to which they are allergic are in the air. For example, in most parts of the United States, grass pollen is present during the spring. Allergic rhinitis caused by pollen, also called "seasonal allergic rhinitis," affects approximately 7 percent of adults and 9 percent of children in the

United States. However, not all seasonal symptoms are due to pollen. Rhinovirus, the cause of the common cold, causes runny noses and triggers asthma attacks in the fall and spring. It is not always easy to figure out whether allergy or a common cold is the cause of these symptoms, although some clues can help tell the two apart. For example, a fever suggests a cold rather than an allergy, and symptoms lasting more than two weeks suggest allergies rather than a cold.

Most of the pollens that generate allergic reactions come from trees, weeds, and grasses. These plants make small, light, and dry pollen grains that are carried by wind. Among North American plants, grasses are the most common cause of allergy. Ragweed is a main culprit among the weeds, but other major sources of weed pollen include sagebrush, pigweed, lamb's quarters, and tumbleweed. Certain species of trees, including birch, cedar, and oak, also produce highly allergenic pollen. Plants that are pollinated with the help of insects, such as roses and ornamental flowering trees like cherry and pear trees, usually do not cause allergic rhinitis or asthma.

A pollen count, often reported by local weather broadcasts or allergy websites, is a measure of how much pollen is in the air. Pollen counts tend to be highest early in the morning on warm, dry, breezy days and lowest during chilly, wet periods. Although pollen counts reflect the past 24 hours, they are useful as a general guide for when it may be wise to stay indoors with windows closed to avoid contact with a certain pollen.

Mold

Molds are found both indoors and outdoors. Outdoor molds are carried by the wind, like pollens. There are many different types of molds, but only some seem to cause health problems. High levels of the mold Alternaria have been associated with severe asthma in the late summer in the upper Midwest of the United States. Aspergillus, another type of mold, is associated with a severe and chronic form of asthma.

Indoor molds may cause allergy as well as other health effects. Some people report not feeling well when living in a moldy or damp environment, even if they do not have allergies. However, there has been little research examining the health effects of indoor molds.

Other Indoor Allergens

Allergic rhinitis and asthma also can be triggered by exposure to house dust, for example, during household chores such as vacuuming or sweeping. Dust is a mixture of substances and may contain allergens from house dust mites, pets, mold, cockroaches, and rodents. Cockroach and mouse allergy are common in low-income, urban areas and are key causes of asthma-related illness among children, as NIAID-funded research has shown. For example, in 1997, NIAID-supported scientists reported that the combination of cockroach allergy and exposure to the insects is an important cause of asthma-related illness and hospitalizations among inner-city children.

While exposure to animals like cats and dogs can cause symptoms of allergic rhinitis and asthma in sensitive people, exposure in early life may have a protective effect. NIAID-funded scientists found that exposure to dust from homes with dogs may protect against allergies and asthma.

Symptoms of Environmental Allergies

Symptoms of allergic rhinitis and asthma include the following:

- Runny nose and mucus production
- Sneezing
- Itchy nose, eyes, ears, and mouth
- Stuffy nose
- Red and watery eyes
- Swelling around the eyes
- Coughing
- Wheezing
- Chest tightness
- Shortness of breath

Diagnosis of Environmental Allergies

A healthcare professional may perform skin, blood, or allergy component tests to help diagnose environmental allergies.

Skin Tests

A skin prick test can detect if a person is sensitive to a specific allergen. Being "sensitive" means that the immune system produces a type of antibody called IgE against that allergen. IgE attaches to specialized cells called mast cells. This happens throughout the body, including the lining of the nose and the airways, as well as the skin.

During a skin prick test, a healthcare professional uses a piece of plastic to prick the skin on the arm or back and place a tiny amount of allergen extract just below the skin's surface. In sensitive people, the allergen binds to IgE on mast cells in the skin and causes them to release histamine and other chemicals that produce itching, redness, and minor swelling.

A positive skin test to a particular allergen does not necessarily indicate that a person has allergic rhinitis or asthma caused by that allergen. Up to 50 percent of the U.S. population may have at least one positive skin test to a common allergen, but less than half of those people have allergic rhinitis or asthma. Therefore, healthcare professionals often will try to match skin test results with the kind of allergen exposures person may have had.

Blood Tests

Instead of performing a skin test, doctors may take a blood sample to measure levels of allergen-specific IgE antibodies. Most people who are sensitive to a particular allergen will have IgE antibodies detectable by both skin and blood tests.

As with skin testing, a positive blood test to an allergen does not necessarily mean that a person's symptoms are caused by that allergen.

Allergy Component Tests

One reason why a positive skin or blood test does not always indicate that a person's symptoms are caused by a particular allergen is that allergens comprise many different components, some of which are more likely to cause symptoms than others. For example, birch tree pollen contains proteins, sugars, and fats. IgE antibodies to birch pollen proteins are likely to cause allergic reactions, but IgE antibodies to the sugars in birch pollen, although common, are less likely to cause allergic reactions. Allergy component tests are blood tests that can determine exactly which component of an allergen the IgE in a person's blood recognizes. This can help a health professional determine whether the allergen is likely to cause symptoms.

Section 34.2

Testing for Pollen Allergy

Text in this section is excerpted from "Pollen Allergy," National
Institute of Allergy and Infectious Diseases (NIAID), July 2015.

Pollen is one of the most common triggers of seasonal allergies.
Many people know pollen allergy as "hay fever," but health experts
usually refer to it as "seasonal allergic rhinitis." Pollen allergy affects
approximately 7 percent of adults and 9 percent of children in the
United States.

An allergic reaction is a specific response of the body's immune
system to a normally harmless substance called an allergen. People
who have allergies often are sensitive to more than one allergen. In
addition to pollen, other airborne allergens that can cause allergic
reactions include materials from house dust mites, animal dander,
and cockroaches.

Pollen Overview

Each spring, summer, and fall, plants release tiny pollen grains
to fertilize other plants of the same species. Most of the pollens that
cause allergic reactions come from trees, weeds, and grasses. These
plants make small, light, and dry pollen grains that are carried by
the wind. Among North American plants, grasses are the most common cause of allergy. Ragweed is a main culprit among the weeds,
but other major sources of weed pollen include sagebrush, pigweed,
lamb's quarters, and tumbleweed. Certain species of trees, including
birch, cedar, and oak, also produce highly allergenic pollen. Plants
that are pollinated with the help of insects, such as roses and ornamental flowering trees like cherry and pear trees, usually do not cause
allergic rhinitis.

People with pollen allergy only have symptoms for the period or
season when the pollen grains to which they are allergic are in the
air. For example, in most parts of the United States, grass pollen is
present during the spring.

What Is a Pollen Count?

A pollen count, which is often reported by local weather broadcasts or allergy websites, is a measure of how much pollen is in the air. Pollen counts tend to be highest early in the morning on warm, dry, breezy days and lowest during chilly, wet periods. Although pollen counts reflect the last 24 hours, they are useful as a general guide for when it may be wise to stay indoors with windows closed to avoid contact with a certain pollen.

Symptoms

Pollen allergy can cause symptoms such as a runny nose and watery eyes. Reactions to allergens often also play an important role in asthma. Common symptoms of allergic rhinitis and asthma include

- Runny nose and mucus production
- Sneezing
- Itchy nose, eyes, ears, and mouth
- Stuffy nose
- Red and watery eyes
- Swelling around the eyes
- Coughing
- Wheezing
- Chest tightness
- Shortness of breath

However, not all of these seasonal symptoms are due to pollen. Rhinovirus, the cause of the common cold, also can cause runny noses in the fall and spring. It is not always easy to figure out whether an allergy or a common cold is the cause of these symptoms, although some clues can help distinguish between the two. For example, a fever suggests a cold rather than an allergy, and symptoms lasting more than 2 weeks suggest allergies rather than a cold.

Diagnosis

Skin Tests

A skin prick test can detect if a person is sensitive to a specific allergen. Being "sensitive" means that the immune system produces a type of antibody called immunoglobulin E (IgE) that recognizes that allergen. IgE attaches to specialized cells called mast cells. This happens throughout the body, including the skin.

During a skin prick test, a health care provider uses a piece of plastic to prick the skin on a person's arm or back and places a tiny amount of allergen extract just below the skin's surface. In sensitive people, the allergen binds to IgE on mast cells in the skin and causes them to release histamine and other chemicals that produce itching, redness, and minor swelling.

A positive skin prick test to a particular pollen allergen does not necessarily indicate that a person has allergic rhinitis caused by that allergen. Therefore, health care providers must compare the skin test results with the time and place of a person's symptoms to see if they match.

Blood Tests

Instead of performing a skin test, doctors may take a blood sample to measure levels of allergen-specific IgE antibodies. Most people who are sensitive to a particular allergen will have IgE antibodies detectable by both skin and blood tests. As with skin testing, a positive blood test to an allergen does not necessarily mean that a person's symptoms are caused by that allergen.

One reason why a positive skin or blood test does not always indicate that a person's symptoms are caused by a particular allergen is that allergens include many different components, some of which are more likely to cause symptoms than others. For example, birch tree pollen contains proteins, sugars, and fats. IgE antibodies to birch pollen proteins are likely to cause allergic reactions, but IgE antibodies to the sugars in birch pollen, although common, are less likely to cause allergic reactions.

Section 34.3

Testing for Food Allergy

Text in this section begins with excerpts from "Food Allergies: What
You Need to Know," U.S. Food and Drug Administration (FDA),
September 2, 2015.

Text in this section beginning with "Detailed History" is excerpted
from "Food Allergy Diagnosis," National Institute of Allergy and
Infectious Diseases (NIAID), February 29, 2012.

Each year, millions of Americans have allergic reactions to food.
Although most food allergies cause relatively mild and minor symptoms, some food allergies can cause severe reactions, and may even
be life-threatening.

There is no cure for food allergies. Strict avoidance of food allergens—and early recognition and management of allergic reactions to
food—are important measures to prevent serious health consequences.

FDA's Role:

Labeling

To help Americans avoid the health risks posed by food allergens,
Congress passed the **Food Allergen Labeling and consumer Protection Act of 2004 (FALCPA)**. The law applies to all foods whose
labeling is regulated by FDA, both domestic and imported. (FDA regulates the labeling of all foods, except for poultry, most meats, certain
egg products, and most alcoholic beverages.)

- Before FALCPA, the labels of foods made from two or more
  ingredients were required to list all **ingredients** by their common or usual names. The names of some ingredients, however,
  do not clearly identify their food source.

- Now, the law requires that labels must clearly identify the **food
  source names** of all ingredients that are—or contain any protein derived from—the **eight most common food allergens**,
  which FALCPA defines as **"major food allergens."**

433

As a result, food labels help allergic consumers to identify offending foods or ingredients so they can more easily avoid them.

About Foods Labeled before January 1, 2006

FALCPA did not require relabeling of food products labeled before January 1, 2006, which were made with a major food allergen that did not identify its food source name in the ingredient list. Although it is unlikely that any of these foods are still on store shelves, always use special care to read the complete ingredient list on food labels when you go shopping.

Food Allergies

What to Do If Symptoms Occur

The appearance of symptoms after eating food may be a sign of a food allergy. The food(s) that caused these symptoms should be avoided, and the affected person, should contact a doctor or health care provider for appropriate testing and evaluation.

- Persons found to have a food allergy should be taught to **read labels** and **avoid the offending foods**. They should also be taught, in case of accidental ingestion, to **recognize the early symptoms** of an allergic reaction, and be properly educated on—and armed with—appropriate treatment measures.

- Persons with a known food allergy who begin experiencing symptoms while, or after, eating a food should **initiate treatment immediately**, and go to a **nearby emergency room** if symptoms progress.

The Hard Facts: Severe Food Allergies Can Be Life-Threatening

Following ingestion of a food allergen(s), a person with food allergies can experience a severe, life-threatening allergic reaction called anaphylaxis.

This can lead to:

- constricted airways in the lungs

- severe lowering of blood pressure and shock (**"anaphylactic shock"**)

- suffocation by swelling of the throat

Each year in the U.S., it is estimated that anaphylaxis to food results in:

- 30,000 emergency room visits

- 2,000 hospitalizations

- 150 deaths

Prompt administration of epinephrine by autoinjector (e.g., Epipen) during early symptoms of anaphylaxis may help prevent these serious consequences.

What Are *Major Food Allergens*?

While more than 160 foods can cause allergic reactions in people with food allergies, the law identifies the eight most common allergenic foods. These foods account for 90 percent of food allergic reactions, and are the food sources from which many other ingredients are derived.

The eight foods identified by the law are:

Milk

Eggs

Fish (e.g., bass, flounder, cod)

Crustacean shellfish (e.g. crab, lobster, shrimp)

Tree nuts (e.g., almonds, walnuts, pecans)

Peanuts

Wheat

Soybeans

These eight foods, and any ingredient that contains protein derived from one or more of them, are designated as "major food allergens" by FALCPA.

How *Major Food Allergens* Are Listed

The law requires that food labels identify the food source names of all major food allergens used to make the food. This requirement is met if the common or usual name of an ingredient (e.g., buttermilk) that is a major food allergen already identifies that allergen's food source name (i.e., milk). Otherwise, the allergen's food source name must be declared at least once on the food label in one of two ways.

The name of the food source of a major food allergen must appear:

In parentheses following the name of the ingredient.

Examples: "lecithin (soy)," "flour (wheat)," and "whey (milk)

– OR –

Immediately after or next to the list of ingredients in a "contains" statement.

Example: "Contains Wheat, Milk, and Soy."

Know the Symptoms

Symptoms of food allergies typically appear from within a few minutes to two hours after a person has eaten the food to which he or she is allergic.

Allergic reactions can include:

- Hives
- Flushed skin or rash
- Tingling or itchy sensation in the mouth
- Face, tongue, or lip swelling
- Vomiting and/or diarrhea
- Abdominal cramps
- Coughing or wheezing
- Dizziness and/or lightheadedness
- Swelling of the throat and vocal cords
- Difficulty breathing
- Loss of consciousness

About Other Allergens

Persons may still be allergic to—and have serious reactions to—foods other than the eight foods identified by the law. So, always be sure to read the food label's ingredient list carefully to avoid the food allergens in question.

Food Allergen "Advisory" Labeling

FALCPA's labeling requirements do not apply to the potential or unintentional presence of major food allergens in foods resulting from "cross-contact" situations during manufacturing, e.g., because of shared equipment or processing lines. In the context of food allergens, "cross-contact" occurs when a residue or trace amount of an allergenic food becomes incorporated into another food not intended to contain it. FDA guidance for the food industry states that food allergen advisory statements, e.g., "may contain [allergen]" or "produced in a facility that also uses [allergen]" should not be used as a substitute for adhering to current good manufacturing practices and must be truthful and not misleading. FDA is considering ways to best manage the use of these types of statements by manufacturers to better inform consumers.

Allergy Alert: Mild Symptoms Can Become More Severe

Initially mild *symptoms* that occur after ingesting a food allergen are not always a measure of mild *severity*. In fact, if not treated promptly, these symptoms can become more serious in a very short amount of time, and could lead to **anaphylaxis**.

Detailed History

Your healthcare professional will begin by taking a detailed medical history to find out if your symptoms are caused by an allergy to specific foods, food intolerance, or other health problems.

A detailed history is the most valuable tool used for diagnosing food allergy. Your healthcare professional will ask you several questions, including the following:

- Did your reaction come on quickly, usually within several minutes after eating the food?

- Is your reaction always associated with a certain food?

- How much of this potentially allergenic food did you eat before you had a reaction?

- Have you eaten this food before and had a reaction?

- Did anyone else who ate the same food get sick?

- Did you take allergy medicines, and if so, did they help? (Antihistamines should relieve hives, for example.)

Diet diary

Sometimes your healthcare professional cannot make a diagnosis based only on your history. You may be asked to keep a diet diary containing details about the foods you eat and whether you have a reaction. Based on the diary record, you and your healthcare professional may be able to identify a consistent pattern in your reactions.

Elimination diet

The next step some healthcare professionals use is a limited elimination diet, in which the food that is suspected of causing an allergic reaction is removed from your diet to see whether that stops your allergic reactions. For example, if you suspect you are allergic to egg, your healthcare professional will instruct you to eliminate egg from your diet. The limited elimination diet is done under the direction of your healthcare professional.

Skin prick test

If your history, diet diary, or elimination diet suggests a specific food allergy is likely, then your healthcare professional will use the skin prick test to confirm the diagnosis.

With a skin prick test, your healthcare professional uses a needle to place a tiny amount of food extract just below the surface of the skin on your lower arm or back. If you are allergic, there will be swelling or redness at the test site. This is a positive result. It means that there are immunoglobulin E (IgE) molecules on the skin's mast cells that are specific to the food being tested.

The skin prick test is simple and relatively safe, and results are ready in minutes.

You can have a positive skin test to a food, however, without having an allergic reaction to that food. A healthcare professional often makes a diagnosis of food allergy when someone has both a positive skin test to a specific food and a history of reactions that suggests an allergy to the same food.

Blood test

Instead of the skin prick test, your healthcare professional can take a blood sample to measure the levels of food-specific IgE antibodies.

As with skin testing, positive blood tests do not necessarily mean that you have a food allergy. Your healthcare professionals must combine these test results with information about your history of reactions to food to make an accurate diagnosis of food allergy.

Oral food challenge

An oral food challenge is the final method healthcare professionals use to diagnose food allergy. This method includes the following steps:

- Your healthcare professional gives you individual doses of various foods (masked so that you do not know what food is present), some of which are suspected of starting an allergic reaction.

- Initially, the dose of food is very small, but the amount is gradually increased during the challenge.

- You swallow the individual dose.

- Your healthcare professional watches you to see if a reaction occurs.

To prevent bias, oral food challenges are often double blinded. In a true double-blind challenge, neither you nor your healthcare professional knows whether the substance you eat contains the likely allergen. Another medical professional has made up the individual doses. In a single-blind challenge, your healthcare professional knows what you are eating but you do not.

A reaction only to suspected foods and not to the other foods tested confirms the diagnosis of a food allergy.

Chapter 35

Asthma Testing

What Is Asthma?

Asthma is a chronic (long-term) lung disease that inflames and narrows the airways. Asthma causes recurring periods of wheezing (a whistling sound when you breathe), chest tightness, shortness of breath, and coughing. The coughing often occurs at night or early in the morning.

Asthma affects people of all ages, but it most often starts during childhood. In the United States, more than 25 million people are known to have asthma. About 7 million of these people are children.

Overview

To understand asthma, it helps to know how the airways work. The airways are tubes that carry air into and out of your lungs. People who have asthma have inflamed airways. The inflammation makes the airways swollen and very sensitive. The airways tend to react strongly to certain inhaled substances.

When the airways react, the muscles around them tighten. This narrows the airways, causing less air to flow into the lungs. The swelling also can worsen, making the airways even narrower. Cells in the airways might make more mucus than usual. Mucus is a sticky, thick liquid that can further narrow the airways.

Text in this chapter is excerpted from "Asthma," National Heart, Lung, and Blood Institute (NHLBI), August 4, 2014.

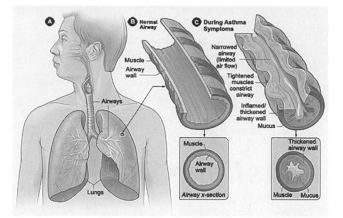

Figure 35.1. Asthma: *"A" shows the location of the lungs and airways in the body. "B" shows a cross-section of a normal airway. "C" shows a cross-section of an airway during asthma symptoms.*

This chain reaction can result in asthma symptoms. Symptoms can happen each time the airways are inflamed.

Sometimes asthma symptoms are mild and go away on their own or after minimal treatment with asthma medicine. Other times, symptoms continue to get worse.

When symptoms get more intense and/or more symptoms occur, you're having an asthma attack. Asthma attacks also are called flareups or exacerbations (eg-zas-er-BA-shuns).

Treating symptoms when you first notice them is important. This will help prevent the symptoms from worsening and causing a severe asthma attack. Severe asthma attacks may require emergency care, and they can be fatal.

Outlook

Asthma has no cure. Even when you feel fine, you still have the disease and it can flare up at any time.

However, with today's knowledge and treatments, most people who have asthma are able to manage the disease. They have few, if any, symptoms. They can live normal, active lives and sleep through the night without interruption from asthma.

If you have asthma, you can take an active role in managing the disease. For successful, thorough, and ongoing treatment, build strong partnerships with your doctor and other health care providers.

What Causes Asthma?

The exact cause of asthma isn't known. Researchers think some genetic and environmental factors interact to cause asthma, most often early in life. These factors include:

- An inherited tendency to develop allergies, called atopy
- Parents who have asthma
- Certain respiratory infections during childhood
- Contact with some airborne allergens or exposure to some viral infections in infancy or in early childhood when the immune system is developing

If asthma or atopy runs in your family, exposure to irritants (for example, tobacco smoke) may make your airways more reactive to substances in the air.

Some factors may be more likely to cause asthma in some people than in others. Researchers continue to explore what causes asthma.

The "Hygiene Hypothesis"

One theory researchers have for what causes asthma is the "hygiene hypothesis." They believe that our Western lifestyle—with its emphasis on hygiene and sanitation—has resulted in changes in our living conditions and an overall decline in infections in early childhood.

Many young children no longer have the same types of environmental exposures and infections as children did in the past. This affects the way that young children's immune systems develop during very early childhood, and it may increase their risk for atopy and asthma. This is especially true for children who have close family members with one or both of these conditions.

Who Is at Risk for Asthma?

Asthma affects people of all ages, but it most often starts during childhood. In the United States, more than 22 million people are known to have asthma. Nearly 6 million of these people are children.

Young children who often wheeze and have respiratory infections—as well as certain other risk factors—are at highest risk of developing asthma that continues beyond 6 years of age. The other risk factors include having allergies, eczema (an allergic skin condition), or parents who have asthma.

Among children, more boys have asthma than girls. But among adults, more women have the disease than men. It's not clear whether or how sex and sex hormones play a role in causing asthma.

Most, but not all, people who have asthma have allergies.

Some people develop asthma because of contact with certain chemical irritants or industrial dusts in the workplace. This type of asthma is called occupational asthma.

What Are the Signs and Symptoms of Asthma?

Common signs and symptoms of asthma include:

- Coughing. Coughing from asthma often is worse at night or early in the morning, making it hard to sleep.

- Wheezing. Wheezing is a whistling or squeaky sound that occurs when you breathe.

- Chest tightness. This may feel like something is squeezing or sitting on your chest.

- Shortness of breath. Some people who have asthma say they can't catch their breath or they feel out of breath. You may feel like you can't get air out of your lungs.

Not all people who have asthma have these symptoms. Likewise, having these symptoms doesn't always mean that you have asthma. The best way to diagnose asthma for certain is to use a lung function test, a medical history (including type and frequency of symptoms), and a physical exam.

The types of asthma symptoms you have, how often they occur, and how severe they are may vary over time. Sometimes your symptoms may just annoy you. Other times, they may be troublesome enough to limit your daily routine.

Severe symptoms can be fatal. It's important to treat symptoms when you first notice them so they don't become severe.

With proper treatment, most people who have asthma can expect to have few, if any, symptoms either during the day or at night.

What Causes Asthma Symptoms to Occur?

Many things can trigger or worsen asthma symptoms. Your doctor will help you find out which things (sometimes called triggers) may cause your asthma to flare up if you come in contact with them. Triggers may include:

- Allergens from dust, animal fur, cockroaches, mold, and pollens from trees, grasses, and flowers

- Irritants such as cigarette smoke, air pollution, chemicals or dust in the workplace, compounds in home décor products, and sprays (such as hairspray)

- Medicines such as aspirin or other nonsteroidal anti-inflammatory drugs and nonselective beta-blockers

- Sulfites in foods and drinks

- Viral upper respiratory infections, such as colds

- Physical activity, including exercise

Other health conditions can make asthma harder to manage. Examples of these conditions include a runny nose, sinus infections, reflux disease, psychological stress, and sleep apnea. These conditions need treatment as part of an overall asthma care plan.

Asthma is different for each person. Some of the triggers listed above may not affect you. Other triggers that do affect you may not be on the list. Talk with your doctor about the things that seem to make your asthma worse.

How Is Asthma Diagnosed?

Your primary care doctor will diagnose asthma based on your medical and family histories, a physical exam, and test results.

Your doctor also will figure out the severity of your asthma—that is, whether it's intermittent, mild, moderate, or severe. The level of severity will determine what treatment you'll start on.

You may need to see an asthma specialist if:

- You need special tests to help diagnose asthma

- You've had a life-threatening asthma attack

- You need more than one kind of medicine or higher doses of medicine to control your asthma, or if you have overall problems getting your asthma well controlled

- You're thinking about getting allergy treatments

Medical and Family Histories

Your doctor may ask about your family history of asthma and allergies. He or she also may ask whether you have asthma symptoms and when and how often they occur.

Let your doctor know whether your symptoms seem to happen only during certain times of the year or in certain places, or if they get worse at night.

Your doctor also may want to know what factors seem to trigger your symptoms or worsen them.

Your doctor may ask you about related health conditions that can interfere with asthma management. These conditions include a runny nose, sinus infections, reflux disease, psychological stress, and sleep apnea.

Physical Exam

Your doctor will listen to your breathing and look for signs of asthma or allergies. These signs include wheezing, a runny nose or swollen nasal passages, and allergic skin conditions (such as eczema).

Keep in mind that you can still have asthma even if you don't have these signs on the day that your doctor examines you.

Diagnostic Tests

Lung Function Test

Your doctor will use a test called spirometry to check how your lungs are working. This test measures how much air you can breathe in and out. It also measures how fast you can blow air out.

Your doctor also may give you medicine and then test you again to see whether the results have improved.

If the starting results are lower than normal and improve with the medicine, and if your medical history shows a pattern of asthma symptoms, your diagnosis will likely be asthma.

Other Tests

Your doctor may recommend other tests if he or she needs more information to make a diagnosis. Other tests may include:

- Allergy testing to find out which allergens affect you, if any.

- A test to measure how sensitive your airways are. This is called a bronchoprovocation test. Using spirometry, this test repeatedly

measures your lung function during physical activity or after
you receive increasing doses of cold air or a special chemical to
breathe in.

- A test to show whether you have another condition with the
  same symptoms as asthma, such as reflux disease, vocal cord
  dysfunction, or sleep apnea.
- A chest X-ray or an EKG (electrocardiogram). These tests will
  help find out whether a foreign object or other disease may be
  causing your symptoms.

Diagnosing Asthma in Young Children

Most children who have asthma develop their first symptoms before
5 years of age. However, asthma in young children (aged 0 to 5 years)
can be hard to diagnose.

Sometimes it's hard to tell whether a child has asthma or another
childhood condition. This is because the symptoms of asthma also occur
with other conditions.

Also, many young children who wheeze when they get colds or respiratory infections don't go on to have asthma after they're 6 years old.

A child may wheeze because he or she has small airways that
become even narrower during colds or respiratory infections. The airways grow as the child grows older, so wheezing no longer occurs when
the child gets colds.

A young child who has frequent wheezing with colds or respiratory
infections is more likely to have asthma if:

- One or both parents have asthma
- The child has signs of allergies, including the allergic skin condition eczema
- The child has allergic reactions to pollens or other airborne
  allergens
- The child wheezes even when he or she doesn't have a cold or
  other infection

The most certain way to diagnose asthma is with a lung function
test, a medical history, and a physical exam. However, it's hard to do
lung function tests in children younger than 5 years. Thus, doctors
must rely on children's medical histories, signs and symptoms, and
physical exams to make a diagnosis.

Doctors also may use a 4–6 week trial of asthma medicines to see
how well a child responds.

Chapter 36

Bladder and Kidney Function Tests

Chapter Contents

Section 36.1

Urodynamic Testing

Text in this section is excerpted from "Urodynamic Testing," National Institute of Diabetes and Digestive and Kidney Diseases (NIDDK), February 5, 2014.

What is the urinary tract?

The urinary tract is the body's drainage system for removing wastes and extra water. The urinary tract includes two kidneys, two ureters, a bladder, and a urethra. Blood flows through the kidneys, and the kidneys filter out wastes and extra water, making urine. The urine travels down two narrow tubes called the ureters. The urine is then stored in a muscular, balloon-like organ called the bladder. The bladder swells into a round shape when it is full and gets smaller as it empties. When the bladder empties, urine flows out of the body through the urethra.

What is the lower urinary tract and how does it work?

The lower urinary tract includes the bladder and urethra. The bladder sits in the pelvis and is attached to other organs, muscles, and the pelvic bones, which hold it in place. The urethra is a tube at the bottom of the bladder that carries urine from the bladder to the outside of the body.

The lower urinary tract works by coordinating the muscles of the bladder wall with the sphincters, which are circular muscles that surround the area of the bladder that opens into the urethra. The muscles of the bladder wall relax as the bladder fills with urine. If the urinary tract is healthy, the bladder can hold up to 2 cups, or 16 ounces, of urine comfortably for 2 to 5 hours. The sphincters close tightly like rubber bands around the bladder to help keep urine from leaking. As the bladder fills, the need to urinate becomes stronger and stronger, until the bladder reaches its limit. Urination is the process of emptying the bladder. To urinate, the brain signals the bladder muscles to tighten, squeezing urine out of the bladder. At the same time, the brain signals the sphincters to relax. As the sphincters relax, urine

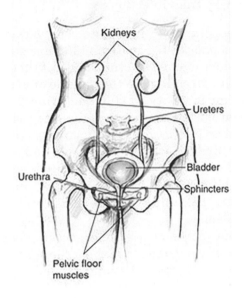

Figure 36.1. *Front view of the urinary tract*

exits the bladder through the urethra. When all the signals occur in the correct order, normal urination occurs.

What is urodynamic testing?

Urodynamic testing is any procedure that looks at how well the bladder, sphincters, and urethra are storing and releasing urine. Most urodynamic tests focus on the bladder's ability to hold urine and empty steadily and completely. Urodynamic tests can also show whether the bladder is having involuntary contractions that cause urine leakage. A health care provider may recommend urodynamic tests if symptoms suggest problems with the lower urinary tract. Lower urinary tract symptoms (LUTS) include

- urine leakage
- frequent urination
- painful urination
- sudden, strong urges to urinate
- problems starting a urine stream
- problems emptying the bladder completely

- recurrent urinary tract infections

Urodynamic tests range from simple observation to precise measurements using sophisticated instruments. For simple observation, a health care provider may record the length of time it takes a person to produce a urinary stream, note the volume of urine produced, and record the ability or inability to stop the urine flow in midstream. For precise measurements, imaging equipment takes pictures of the bladder filling and emptying, pressure monitors record the pressures inside the bladder, and sensors record muscle and nerve activity. The health care provider will decide the type of urodynamic test based on the person's health information, physical exam, and LUTS. The urodynamic test results help diagnose the cause and nature of a lower urinary tract problem.

Most urodynamic tests do not involve special preparations, though some tests may require a person to make a change in fluid intake or to stop taking certain medications. Depending on the test, a person may be instructed to arrive for testing with a full bladder.

What are the urodynamic tests?

Urodynamic tests include

- uroflowmetry
- postvoid residual measurement
- cystometric test
- leak point pressure measurement
- pressure flow study
- electromyography
- video urodynamic tests

Uroflowmetry

Uroflowmetry is the measurement of urine speed and volume. Special equipment automatically measures the amount of urine and the flow rate—how fast the urine comes out. Uroflowmetry equipment includes a device for catching and measuring urine and a computer to record the data. During a uroflowmetry test, the person urinates privately into a special toilet or funnel that has a container for collecting the urine and a scale. The equipment creates a graph that shows changes in flow rate from second to second so the health care provider can see when the flow rate is the highest and how many seconds it takes to get there. Results of this test will be abnormal if the bladder muscles are weak or urine flow is blocked. Another approach to measuring flow rate is to record the time it takes to urinate into a special container that accurately measures the volume of urine. Uroflowmetry measurements are performed in a health care provider's office; no anesthesia is needed.

Postvoid Residual Measurement

This urodynamic test measures the amount of urine left in the bladder after urination. The remaining urine is called the postvoid residual. Postvoid residual can be measured with ultrasound equipment that uses harmless sound waves to create a picture of the bladder. Bladder ultrasounds are performed in a health care provider's office, radiology center, or hospital by a specially trained technician and interpreted by a doctor, usually a radiologist. Anesthesia is not needed. Postvoid residual can also be measured using a catheter—a thin flexible tube. A health care provider inserts the catheter through the urethra up into the bladder to remove and measure the amount of remaining urine. A postvoid residual of 100 milliliters or more is a sign that the bladder is not emptying completely. Catheter measurements are performed in a health care provider's office, clinic, or hospital with local anesthesia.

Cystometric Test

A cystometric test measures how much urine the bladder can hold, how much pressure builds up inside the bladder as it stores urine, and how full it is when the urge to urinate begins. A catheter is used to empty the bladder completely. Then a special, smaller catheter is placed in the bladder. This catheter has a pressure-measuring device called a manometer. Another catheter may be placed in the rectum to record pressure there.

Once the bladder is emptied completely, the bladder is filled slowly with warm water. During this time, the person is asked to describe how the bladder feels and indicate when the need to urinate arises. When the urge to urinate occurs, the volume of water and the bladder pressure are recorded. The person may be asked to cough or strain during this procedure to see if the bladder pressure changes. A cystometric test can also identify involuntary bladder contractions. Cystometric tests are performed in a health care provider's office, clinic, or hospital with local anesthesia.

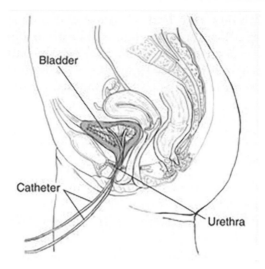

Figure 36.2. *Cystometric test*

Leak Point Pressure Measurement

This urodynamic test measures pressure at the point of leakage during a cystometric test. While the bladder is being filled for the cystometric test, it may suddenly contract and squeeze some water out without warning. The manometer measures the pressure inside the bladder when this leakage occurs. This reading may provide information about the kind of bladder problem that exists. The person may be asked to apply abdominal pressure to the bladder by coughing, shifting position, or trying to exhale while holding the nose and mouth. These actions help the health care provider evaluate the sphincters.

Pressure Flow Study

A pressure flow study measures the bladder pressure required to urinate and the flow rate a given pressure generates. After the cystometric test, the person empties the bladder, during which time a manometer is used to measure bladder pressure and flow rate. This pressure flow study helps identify bladder outlet blockage that men may experience with prostate enlargement. Bladder outlet blockage is less common in women but can occur with a cystocele or, rarely, after a surgical procedure for urinary incontinence. Pressure flow studies are performed in a health care provider's office, clinic, or hospital with local anesthesia.

Electromyography

Electromyography uses special sensors to measure the electrical activity of the muscles and nerves in and around the bladder and the sphincters. If the health care provider thinks the urinary problem is related to nerve or muscle damage, the person may be given an electromyography. The sensors are placed on the skin near the urethra and rectum or on a urethral or rectal catheter. Muscle and nerve activity is recorded on a machine. The patterns of the nerve impulses show whether the messages sent to the bladder and sphincters are coordinated correctly. Electromyography is performed by a specially trained technician in a health care provider's office, outpatient clinic, or hospital. Anesthesia is not needed if sensors are placed on the skin. Local anesthesia is needed if sensors are placed on a urethral or rectal catheter.

Video Urodynamic Tests

Video urodynamic tests take pictures and videos of the bladder during filling and emptying. The imaging equipment may use X-rays or ultrasound. If X-ray equipment is used, the bladder will be filled with a special fluid, called contrast medium, that shows up on X-rays. X-rays are performed by an X-ray technician in a health care provider's office, outpatient facility, or hospital; anesthesia is not needed. If ultrasound equipment is used, the bladder is filled with warm water and harmless sound waves are used to create a picture of the bladder. The pictures and videos show the size and shape of the bladder and help the health care provider understand the problem. Bladder ultrasounds are performed in a health care provider's office, radiology center, or hospital by a specially trained technician and interpreted by a doctor, usually a radiologist. Although anesthesia is not needed for the ultrasound, local anesthesia is needed to insert the catheter to fill the bladder

What happens after urodynamic tests?

After having urodynamic tests, a person may feel mild discomfort for a few hours when urinating. Drinking an 8-ounce glass of water every half-hour for 2 hours may help to reduce the discomfort. The health care provider may recommend taking a warm bath or holding a warm, damp washcloth over the urethral opening to relieve the discomfort.

An antibiotic may be prescribed for 1 or 2 days to prevent infection, but not always. People with signs of infection—including pain, chills, or fever—should call their health care provider immediately.

How soon will test results be available?

Results for simple tests such as cystometry and uroflowmetry are often available immediately after the test. Results of other tests such as electromyography and video urodynamic tests may take a few days to come back. A health care provider will talk with the patient about the results and possible treatments.

Section 36.2

Testing for Kidney Disease

Text in this section is excerpted from "Testing for Kidney Disease," National Kidney Disease Education Program (NKDEP), September 17, 2014.

Early kidney disease usually does not have signs (a change in your body) or symptoms (a change in how you feel). Testing is the only way to know how your kidneys are doing. It is important for you to get checked for kidney disease if you have the key risk factors – diabetes, high blood pressure, heart disease, or a family history of kidney failure.

Two tests are needed to check for kidney disease.

1. A blood test checks your GFR, which tells how well your kidneys are filtering. GFR stands for glomerular filtration rate.

2. A urine test checks for albumin in your urine. Albumin is a protein that can pass into the urine when the kidneys are damaged.

It is also important to have your blood pressure checked. High blood pressure can be a sign of kidney disease. Keep your blood pressure at or below the target set by your health care provider. For most people, the blood pressure target is less than 140/90 mm Hg.

The sooner you know you have kidney disease, the sooner you can get treatment to help delay or prevent kidney failure. If you have diabetes, get checked every year. If you have other risk factors, such as high blood pressure, heart disease, or a family history of kidney failure, talk to your provider about how often you should be tested.

Understanding GFR

GFR stands for glomerular filtration rate. A blood test checks your GFR, which tells how well your kidneys are filtering.

It's important to know your GFR if you are at risk for kidney disease. A urine test will also be used to check your kidneys.

GFR is reported as a number.

- **A GFR of 60 or higher** is in the normal range.

- **A GFR below 60** may mean you have kidney disease.

- **A GFR of 15 or lower** may mean kidney failure.

You can't raise your GFR, but you can try to keep it from going lower. Learn more about what you can do to keep your kidneys healthy.

The graphic below can help you understand the meaning of your GFR result. Please remember that this information should not take the place of talking with your health care provider.

If you have a:

GFR of 60 or higher*: Your kidney function is in the normal range. Ask your provider when your GFR should be checked again. You still need to get your urine checked for kidney damage.

* If your lab report shows an actual number that is higher than 60, such as 75,90, 100, consider your result as "60 or higher" and in the normal range.

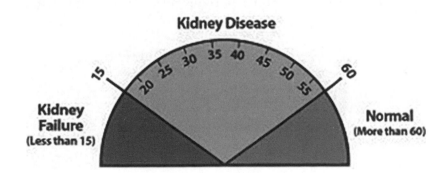

Figure 36.3. *GFR*

GFR below 60: This may mean kidney disease. Talk to your provider about treatment to keep your kidney health at this level. Ask about:

- medicines you should take,

- medicines to stay away from,

- changes to your diet,

- other lifestyle changes,

- whether your kidney disease is likely to get worse,

- ways to treat kidney failure, and

- if you should begin preparing for dialysis.

GFR of 15 or lower: This is usually referred to as kidney failure. Most people at this point may need dialysis or a kidney transplant. Talk to your provider about your treatment options.

Understanding Urine Albumin

Albumin (al-BYOO-min) is a protein found in the blood. A healthy kidney does not let albumin pass into the urine. A damaged kidney lets some albumin pass into the urine. The less albumin in your urine, the better.

If you are at risk for kidney disease, your provider should check your urine for albumin along with checking your GFR.

Testing for Urine Albumin

Your provider may send your urine sample to the lab to see if albumin, a type of protein, is in your urine.

- If you have albumin in your urine, your provider may want to test it one or two more times to confirm the result. Measuring

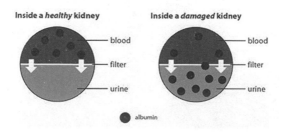
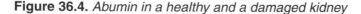

Figure 36.4. *Abumin in a healthy and a damaged kidney*

When your results come back, you may hear terms such as "microalbuminuria," "macroalbuminuria," "urine protein," "proteinuria," "albuminuria," or "urine-to-creatinine ratio," which are all used to describe how much albumin was found.

the albumin level in your urine helps your provider know which treatment is best for you.

Understanding a Urine Albumin Result

- A urine albumin result below 30 is normal.

- A urine albumin result above 30 is abnormal and may mean kidney disease.

In addition to your urine albumin test, your provider should also check your GFR.

If you do not understand your lab results, ask your health care provider to explain them to you. Please remember that the information on this website should not take the place of talking with your health care provider.

You should also ask your provider what you can do to keep your kidneys healthy.

Chapter 37

Cancer Screening Tests

Chapter Contents

Section 37.1

Cancer Screening Overview

Text in this section is excerpted from "Cancer Screening Overview (PDQ®)," National Cancer Institute (NCI), July 2, 2014.

What Is Cancer Screening?

Screening is looking for cancer before a person has any symptoms. This can help find cancer at an early stage. When abnormal tissue or cancer is found early, it may be easier to treat. By the time symptoms appear, cancer may have begun to spread.

Scientists are trying to better understand which people are more likely to get certain types of cancer. They also study the things we do and the things around us to see if they cause cancer. This information helps doctors recommend who should be screened for cancer, which screening tests should be used, and how often the tests should be done.

It is important to remember that your doctor does not necessarily think you have cancer if he or she suggests a screening test. Screening tests are given when you have no cancer symptoms.

If a screening test result is abnormal, you may need to have more tests done to find out if you have cancer. These are called diagnostic tests.

There are different kinds of screening tests.

Screening tests include the following:

- Physical exam and history: An exam of the body to check general signs of health, including checking for signs of disease, such as lumps or anything else that seems unusual. A history of the patient's health habits and past illnesses and treatments will also be taken.

- Laboratory tests: Medical procedures that test samples of tissue, blood, urine, or other substances in the body.

- Imaging procedures: Procedures that make pictures of areas inside the body.

- Genetic tests: Tests that look for certain gene mutations (changes) that are linked to some types of cancer.

Screening tests have risks.

Not all screening tests are helpful and most have risks. It is important to know the risks of the test and whether it has been proven to decrease the chance of dying from cancer.

Some screening tests can cause serious problems.

Some screening procedures can cause bleeding or other problems. For example, colon cancer screening with sigmoidoscopy or colonoscopy can cause tears in the lining of the colon.

False-positive test results are possible.

Screening test results may appear to be abnormal even though there is no cancer. A false-positive test result (one that shows there is cancer when there really isn't) can cause anxiety and is usually followed by more tests and procedures, which also have risks.

False-negative test results are possible.

Screening test results may appear to be normal even though there is cancer. A person who receives a false-negative test result (one that shows there is no cancer when there really is) may delay seeking medical care even if there are symptoms.

Finding the cancer may not improve the person's health or help the person live longer.

Some cancers never cause symptoms or become life-threatening, but if found by a screening test, the cancer may be treated. There is no way to know if treating the cancer would help the person live longer than if no treatment were given. In both teenagers and adults, there is an increased risk of suicide in the first year after being diagnosed with cancer. Also, treatments for cancer have side effects.

For some cancers, finding and treating the cancer early does not improve the chance of a cure or help the person live longer.

What Are the Goals of Screening Tests?

Screening tests have many goals.

A screening test that works the way it should and is helpful does the following:

- Finds cancer before symptoms appear.

- Screens for a cancer that is easier to treat and cure when found early.

- Has few false-negative test results and false-positive test results.

- Decreases the chance of dying from cancer.

Screening tests are not meant to diagnose cancer.

Screening tests usually do not diagnose cancer. If a screening test result is abnormal, more tests may be done to check for cancer. For example, a screening mammogram may find a lump in the breast. A lump may be cancer or something else. More tests need to be done to find out if the lump is cancer. These are called diagnostic tests. Diagnostic tests may include a biopsy, in which cells or tissues are removed so a pathologist can check them under a microscope for signs of cancer.

Who Needs to Be Screened?

Certain screening tests may be suggested only for people who have a high risk for certain cancers.

Anything that increases the chance of cancer is called a cancer risk factor. Having a risk factor does not mean that you will get cancer; not having risk factors doesn't mean that you will not get cancer.

Some screening tests are used only for people who have known risk factors for certain types of cancer. People known to have a higher risk of cancer than others include those who:

- Have had cancer in the past; or

- Have two or more first-degree relatives (a parent, brother, or sister) who have had cancer; or

- Have certain gene mutations (changes) that have been linked to cancer.

People who have a high risk of cancer may need to be screened more often or at an earlier age than other people.

Cancer screening research includes finding out who has an increased risk of cancer.

Scientists are trying to better understand who is likely to get certain types of cancer. They study the things we do and the things around us to see if they cause cancer. This information helps doctors figure out who should be screened for cancer, which screening tests should be used, and how often the tests should be done.

Since 1973, the Surveillance, Epidemiology, and End Results (SEER) Program of the National Cancer Institute has been collecting information on people with cancer from different parts of the United States. Information from SEER, research studies, and other sources is used to study who is at risk.

How is Cancer Risk Measured?

Cancer risk is measured in different ways. The findings from surveys and studies about cancer risk are studied and the results are explained in different ways. Some of the ways risk is explained include *absolute risk*, *relative risk*, and *odds ratios*.

- **Absolute risk**

This is the risk a person has of developing a disease, in a given population (for example, the entire U.S. population) over a certain period of time. Researchers estimate the absolute risk by studying a large number of people that are part of a certain population (for example, women in a given age group). Researchers count the number of people in the group who get a certain disease over a certain period of time. For example, a group of 100,000 women between the ages of 20 and 29 are observed for one year, and 4 of them get breast cancer during that time. This means that the one-year absolute risk of breast cancer for a woman in this age group is 4 in 100,000, or 4 chances in 100,000.

- **Relative risk**

This is often used in research studies to find out whether a trait or a factor can be linked to the risk of a disease. Researchers compare two groups of people who are a lot alike. However, the people in one of the groups must have the trait or factor being studied (they have been "exposed"). The people in the other group do not have it (they have not been exposed). To figure out relative risk, the percentage of people in the exposed group who have the disease is divided by the percentage of people in the unexposed group who have the disease.

Relative risks can be:

- Larger than 1: The trait or factor is linked to an increase in risk.

- Equal to 1: The trait or factor is not linked to risk.

- Less than 1: The trait or factor is linked to a decrease in risk.

Relative risks are also called risk ratios.

- **Odds ratio**

In some types of studies, researchers don't have enough information to figure out relative risks. They use something called an odds ratio instead. An odds ratio can be an estimate of relative risk.

One type of study that uses an odds ratio instead of relative risk is called a case-control study. In a case-control study, two groups of people are compared. However, the individuals in each group are chosen based on whether or not they have a certain disease. Researchers look at the odds that the people in each group were exposed to something (a trait or factor) that might have caused the disease. Odds describes the number of times the trait or factor was present or happened, divided by the number of times it wasn't present or didn't happen. To get an odds ratio, the odds for one group are divided by the odds for the other group.

Odds ratios can be:

- Larger than 1: The trait or factor is linked to an increase in risk.

- Equal to 1: The trait or factor is not linked to risk.

- Less than 1: The trait or factor is linked to a decrease in risk.

Looking at traits and exposures in people with and without cancer can help find possible risk factors. Knowing who is at an increased risk for certain types of cancer can help doctors decide when and how often they should be screened.

Does Screening Help People Live Longer?

Finding some cancers at an early stage (before symptoms appear) may help decrease the chance of dying from those cancers.

For many cancers, the chance of recovery depends on the stage (the amount or spread of cancer in the body) of the cancer when it was diagnosed. Cancers that are diagnosed at earlier stages are often easier to treat or cure.

Studies of cancer screening compare the death rate of people screened for a certain cancer with the death rate from that cancer in people who were not screened. Some screening tests have been shown to be helpful both in finding cancers early and in decreasing the chance of dying from those cancers. Other tests are used because they have been shown to find a certain type of cancer in some people before symptoms appear, but they have not been proven to decrease the risk of dying from that cancer. If a cancer is fast-growing and spreads quickly, finding it early may not help the person survive the cancer.

Screening studies are done to see whether deaths from cancer decrease when people are screened.

When collecting information on how long cancer patients live, some studies define survival as living 5 years after the diagnosis. This is often used to measure how well cancer treatments work. However, to see if screening tests are useful, studies usually look at whether deaths from the cancer decrease in people who were screened. Over time, signs that a cancer screening test is working include:

- An increase in the number of early-stage cancers found.

- A decrease in the number of late-stage cancers found.

- A decrease in the number of deaths from the cancer.

The number of deaths from cancer is lower today than it was in the past. It is not always clear if this is because screening tests found the cancers earlier or because cancer treatments have gotten better, or both. The Surveillance, Epidemiology, and End Results (SEER) Program of the National Cancer Institute collects and reports information on survival times of people with cancer in the United States. This information is studied to see if finding cancer early affects how long these people live.

Certain factors may cause survival times to look like they are getting better when they are not.

These factors include lead-time bias and overdiagnosis.

- **Lead-time bias**

Survival time for cancer patients is usually measured from the day the cancer is diagnosed until the day they die. Patients are often diagnosed after they have signs and symptoms of cancer. If a screening test leads to a diagnosis before a patient has any symptoms, the patient's survival time is increased because the date of diagnosis is earlier. This increase in survival time makes it seem as though screened patients are living longer when that may not be happening. This is called lead-time bias. It could be that the only reason the survival time appears to be longer is that the date of diagnosis is earlier for the screened patients. But the screened patients may die at the same time they would have without the screening test.

- **Overdiagnosis**

Sometimes, screening tests find cancers that don't matter because they would have gone away on their own or never caused any symptoms. These cancers would never have been found if not for the screening test. Finding these cancers is called overdiagnosis. Overdiagnosis can make it seem like more people are surviving cancer longer, but in reality, these are people who would not have died from cancer anyway.

Section 37.2

Screening for Bladder and Other Urothelial Cancers

Text in this section is excerpted from "Bladder and Other Urothelial Cancers Screening (PDQ®)," National Cancer Institute (NCI), August 7, 2015.

General Information about Bladder and Other Urothelial Cancers

Bladder and other urothelial cancers are diseases in which malignant (cancer) cells form in the urothelium.

The bladder is a hollow organ in the lower part of the abdomen. It is shaped like a small balloon and has a muscle wall that allows it to get larger or smaller to store urine made by the kidneys. There are two kidneys, one on each side of the backbone, above the waist. Tiny tubules in the kidneys filter and clean the blood. They take out waste products and make urine. The urine passes from each kidney through a long tube called a ureter into the bladder. The bladder holds the urine until it passes through the urethra and leaves the body.

The urothelium is a layer of tissue that lines the urethra, bladder, ureters, prostate, and renal pelvis. Cancer that begins in the urothelium of the bladder is much more common than cancer that begins in the urothelium of the urethra, ureters, prostate, or renal pelvis. Because it is the most common form of urothelial cancer, bladder cancer is the focus of this summary.

There are 3 types of cancer that begin in the urothelial cells of the bladder. These cancers are named for the type of cells that become malignant (cancerous):

- Transitional cell carcinoma: Cancer that begins in cells in the innermost layer of the bladder urothelium. These cells are able to stretch when the bladder is full and shrink when it is emptied. Most bladder cancers begin in the transitional cells.

- Squamous cell carcinoma: Cancer that forms in squamous cells, which are thin, flat cells that may form in the bladder urothelium after long-term infection or irritation.

- Adenocarcinoma: Cancer that begins in glandular (secretory) cells. Glandular cells in the bladder urothelium make substances such as mucus.

The risk of bladder cancer increases with age.

In the United States, bladder cancer occurs more often in men than in women, and more often in Whites than in Blacks. As the U.S. population has gotten older, the number of people diagnosed with bladder cancer has increased, but the number of deaths from bladder cancer has decreased. This is true for men and women of all races over the last 30 years.

Smoking can affect the risk of bladder cancer.

Anything that increases your chance of getting a disease is called a risk factor. Having a risk factor does not mean that you will get cancer; not having risk factors doesn't mean that you will not get cancer. Talk to your doctor if you think you may be at risk for bladder cancer. Risk factors for bladder cancer include:

- Using tobacco, especially smoking cigarettes.

- Having a family history of bladder cancer.

- Having certain changes in the genes.

- Being exposed to paints, dyes, metals or petroleum products in the workplace.

- Past treatment with radiation therapy to the pelvis or with certain anticancer drugs, such as cyclophosphamide or ifosfamide.

- Taking *Aristolochia fangchi*, a Chinese herb.

- Drinking well water that has high levels of arsenic.

- Drinking water that has been treated with chlorine.

- Having a history of bladder infections, including bladder infections caused by *Schistosoma haematobium*.

- Using urinary catheters for a long time.

Screening for Bladder and Other Urothelial Cancers

Tests are used to screen for different types of cancer.

Some screening tests are used because they have been shown to be helpful both in finding cancers early and in decreasing the chance of dying from these cancers. Other tests are used because they have been shown to find cancer in some people; however, it has not been proven in clinical trials that use of these tests will decrease the risk of dying from cancer.

Scientists study screening tests to find those with the fewest risks and most benefits. Cancer screening trials also are meant to show whether early detection (finding cancer before it causes symptoms) decreases a person's chance of dying from the disease. For some types of cancer, finding and treating the disease at an early stage may result in a better chance of recovery.

There is no standard or routine screening test for bladder cancer.

Screening for bladder cancer is under study and there are screening clinical trials taking place in many parts of the country.

Two tests may be used to screen for bladder cancer in patients who have had bladder cancer in the past:

Cystoscopy

Cystoscopy is a procedure to look inside the bladder and urethra to check for abnormal areas. A cystoscope (a thin, lighted tube) is inserted through the urethra into the bladder. Tissue samples may be taken for biopsy.

Urine cytology

Urine cytology is a laboratory test in which a sample of urine is checked under a microscope for abnormal cells.

Hematuria tests may also be used to screen for bladder cancer.

Hematuria (red blood cells in the urine) may be caused by cancer or by other conditions. A hematuria test is used to check for blood in a sample of urine by viewing it under a microscope or using a special test strip. The test may be repeated over time.

Risks of Screening for Bladder and Other Urothelial Cancers

Screening tests have risks.

Decisions about screening tests can be difficult. Not all screening tests are helpful and most have risks. Before having any screening test, you may want to discuss the test with your doctor. It is important to know the risks of the test and whether it has been proven to reduce the risk of dying from cancer.

False-positive test results can occur.

Screening test results may appear to be abnormal even though no cancer is present. A false-positive test result (one that shows there is cancer when there really isn't) can cause anxiety and is usually followed by more tests (such as cystoscopy or other invasive procedures), which also have risks. False-positive results often occur with hematuria testing; blood in the urine is usually caused by conditions other than cancer.

False-negative test results can occur.

Screening test results may appear to be normal even though bladder cancer is present. A person who receives a false-negative test result (one that shows there is no cancer when there really is) may delay seeking medical care even if there are symptoms.

Your doctor can advise you about your risk for bladder cancer and your need for screening tests.

Section 37.3

Screening for Colorectal Cancer

Text in this section is excerpted from "Colorectal Cancer Screening
(PDQ®)," National Cancer Institute (NCI), July 23, 2015.

General Information about Colorectal Cancer

Colorectal cancer is a disease in which malignant (cancer) cells form
in the tissues of the colon or the rectum.

The colon and rectum are parts of the body's digestive system. The
digestive system removes and processes nutrients (vitamins, minerals,
carbohydrates, fats, proteins, and water) from foods and helps pass
waste material out of the body. The digestive system is made up of the
mouth, throat, esophagus, stomach, and the small and large intestines.
The colon (large bowel) is the first part of the large intestine and is
about 5 feet long. Together, the rectum and anal canal make up the last
part of the large intestine and are 6-8 inches long. The anal canal ends
at the anus (the opening of the large intestine to the outside of the body).

Cancer that begins in the colon is called colon cancer, and cancer
that begins in the rectum is called rectal cancer. Cancer that begins
in either of these organs may also be called colorectal cancer.

**Colorectal cancer is the second leading cause of death from
cancer in the United States.**

The number of new colorectal cancer cases and the number of
deaths from colorectal cancer are decreasing a little bit each year.
But in adults younger than 50 years, there has been a small increase
in the number of new cases each year since 1998. Colorectal cancer is
found more often in men than in women.

**Age and health history can affect the risk of developing colon
cancer.**

Anything that increases a person's chance of getting a disease
is called a risk factor. Risk factors for colorectal cancer include the
following:

• Being older than 50 years of age.

472

- Having a personal history of any of the following:

- Colorectal cancer.

- Polyps in the colon or rectum.

- Cancer of the ovary, endometrium, or breast.

- Ulcerative colitis or Crohn disease.

- Having a parent, brother, sister, or child with colorectal cancer.

- Having certain hereditary conditions, such as familial adenomatous polyposis (FAP) and hereditary nonpolyposis colon cancer (HNPCC; Lynch Syndrome).

Colorectal Cancer Screening

Tests are used to screen for different types of cancer.

Some screening tests are used because they have been shown to be helpful both in finding cancers early and decreasing the chance of dying from these cancers. Other tests are used because they have been shown to find cancer in some people; however, it has not been proven in clinical trials that use of these tests will decrease the risk of dying from cancer.

Scientists study screening tests to find those with the fewest risks and most benefits. Cancer screening trials also are meant to show whether early detection (finding cancer before it causes symptoms) decreases a person's chance of dying from the disease. For some types of cancer, finding and treating the disease at an early stage may result in a better chance of recovery.

Clinical trials that study cancer screening methods are taking place in many parts of the country.

Studies show that screening for colorectal cancer helps decrease the number of deaths from the disease.

Four tests are used to screen for colorectal cancer:

1. **Fecal occult blood test**

A fecal occult blood test (FOBT) is a test to check stool (solid waste) for blood that can only be seen with a microscope. Small samples of stool are placed on special cards and returned to the doctor or laboratory for testing. Blood in the stool may be a sign of polyps or cancer.

A new colorectal cancer screening test called immunochemical FOBT (iFOBT) is being studied to see if it is better at finding advanced polyps or cancer than the FOBT.

2. Sigmoidoscopy

Sigmoidoscopy is a procedure to look inside the rectum and sigmoid (lower) colon for polyps, abnormal areas, or cancer. A sigmoidoscope is inserted through the rectum into the sigmoid colon. A sigmoidoscope is a thin, tube-like instrument with a light and a lens for viewing. It may also have a tool to remove polyps or tissue samples, which are checked under a microscope for signs of cancer.

3. Barium enema

A barium enema is a series of X-rays of the lower gastrointestinal tract. A liquid that contains barium (a silver-White metallic compound) is put into the rectum. The barium coats the lower gastrointestinal tract and X-rays are taken. This procedure is also called a lower GI series.

4. Colonoscopy

Colonoscopy is a procedure to look inside the rectum and colon for polyps, abnormal areas, or cancer. A colonoscope is inserted through the rectum into the colon. A colonoscope is a thin, tube-like instrument with a light and a lens for viewing. It may also have a tool to remove polyps or tissue samples, which are checked under a microscope for signs of cancer.

Studies have not shown that screening for colorectal cancer using digital rectal exam helps decrease the number of deaths from the disease.

A digital rectal exam (DRE) may be done as part of a routine physical exam. A digital rectal exam is an exam of the rectum. A doctor or nurse inserts a lubricated, gloved finger into the lower part of the rectum to feel for lumps or anything else that seems unusual. Study results have shown that there is no evidence to support DRE as a screening method for colorectal cancer.

New screening tests are being studied in clinical trials.

Virtual colonoscopy

Virtual colonoscopy is a procedure that uses a series of X-rays called computed tomography to make a series of pictures of the colon. A computer puts the pictures together to create detailed images that may show polyps and anything else that seems unusual on the inside surface of the colon. This test is also called colonography or CT colonography. Clinical trials are comparing virtual colonoscopy with commonly used colorectal cancer screening tests. Other clinical trials are testing whether drinking a contrast material that coats the stool, instead of using laxatives to clear the colon, shows polyps clearly.

DNA stool test

This test checks DNA in stool cells for genetic changes that may be a sign of colorectal cancer.

Risks of Colorectal Cancer Screening

Screening tests have risks.

Decisions about screening tests can be difficult. Not all screening tests are helpful and most have risks. Before having any screening test, you may want to discuss the test with your doctor. It is important to know the risks of the test and whether it has been proven to reduce the risk of dying from cancer.

False-negative test results can occur.

Screening test results may appear to be normal even though colorectal cancer is present. A person who receives a false-negative test result (one that shows there is no cancer when there really is) may delay seeking medical care even if there are symptoms.

False-positive test results can occur.

Screening test results may appear to be abnormal even though no cancer is present. A false-positive test result (one that shows there is cancer when there really isn't) can cause anxiety and is usually followed by more tests (such as biopsy), which also have risks.

The following colorectal cancer screening tests have risks:

Fecal occult blood testing

The results of fecal occult blood testing may appear to be abnormal even though no cancer is present. A false-positive test result can cause anxiety and lead to more testing, including colonoscopy or barium enema with sigmoidoscopy.

Sigmoidoscopy

There can be discomfort or pain during sigmoidoscopy. Women may have more pain during the procedure, which may lead them to avoid future screening. Tears in the lining of the colon and bleeding also may occur.

Colonoscopy

Serious complications from colonoscopy are rare, but can include tears in the lining of the colon, bleeding, and problems with the heart or blood vessels. These complications may occur more often in older patients.

Virtual colonoscopy

Virtual colonoscopy often finds problems with organs other than the colon, including the kidneys, chest, liver, ovaries, spleen, and pancreas. Some of these findings lead to more testing. The risks and benefits of this follow-up testing are being studied.

Your doctor can advise you about your risk for colorectal cancer and your need for screening tests.

Section 37.4

Screening for Esophageal Cancer

Text in this section is excerpted from "Esophageal Cancer Screening (PDQ®)," National Cancer Institute (NCI), July 27, 2015.

General Information about Esophageal Cancer

Esophageal cancer is a disease in which malignant (cancer) cells form in the tissues of the esophagus.

The esophagus is the hollow, muscular tube that moves food and liquid from the throat to the stomach. The wall of the esophagus is made up of several layers of tissue, including mucous membrane, muscle, and connective tissue. Esophageal cancer starts in the inside lining of the esophagus and spreads outward through the other layers as it grows.

The two most common types of esophageal cancer are named for the type of cells that become malignant (cancerous):

- Squamous cell carcinoma: Cancer that begins in squamous cells, the thin, flat cells lining the esophagus. This cancer is most often found in the upper and middle part of the esophagus but can occur anywhere along the esophagus. This is also called epidermoid carcinoma.

- Adenocarcinoma: Cancer that begins in glandular (secretory) cells. Glandular cells in the lining of the esophagus produce and release fluids such as mucus. Adenocarcinomas usually form in the lower part of the esophagus, near the stomach.

Esophageal cancer is found more often in men.

Men are about three times more likely than women to have esophageal cancer. There are more new cases of esophageal adenocarcinoma each year and fewer new cases of squamous cell carcinoma. Squamous cell carcinoma of the esophagus is found more often in Blacks than in Whites. The chance of developing esophageal cancer increases with age.

Smoking, heavy alcohol use, and Barrett esophagus can affect the risk of developing esophageal cancer.

Anything that increases the chance of getting a disease is called a risk factor. Having a risk factor does not mean that you will get cancer; not having risk factors doesn't mean that you will not get cancer. People who think they may be at risk should discuss this with their doctor.

Risk factors for squamous cell esophageal cancer include the following:

- Using tobacco.
- Drinking a lot of alcohol.
- Being malnourished (lacking nutrients and/or calories).
- Being infected with human papillomavirus (HPV).
- Having tylosis.
- Having achalasia.
- Having swallowed lye (a chemical found in some cleaning fluids).
- Drinking very hot liquids on a regular basis.

Risk factors for esophageal adenocarcinoma include the following:
- Having gastroesophageal reflux disease (GERD).
- Having Barrett esophagus.
- Having a history of using drugs that relax the lower esophageal sphincter (the ring of muscle that opens and closes the opening between the esophagus and the stomach).
- Being overweight.

Esophageal Cancer Screening

Tests are used to screen for different types of cancer.

Some screening tests are used because they have been shown to be helpful both in finding cancers early and in decreasing the chance of dying from these cancers. Other tests are used because they have been shown to find cancer in some people; however, it has not been proven in clinical trials that use of these tests will decrease the risk of dying from cancer.

Scientists study screening tests to find those with the fewest risks and most benefits. Cancer screening trials also are meant to show whether early detection (finding cancer before it causes symptoms) decreases a person's chance of dying from the disease. For some types of cancer, the chance of recovery is better if the disease is found and treated at an early stage.

There is no standard or routine screening test for esophageal cancer.

Screening for esophageal cancer is under study with screening clinical trials taking place in many parts of the country.

Tests that may detect (find) esophageal cancer are being studied:

Esophagoscopy

A procedure to look inside the esophagus to check for abnormal areas. An esophagoscope is inserted through the mouth or nose and down the throat into the esophagus. An esophagoscope is a thin, tube-like instrument with a light and a lens for viewing. It may also have a tool to remove tissue samples, which are checked under a microscope for signs of cancer.

Biopsy

The removal of cells or tissues so they can be viewed under a microscope by a pathologist to check for signs of cancer. Taking biopsy samples from several different areas in the lining of the lower part of the esophagus may detect early Barrett esophagus. This procedure may be used for patients who have risk factors for Barrett esophagus.

Brush cytology

A procedure in which cells are brushed from the lining of the esophagus and viewed under a microscope to see if they are abnormal. This may be done during an esophagoscopy.

Balloon cytology

A procedure in which cells are collected from the lining of the esophagus using a deflated balloon that is swallowed by the patient. The balloon is then inflated and pulled out of the esophagus. Esophageal cells on the balloon are viewed under a microscope to see if they are abnormal.

Chromoendoscopy

A procedure in which a dye is sprayed onto the lining of the esophagus during esophagoscopy. Increased staining of certain areas of the lining may be a sign of early Barrett esophagus.

Fluorescence spectroscopy

A procedure that uses a special light to view tissue in the lining of the esophagus. The light probe is passed through an endoscope and shines on the lining of the esophagus. The light given off by the cells lining the esophagus is then measured. Malignant tissue gives off less light than normal tissue.

Risks of Esophageal Cancer Screening

Screening tests have risks.

Decisions about screening tests can be difficult. Not all screening tests are helpful and most have risks. Before having any screening test, you may want to discuss the test with your doctor. It is important to know the risks of the test and whether it has been proven to reduce the risk of dying from cancer.

The risks of esophageal cancer screening tests include the following:

Finding esophageal cancer may not improve health or help a person live longer.

Screening may not improve your health or help you live longer if you have advanced esophageal cancer or if it has already spread to other places in your body.

Some cancers never cause symptoms or become life-threatening, but if found by a screening test, the cancer may be treated. It is not known if treatment of these cancers will help you live longer than if no treatment were given, and treatments for cancer may have serious side effects.

False-negative test results can occur.

Screening test results may appear to be normal even though esophageal cancer is present. A person who receives a false-negative test result (one that shows there is no cancer when there really is) may delay seeking medical care even if there are symptoms.

479

False-positive test results can occur.

Screening test results may appear to be abnormal even though no cancer is present. A false-positive test result (one that shows there is cancer when there really isn't) can cause anxiety and is usually followed by more tests (such as biopsy), which also have risks.

Side effects may be caused by the test itself.

There are rare but serious side effects that may occur with esophagoscopy and biopsy. These include the following:

- A small hole (puncture) in the esophagus.

- Problems with breathing.

- Heart attack.

- Passage of food, water, stomach acid or vomit into the airway.

- Severe bleeding that may need to be treated in a hospital.

Screening tests have risks.

Decisions about screening tests can be difficult. Not all screening tests are helpful and most have risks. Before having any screening test, you may want to discuss the test with your doctor. It is important to know the risks of the test and whether it has been proven to reduce the risk of dying from cancer.

The risks of esophageal cancer screening tests include the following:

Finding esophageal cancer may not improve health or help a person live longer.

Screening may not improve your health or help you live longer if you have advanced esophageal cancer or if it has already spread to other places in your body.

Some cancers never cause symptoms or become life-threatening, but if found by a screening test, the cancer may be treated. It is not known if treatment of these cancers will help you live longer than if no treatment were given, and treatments for cancer may have serious side effects.

False-negative test results can occur.

Screening test results may appear to be normal even though esophageal cancer is present. A person who receives a false-negative test result(one that shows there is no cancer when there really is) may delay seeking medical care even if there are symptoms.

False-positive test results can occur.

Screening test results may appear to be abnormaleven though no cancer is present. A false-positive test result (one that shows there is cancer when there really isn't) can cause anxiety and is usually followed by more tests (such as biopsy), which also have risks.

Side effects may be caused by the test itself.

There are rare but serious side effects that may occur with esophagoscopy and biopsy. These include the following:

- A small hole (puncture) in the esophagus.

- Problems with breathing.

- Heart attack.

- Passage of food, water, stomach acid or vomitinto the airway.

- Severe bleeding that may need to be treated in a hospital.

Section 37.5

Screening for Liver (Hepatocellular) Cancer

Text in this section is excerpted from "Liver (Hepatocellular) Cancer Screening (PDQ®)," National Cancer Institute (NCI), July 31, 2015.

General Information about Liver (Hepatocellular) Cancer

Liver cancer is a disease in which malignant (cancer) cells form in the tissues of the liver.

The liver is one of the largest organs in the body. It has four lobes and fills the upper right side of the abdomen inside the rib cage. Three of the many important functions of the liver are:

- To filter harmful substances from the blood so they can be passed from the body in stools and urine.

- To make bile to help digest fats from food.

- To store glycogen (sugar), which the body uses for energy.

Liver cancer is less common in the United States than in other parts of the world.

Liver cancer is uncommon in the United States, but is the fourth most common cancer in the world. In the United States, men, especially Chinese American men, have a greater risk of developing liver cancer.

Having hepatitis or cirrhosis can increase the risk of developing liver cancer.

Anything that increases the chance of getting a disease is called a risk factor. Having a risk factor does not mean that you will get cancer; not having risk factors doesn't mean that you will not get cancer. People who think they may be at risk should discuss this with their doctor. Risk factors for liver cancer include:

- Having hepatitis B or hepatitis C; having both hepatitis B and hepatitis C increases the risk even more.

- Having cirrhosis, which can be caused by:

- hepatitis (especially hepatitis C); or

- drinking large amounts of alcohol for many years or being an alcoholic.

- Eating foods tainted with aflatoxin (poison from a fungus that can grow on foods, such as grains and nuts, that have not been stored properly).

Liver (Hepatocellular) Cancer Screening

Tests are used to screen for different types of cancer.

Some screening tests are used because they have been shown to be helpful both in finding cancers early and in decreasing the chance of dying from these cancers. Other tests are used because they have been shown to find cancer in some people; however, it has not been proven in clinical trials that use of these tests will decrease the risk of dying from cancer.

Scientists study screening tests to find those with the fewest risks and most benefits. Cancer screening trials also are meant to show whether early detection (finding cancer before it causes symptoms) decreases a person's chance of dying from the disease. For some types of cancer, the chance of recovery is better if the disease is found and treated at an early stage.

Clinical trials that study cancer screening methods are taking place in many parts of the country.

There is no standard or routine screening test for liver cancer.

Although there are no standard or routine screening tests for liver cancer, the following tests are being used or studied to screen for it:

Ultrasound

Ultrasound is a procedure in which high-energy sound waves (ultrasound) are bounced off the liver and make echoes. The echoes form a picture of the liver called a sonogram. The picture can be printed to be looked at later.

CT scan

CT scan is a procedure that makes a series of detailed pictures of the liver, taken from different angles. The pictures are made by a computer linked to an X-ray machine. A dye may be injected into a vein or swallowed to help the liver show up more clearly. This procedure is also called CAT scan or computed tomography.

Tumor markers

Tumor markers, also called biomarkers, are substances made by the tumor that may be found in the blood, other body fluids, or tissues. A high level of a specific tumor marker may mean that a certain type of cancer is present in the body.

Alpha-fetoprotein (AFP) is the most widely used tumor marker for detecting liver cancer. However, other cancers and certain conditions, including pregnancy, hepatitis, and other types of cancer, may also increase AFP levels.

Specific tumor markers that may lead to early detection of liver cancer are being studied.

Risks of Liver (Hepatocellular) Cancer Screening

Screening tests have risks.

Decisions about screening tests can be difficult. Not all screening tests are helpful and most have risks. Before having any screening test, you may want to discuss the test with your doctor. It is important to know the risks of the test and whether it has been proven to reduce the risk of dying from cancer.

The risks of liver cancer screening include the following:

False-negative test results can occur.

Screening test results may appear to be normal even though liver cancer is present. A person who receives a false-negative test result (one that shows there is no cancer when there really is) may delay seeking medical care even if there are symptoms.

False-positive test results can occur.

Screening test results may appear to be abnormal even though no cancer is present. A false-positive test result (one that shows there is cancer when there really isn't) can cause anxiety and is usually followed by diagnostic tests and procedures, such as a liver biopsy, which also have risks.

Side effects may be caused by procedures to diagnose liver cancer.

Abnormal screening results may lead to a liver biopsy to diagnose liver cancer. Liver biopsy may cause the following rare, but serious, side effects:

- Hemorrhage.

- Trouble breathing.

- Leakage of bile, which can cause an infection of the lining of the abdomen.

- A small puncture (hole) in an organ in the abdomen.

- Spread of cancer cells along the needle path when the biopsy needle is inserted and withdrawn (taken out).

Your doctor can advise you about your risk for liver cancer and your need for screening tests.

Section 37.6

Screening for Neuroblastoma

Text in this section is excerpted from "Neuroblastoma Screening (PDQ®)," National Cancer Institute (NCI), August 28, 2014.

General Information about Neuroblastoma Cancer

Neuroblastoma is a disease in which malignant (cancer) cells form in nerve tissue.

Neuroblastoma often begins in the nerve tissue of the adrenal glands. There are two adrenal glands, one on top of each kidney, in the back of the upper abdomen. The adrenal glands make important hormones that help control heart rate, blood pressure, blood sugar, and the way the body reacts to stress. Neuroblastoma may also begin in the abdomen, chest, spinal cord, or in nerve tissue near the spine in the neck.

Neuroblastoma most often begins during early childhood, usually in children younger than 5 years of age. **Most cases of neuroblastoma are diagnosed before 1 year of age.**

Neuroblastoma is the most common type of cancer in infants. The number of new cases of neuroblastoma is greatest among children under 1 year of age. As children get older, the number of new cases decreases. Neuroblastoma is slightly more common in males than females.

Neuroblastoma sometimes forms before birth but is usually found later, when the tumor begins to grow and cause symptoms. In rare cases, neuroblastoma may be found before birth, by fetal ultrasound.

Neuroblastoma Screening

Tests are used to screen for different types of cancer.

Some screening tests are used because they have been shown to be helpful both in finding cancers early and in decreasing the chance of dying from these cancers. Other tests are used because they have been shown to find cancer in some people; however, it has not been proven in clinical trials that use of these tests will decrease the risk of dying from cancer.

Scientists study screening tests to find those with the fewest risks and most benefits. Cancer screening trials also are meant to show whether early detection (finding cancer before it causes symptoms) decreases a person's chance of dying from the disease. For some types of cancer, the chance of recovery is better if the disease is found and treated at an early stage.

Clinical trials that study cancer screening methods are taking place in many parts of the country.

There is no standard or routine screening test for neuroblastoma.

There is no standard or routine screening test used to find neuroblastoma. A urine test is sometimes used to check for neuroblastoma, usually when the child is 6 months old. This is a test in which urine is collected for 24 hours to measure the amounts of certain substances. An unusual (higher or lower than normal) amount of a substance can be a sign of disease in the organ or tissue that makes it. A higher than normal amount of homovanillic acid (HMA) and vanillylmandelic acid (VMA) may be a sign of neuroblastoma.

Screening for neuroblastoma may not help the child live longer.

Studies have shown that screening for neuroblastoma does not decrease the chance of dying from the disease. Almost all neuroblastomas that are found by screening children at 6 months of age are the type that have a good prognosis (chance of recovery).

Risks of Neuroblastoma Screening

Screening tests have risks.

Decisions about screening tests can be difficult. Not all screening tests are helpful and most have risks. Before having any screening test, you may want to discuss the test with your doctor. It is important to know the risks of the test and whether it has been proven to reduce the risk of dying from cancer.

The risks of neuroblastoma screening include the following:

Neuroblastoma may be overdiagnosed.

When a screening test result leads to the diagnosis and treatment of a disease that may never have caused symptoms or become life-threatening, it is called overdiagnosis. For example, when a urine test result shows a higher than normal amount of homovanillic acid (HMA) or vanillylmandelic acid (VMA), tests and treatments for neuroblastoma are likely to be done, but may not be needed. At this time, it is not possible to know which neuroblastomas found by a screening test will cause symptoms and which neuroblastomas will not. Diagnostic tests (such as biopsies) and cancer treatments (such as surgery, radiation therapy, and chemotherapy) can have serious risks, including physical and emotional problems.

False-negative test results can occur.

Screening test results may appear to be normal even though neuroblastoma is present. A person who receives a false-negative test result (one that shows there is no cancer when there really is) may delay seeking medical care even if there are symptoms.

False-positive test results can occur.

Screening test results may appear to be abnormal even though no cancer is present. A false-positive test result (one that shows there is cancer when there really isn't) can cause anxiety and is usually followed by more tests and procedures, which also have risks.

Section 37.7

Screening for Oral Cavity and Oropharyngeal Cancer

Text in this section is excerpted from "Oral Cavity and Oropharyngeal Cancer Screening (PDQ®)," National Cancer Institute (NCI), July 23, 2015.

General Information about Oral Cavity and Oropharyngeal Cancer

Oral cancer is a disease in which malignant (cancer) cells form in the lips, oral cavity, or oropharynx.

Oral cancer may develop in any of the following areas:

• Lips.

- Oral cavity:
  - The front two thirds of the tongue.
  - The gingiva (gums).
  - The buccal mucosa (the lining of the inside of the cheeks).
  - The floor (bottom) of the mouth under the tongue.
  - The hard palate (the front of the roof of the mouth).
  - The retromolar trigone (the small area behind the wisdom teeth).
- Oropharynx:
  - The middle part of the pharynx (throat) behind the mouth.
  - The back one third of the tongue.
  - The soft palate (the back of the roof of the mouth).
  - The side and back walls of the throat.
  - The tonsils.

Most oral cancers start in squamous cells, the thin, flat cells that line the lips, oral cavity, and oropharynx. Cancer that forms in squamous cells is called squamous cell carcinoma.

The number of new cases of oral cancer and the number of deaths from oral cancer have been decreasing slowly.

The number of new cases and deaths from oral cancer has slowly decreased over the past 30 years. However, the number of new cases of oral cancer caused by certain types of human papillomavirus (HPV) infection has increased. One kind of HPV, called HPV 16, is often passed from one person to another during sexual activity.

Although oral cancer occurs in all adults, it occurs most commonly in older adults. Also, oral cancer occurs more often in Blacks than in Whites and in men than in women.

Tobacco and alcohol use can affect the risk of developing oral cancer.

Anything that increases the chance of getting a disease is called a risk factor. Having a risk factor does not mean that you will get cancer;

not having risk factors doesn't mean that you will not get cancer. People who think they may be at risk should discuss this with their doctor. Risk factors for oral cancer include the following:

- Using tobacco products (includes cigarettes, cigars, pipes, and smokeless and chewing tobacco).

- Heavy alcohol use.

- Chewing betel nuts.

- Being infected with a certain type of human papillomavirus (HPV).

- Being exposed to sunlight (lip cancer only).

- Being male.

Oral Cavity and Oropharyngeal Cancer Screening

Tests are used to screen for different types of cancer.

Some screening tests are used because they have been shown to be helpful both in finding cancers early and in decreasing the chance of dying from these cancers. Other tests are used because they have been shown to find cancer in some people; however, it has not been proven in clinical trials that use of these tests will decrease the risk of dying from cancer.

Scientists study screening tests to find those with the fewest risks and most benefits. Cancer screening trials also are meant to show whether early detection (finding cancer before it causes symptoms) decreases a person's chance of dying from the disease. For some types of cancer, the chance of recovery is better if the disease is found and treated at an early stage.

Clinical trials that study cancer screening methods are taking place in many parts of the country.

There is no standard or routine screening test for oral cancer.

Screening for oral cancer may be done during a routine check-up by a dentist or medical doctor. The exam will include looking for lesions, including areas of leukoplakia (an abnormal White patch of cells) and erythroplakia (an abnormal red patch of cells). Leukoplakia and erythroplakia lesions on the mucous membranes may become cancerous.

If lesions are seen in the mouth, the following procedures may be used to find abnormal tissue that might develop into oral cancer:

- Toluidine blue stain: A procedure in which lesions in the mouth are coated with a blue dye. Areas that stain darker are more likely to be cancer or become cancer.

- Fluorescence staining: A procedure in which lesions in the mouth are viewed using a special light. After the patient uses a fluorescent mouth rinse, normal tissue looks different from abnormal tissue when seen under the light.

- Exfoliative cytology: A procedure to collect cells from the lip or oral cavity. A piece of cotton, a brush, or a small wooden stick is used to gently scrape cells from the lips, tongue, mouth, or throat. The cells are viewed under a microscope to find out if they are abnormal.

- Brush biopsy: The removal of cells using a brush that is designed to collect cells from all layers of a lesion. The cells are viewed under a microscope to find out if they are abnormal.

More than half of oral cancers have already spread to lymph nodes or other areas by the time they are found. No studies have shown that screening would decrease the risk of dying from this disease.

Risks of Oral Cavity and Oropharyngeal Cancer Screening

Screening tests have risks.

Decisions about screening tests can be difficult. Not all screening tests are helpful and most have risks. Before having any screening test, you may want to discuss the test with your doctor. It is important to know the risks of the test and whether it has been proven to reduce the risk of dying from cancer.

The risks of oral cancer screening include the following:

Finding oral cancer may not improve health or help a person live longer.

Some cancers never cause symptoms or become life-threatening, but if found by a screening test, the cancer may be treated. Finding these cancers is called overdiagnosis. It is not known if treatment of these cancers would help you live longer than if no treatment were given, and treatments for cancer, such as surgery and radiation therapy, may have serious side effects.

Screening may also find oral cancers that have already spread and cannot be cured. When these cancers are found, treatment may cause serious side effects and not help a person live longer.

False-negative test results can occur.

Screening test results may appear to be normal even though oral cancer is present. A person who receives a false-negative test result (one that shows there is no cancer when there really is) may delay seeking medical care even if there are symptoms.

False-positive test results can occur.

Screening test results may appear to be abnormal even though no cancer is present. A false-positive test result (one that shows there is cancer when there really isn't) can cause anxiety and is usually followed by more tests and procedures (such as biopsy) which also have risks.

Misdiagnosis can occur.

A biopsy is needed to diagnose oral cancer. Cells or tissues are removed from the lips, oral cavity, or oropharynx and viewed under a microscope by a pathologist to check for signs of cancer. When the cells are cancer and the pathologist reports them as not being cancer, the cancer is misdiagnosed. Cancer is also misdiagnosed when the cells are not cancer and the pathologist reports there is cancer. When cancer is misdiagnosed, treatment that is needed may not be given or treatment may be given that is not needed.

Section 37.8

Screening for Skin Cancer

Text in this section is excerpted from "Skin Cancer Screening (PDQ®)," National Cancer Institute (NCI), May 14, 2015.

General Information about Skin Cancer

Skin cancer is a disease in which malignant (cancer) cells form in the tissues of the skin.

The skin is the body's largest organ. It protects against heat, sunlight, injury, and infection. Skin also helps control body temperature and stores water, fat, and vitamin D. The skin has several layers, but the two main layers are the epidermis (top or outer layer) and the dermis (lower or inner layer). Skin cancer begins in the epidermis, which is made up of three kinds of cells:

- Squamous cells: Thin, flat cells that form the top layer of the epidermis. Cancer that forms in squamous cells is called squamous cell carcinoma.

- Basal cells: Round cells under the squamous cells. Cancer that forms in basal cells is called basal cell carcinoma.

- Melanocytes: Found in the lower part of the epidermis, these cells make melanin, the pigment that gives skin its natural color. When skin is exposed to the sun, melanocytes make more pigment and cause the skin to tan, or darken. Cancer that forms in melanocytes is called melanoma.

Nonmelanoma skin cancer is the most common cancer in the United States.

Basal cell carcinoma and squamous cell carcinoma are also called nonmelanoma skin cancer and are the most common forms of skin cancer. Most basal cell and squamous cell skin cancers can be cured.

Melanoma is more likely to spread to nearby tissues and other parts of the body and can be harder to cure. Melanoma is easier to cure if the tumor is found before it spreads to the dermis (inner layer of skin). Melanoma is less likely to cause death when it is found and treated early.

In the United States, the number of cases of nonmelanoma skin cancer seems to have increased in recent years. The number of cases of melanoma has increased over the last 30 years. Part of the reason for these increases may be that people are more aware of skin cancer. They are more likely to have skin exams and biopsies and to be diagnosed with skin cancer.

Over the past 20 years, the number of deaths from melanoma has decreased slightly among White men and women younger than 50 years. During that time, the number of deaths from melanoma has increased slightly among White men older than 50 years and stayed about the same among White women older than 50 years.

The number of cases of childhood melanoma diagnosed in the United States is low, but increasing over time. The number of childhood deaths from melanoma has stayed about the same.

Being exposed to ultraviolet radiation may increase the risk of skin cancer.

Anything that increases your chance of getting a disease is called a risk factor. Having a risk factor does not mean that you will get cancer; not having risk factors doesn't mean that you will not get cancer. People who think they may be at risk should discuss this with their doctor.

Being exposed to ultraviolet (UV) radiation and having skin that is sensitive to UV radiation are risk factors for skin cancer. UV radiation is the name for the invisible rays that are part of the energy that comes from the sun. Sunlamps and tanning beds also give off UV radiation.

Risk factors for nonmelanoma and melanoma cancers are not the same.

Nonmelanoma skin cancer risk factors include:

- Being exposed to natural sunlight or artificial sunlight (such as from tanning beds) over long periods of time.

- Having a fair complexion, which includes the following:

- Fair skin that freckles and burns easily, does not tan, or tans poorly.

- Blue or green or other light-colored eyes.

- Red or blond hair.

- Having actinic keratosis.

- Past treatment with radiation.

- Having a weakened immune system.

- Being exposed to arsenic.

Melanoma skin cancer risk factors include:

- Having a fair complexion, which includes the following:

- Fair skin that freckles and burns easily, does not tan, or tans poorly.

- Blue or green or other light-colored eyes.

- Red or blond hair.

- Being exposed to natural sunlight or artificial sunlight (such as from tanning beds) over long periods of time.

493

- Having a history of many blistering sunburns, especially as a child or teenager.

- Having several large or many small moles.

- Having a family history of unusual moles (atypical nevus syndrome).

- Having a family or personal history of melanoma.

- Being White.

Skin Cancer Screening

Tests are used to screen for different types of cancer.

Some screening tests are used because they have been shown to be helpful both in finding cancers early and in decreasing the chance of dying from these cancers. Other tests are used because they have been shown to find cancer in some people; however, it has not been proven in clinical trials that use of these tests will decrease the risk of dying from cancer.

Scientists study screening tests to find those with the fewest risks and most benefits. Cancer screening trials also are meant to show whether early detection (finding cancer before it causes symptoms) decreases a person's chance of dying from the disease. For some types of cancer, finding and treating the disease at an early stage may result in a better chance of recovery.

Clinical trials that study cancer screening methods are taking place in many parts of the country.

Skin exams are used to screen for skin cancer.

If you find a worrisome change, you should report it to your doctor. Regular skin checks by a doctor are important for people who have already had skin cancer.

If an area on the skin looks abnormal, a biopsy is usually done. The doctor will remove as much of the suspicious tissue as possible with a local excision. A pathologist then looks at the tissue under a microscope to check for cancer cells. Because it is sometimes difficult to tell if a skin growth is benign (not cancer) or malignant (cancer), you may want to have the biopsy sample checked by a second pathologist.

Most melanomas in the skin can be seen by the naked eye. Usually, melanoma grows for a long time under the top layer of skin (the epidermis) but does not grow into the deeper layer of skin (the dermis).

This allows time for skin cancer to be found early. Melanoma is easier to cure if it is found before it spreads.

Other screening tests are being studied in clinical trials.

Screening clinical trials are taking place in many parts of the country.

Risks of Skin Cancer Screening

Screening tests have risks.

Decisions about screening tests can be difficult. Not all screening tests are helpful and most have risks. Before having any screening test, you may want to discuss the test with your doctor. It is important to know the risks of the test and whether it has been proven to reduce the risk of dying from cancer.

The risks of skin cancer screening tests include the following:

Finding skin cancer does not always improve health or help you live longer.

Screening may not improve your health or help you live longer if you have advanced skin cancer.

Some cancers never cause symptoms or become life-threatening, but if found by a screening test, the cancer may be treated. Treatments for cancer may have serious side effects.

False-negative test results can occur.

Screening test results may appear to be normal even though cancer is present. A person who receives a false-negative test result (one that shows there is no cancer when there really is) may delay getting medical care even if there are symptoms.

False-positive test results can occur.

Screening test results may appear to be abnormal even though no cancer is present. A false-positive test result (one that shows there is cancer when there really isn't) can cause anxiety and is usually followed by more tests (such as a biopsy), which also have risks.

A biopsy may cause scarring.

When a skin biopsy is done, the doctor will try to leave the smallest scar possible, but there is a risk of scarring and infection.

Talk to your doctor about your risk for skin cancer and your need for screening tests.

Section 37.9

Screening for Stomach (Gastric) Cancer

Text in this section is excerpted from "Stomach (Gastric)
Cancer Screening (PDQ®)," National Cancer Institute (NCI),
August 22, 2013.

General Information about Stomach (Gastric) Cancer

*Stomach cancer is a disease in which malignant (cancer) cells form in
the lining of the stomach.*

The stomach is a J-shaped organ in the upper abdomen. It is part
of the digestive system, which processes nutrients (vitamins, minerals,
carbohydrates, fats, proteins, and water) in foods that are eaten and
helps pass waste material out of the body. Food moves from the throat
to the stomach through a hollow, muscular tube called the esophagus.
After leaving the stomach, partly-digested food passes into the small
intestine and then into the large intestine.

The wall of the stomach is made up of 3 layers of tissue: the mucosal
(innermost) layer, the muscularis (middle) layer, and the serosal (out-
ermost) layer. Stomach cancer begins in the cells lining the mucosal
layer and spreads through the outer layers as it grows.

Stomach cancer is not common in the United States.

Stomach cancer is less common in the United States than in many
parts of Asia, Europe, and Central and South America. Stomach cancer
is a major cause of death in these parts of the world.

In the United States, the number of new cases of stomach cancer
has greatly decreased since 1930. The reasons for this are not clear,
but may have to do with better food storage and changes in the diet,
such as lower salt intake.

*Older age and certain chronic conditions increase the risk of stomach
cancer.*

Anything that increases the chance of getting a disease is called a
risk factor. Having a risk factor does not mean that you will get cancer;

not having risk factors doesn't mean that you will not get cancer. Talk to your doctor if you think you may be at risk for stomach cancer. Risk factors for stomach cancer include the following:

- Having any of the following medical conditions:

- Helicobacter pylori (H. pylori) infection of the stomach.

- Chronic gastric atrophy (thinning of the stomach lining caused by long-term inflammation of the stomach).

- Pernicious anemia (a type of anemia caused by a vitamin B12 deficiency).

- Intestinal metaplasia (a condition in which the cells that line the stomach are replaced by the cells that normally line the intestines).

- Polyps in the stomach.

- Familial adenomatous polyposis (FAP).

- Hereditary nonpolyposis colon cancer (HNPCC).

- Having a mother, father, sister, or brother who has had stomach cancer.

- Having had a partial gastrectomy.

- Eating a diet high in salted, smoked foods or low in fruits and vegetables.

- Eating foods that have not been prepared or stored the way they should be.

- Smoking cigarettes.

The risk of stomach cancer is increased in people who come from countries where stomach cancer is common.

Stomach (Gastric) Cancer Screening

Tests are used to screen for different types of cancer.

Some screening tests are used because they have been shown to be helpful both in finding cancers early and in decreasing the chance of dying from these cancers. Other tests are used because they have been shown to find cancer in some people; however, it has not been proven in clinical trials that use of these tests will decrease the risk of dying from cancer.

Scientists study screening tests to find those with the fewest risks and most benefits. Cancer screening trials also are meant to show whether early detection (finding cancer before it causes symptoms) decreases a person's chance of dying from the disease. For some types of cancer, the chance of recovery is better if the disease is found and treated at an early stage.

Clinical trials that study cancer screening methods are taking place in many parts of the country.

There is no standard or routine screening test for stomach cancer.

Several types of screening tests have been studied to find stomach cancer at an early stage. These screening tests include the following:

- Barium-meal photofluorography: A series of X-rays of the esophagus and stomach. The patient drinks a liquid that contains barium (a silver-White metallic compound) which coats the esophagus and stomach as it is swallowed. Photographs are taken of the X-ray images. The photographs are processed to make the organs easier to see and then made into a film. This makes it possible to see the motion of the organs while exposing the patient to less radiation.

- Upper endoscopy: A procedure to look inside the esophagus, stomach, and duodenum (first part of the small intestine) to check for abnormal areas. An endoscope is passed through the mouth and down the throat into the esophagus. An endoscope is a thin, tube-like instrument with a light and a lens for viewing. It may also have a tool to remove tissue, which is checked under a microscope for signs of disease.

- Serum pepsinogen levels: A test that measures the levels of pepsinogen in the blood. Low levels of pepsinogen are a sign of chronic gastric atrophy which may lead to stomach cancer.

Studies showed that screening a large number of people for stomach cancer using these tests did not decrease the risk of dying from stomach cancer.

More studies are needed to find out if it would be worthwhile to screen people in the United States who do have a high risk for stomach cancer. Scientists believe that people with certain risk factors may benefit from stomach cancer screening. These include:

- Older people with chronic gastric atrophy or pernicious anemia.

- Patients who have had any of the following:
  - Partial gastrectomy.
  - Polyps in the stomach.
  - Familial adenomatous polyposis (FAP).
  - Hereditary nonpolyposis colon cancer (HNPCC).
- People who come from countries where stomach cancer is more common.

Risks of Stomach (Gastric) Cancer Screening

Screening tests have risks.

Decisions about screening tests can be difficult. Not all screening tests are helpful and most have risks. Before having any screening test, you may want to discuss the test with your doctor. It is important to know the risks of the test and whether it has been proven to reduce the risk of dying from cancer.

The risks of stomach cancer screening include the following:

Finding stomach cancer may not improve health or help you live longer.

Screening may not improve your health or help you live longer if you have advanced stomach cancer.

Some cancers never cause symptoms or become life-threatening, but if found by a screening test, the cancer may be treated. It is not known if treatment of these cancers would help you live longer than if no treatment were given, and treatments for cancer may have serious side effects.

False-negative test results can occur.

Screening test results may appear to be normal even though stomach cancer is present. A person who receives a false-negative result (one that shows there is no cancer when there really is) may delay seeking medical care even if there are symptoms.

False-positive test results can occur.

Screening test results may appear to be abnormal even though no cancer is present. A false-positive test result (one that shows there is cancer when there really isn't) can cause anxiety and is usually followed by more tests and procedures which also have risks.

Side effects may be caused by the screening test itself.

Upper endoscopy may cause the following rare, but serious, side effects:

- A small hole (puncture) in the esophagus or stomach.
- Heart problems.
- Breathing problems.
- Lung infection from inhaling food, fluid, or stomach acid into the lung.
- Severe bleeding that needs to be treated at a hospital.
- Reactions to medicine used during the procedure.

Chapter 38

Cancer Screening Tests for Women

Chapter Contents

Section 38.1

Screening for Breast Cancer

Text in this section is excerpted from "Breast Cancer Screening
(PDQ®)," National Cancer Institute (NCI), April 13, 2015.

General Information about Breast Cancer

*Breast cancer is a disease in which malignant (cancer) cells form in
the tissues of the breast.*

The breast is made up of lobes and ducts. Each breast has 15 to 20
sections called lobes, which have many smaller sections called lobules.
Lobules end in dozens of tiny bulbs that can produce milk. The lobes,
lobules, and bulbs are linked by thin tubes called ducts.

Each breast also contains blood vessels and lymph vessels. The
lymph vessels carry an almost colorless fluid called lymph. Lymph
vessels lead to organs called lymph nodes. Lymph nodes are small
bean-shaped structures that are found throughout the body. They filter
substances in lymph and help fight infection and disease. Clusters of
lymph nodes are found near the breast in the axilla (under the arm),
above the collarbone, and in the chest.

*Breast cancer is the second leading cause of death from cancer in Amer-
ican women.*

Women in the United States get breast cancer more than any other
type of cancer except for skin cancer. Breast cancer is second only to
lung cancer as a cause of cancer death in women.

Breast cancer occurs more often in White women than in Black
women. However, Black women are more likely than White women
to die from the disease.

Breast cancer occurs in men also, but the number of cases is small.

Health history can affect the risk of breast cancer.

Anything that increases your chance of getting a disease is called a
risk factor. Having a risk factor does not mean that you will get cancer;

not having risk factors doesn't mean that you will not get cancer. Talk with your doctor if you think you may be at risk for breast cancer.

Older age is the main risk factor for most cancers. The chance of getting cancer increases as you get older. Other risk factors for breast cancer include the following:

- A family history of breast cancer in a first-degree relative (mother, daughter, or sister) .

- Inherited changes in the BRCA1 and BRCA2 genes or in other genes that increase the risk of breast cancer.

- Drinking alcohol.

- Breast tissue that is dense on a mammogram.

- Exposure of breast tissue to estrogen made by the body:

- Menstruating at an early age.

- Older age at first birth or never having given birth.

- Starting menopause at a later age.

- Taking hormones such as estrogen combined with progestin for symptoms of menopause.

- Taking oral contraceptives ("the pill").

- Obesity.

- A personal history of invasive breast cancer, ductal carcinoma in situ (DCIS), or lobular carcinoma in situ (LCIS).

- A personal history of benign (noncancer) breast disease.

- Being White.

- Treatment with radiation therapy to the breast/chest.

Breast Cancer Screening

Tests are used to screen for different types of cancer.

Some screening tests are used because they have been shown to be helpful both in finding cancers early and in decreasing the chance of dying from these cancers. Other tests are used because they have been shown to find cancer in some people; however, it has not been proven in clinical trials that use of these tests will decrease the risk of dying from cancer.

Scientists study screening tests to find those with the fewest risks and most benefits. Cancer screening trials also are meant to show whether early detection (finding cancer before it causes symptoms) decreases a person's chance of dying from the disease. For some types of cancer, the chance of recovery is better if the disease is found and treated at an early stage.

Clinical trials that study cancer screening methods are taking place in many parts of the country.

Three tests are used by health care providers to screen for breast cancer:

1. **Mammogram**

Mammography is the most common screening test for breast cancer. A mammogram is an X-ray of the breast. This test may find tumors that are too small to feel. A mammogram may also find ductal carcinoma in situ (DCIS). In DCIS, there are abnormal cells in the lining of a breast duct, which may become invasive cancer in some women.

Mammograms are less likely to find breast tumors in women younger than 50 years than in older women. This may be because younger women have denser breast tissue that appears White on a mammogram. Because tumors also appear White on a mammogram, they can be harder to find when there is dense breast tissue.

The following may affect whether a mammogram is able to detect (find) breast cancer:

- The size of the tumor.
- How dense the breast tissue is.
- The skill of the radiologist.

Women aged 40 to 74 years who have screening mammograms have a lower chance of dying from breast cancer than women who do not have screening mammograms.

2. **Clinical breast exam (CBE)**

A clinical breast exam is an exam of the breast by a doctor or other health professional. The doctor will carefully feel the breasts and under the arms for lumps or anything else that seems unusual. It is not known if having clinical breast exams decreases the chance of dying from breast cancer.

Breast self-exams may be done by women or men to check their breasts for lumps or other changes. It is important to know how your breasts usually look and feel. If you feel any lumps or notice any other changes, talk to your doctor. Doing breast self-exams has not been shown to decrease the chance of dying from breast cancer.

504

3. **MRI (magnetic resonance imaging) in women with a high risk of breast cancer**

MRI is a procedure that uses a magnet, radio waves, and a computer to make a series of detailed pictures of areas inside the body. This procedure is also called nuclear magnetic resonance imaging (NMRI). MRI does not use any X-rays.

MRI is used as a screening test for women who have one or more of the following:

- Certain gene changes, such as in the BRCA1 or BRCA2 genes.

- A family history (first degree relative, such as a mother, daughter or sister) with breast cancer.

- Certain genetic syndromes, such as Li-Fraumeni or Cowden syndrome.

MRIs find breast cancer more often than mammograms do, but it is common for MRI results to appear abnormal even when there isn't any cancer.

Other screening tests are being studied in clinical trials.

Thermography

Thermography is a procedure in which a special camera that senses heat is used to record the temperature of the skin that covers the breasts. A computer makes a map of the breast showing the changes in temperature. Tumors can cause temperature changes that may show up on the thermogram.

There have been no clinical trials of thermography to find out how well it detects breast cancer or if having the procedure decreases the risk of dying from breast cancer.

Tissue sampling

Breast tissue sampling is taking cells from breast tissue to check under a microscope. Abnormal cells in breast fluid have been linked to an increased risk of breast cancer in some studies. Scientists are studying whether breast tissue sampling can be used to find breast cancer at an early stage or predict the risk of developing breast cancer. Three ways of taking tissue samples are being studied:

- Fine-needle aspiration: A thin needle is inserted into the breast tissue around the areola (darkened area around the nipple) to take out a sample of cells and fluid.

505

- Nipple aspiration: The use of gentle suction to collect fluid through the nipple. This is done with a device similar to the breast pumps used by women who are breast-feeding.

- Ductal lavage: A hair-size catheter (tube) is inserted into the nipple and a small amount of salt water is released into the duct. The water picks up breast cells and is removed.

Screening clinical trials are taking place in many parts of the country.

Risks of Breast Cancer Screening

Screening tests have risks.

Decisions about screening tests can be difficult. Not all screening tests are helpful and most have risks. Before having any screening test, you may want to discuss the test with your doctor. It is important to know the risks of the test and whether it has been proven to reduce the risk of dying from cancer.

The risks of breast cancer screening tests include the following:

Finding breast cancer may not improve health or help a woman live longer.

Screening may not help you if you have fast-growing breast cancer or if it has already spread to other places in your body. Also, some breast cancers found on a screening mammogram may never cause symptoms or become life-threatening. Finding these cancers is called overdiagnosis. When such cancers are found, treatment would not help you live longer and may instead cause serious side effects. At this time, it is not possible to be sure which breast cancers found by screening will cause problems and which ones will not.

False-negative test results can occur.

Screening test results may appear to be normal even though breast cancer is present. A woman who receives a false-negative test result (one that shows there is no cancer when there really is) may delay seeking medical care even if she has symptoms.

One in 5 cancers may be missed by mammography. False-negative results occur more often in younger women than in older women because the breast tissue of younger women is more dense. The chance of a false-negative result is also affected by the following:

- The size of the tumor.

- The rate of tumor growth.

- The level of hormones, such as estrogen and progesterone, in the woman's body.

- The skill of the radiologist.

False-positive test results can occur.

Screening test results may appear to be abnormal even though no cancer is present. A false-positive test result (one that shows there is cancer when there really isn't) is usually followed by more tests (such as biopsy), which also have risks.

Most abnormal test results turn out not to be cancer. False-positive results are more common in the following:

- Younger women.

- Women who have had previous breast biopsies.

- Women with a family history of breast cancer.

- Women who take hormones, such as estrogen and progestin.

The skill of the radiologist also can affect the chance of a false-positive result.

Anxiety from additional testing may result from false positive results.

False-positive results from screening mammograms are usually followed by more testing that can lead to anxiety. In one study, women who had a false-positive screening mammogram followed by more testing reported feeling anxiety 3 months later, even though cancer was not diagnosed. However, several studies show that women who feel anxiety after false-positive test results are more likely to schedule regular breast screening exams in the future.

Mammograms expose the breast to radiation.

Being exposed to radiation is a risk factor for breast cancer. The risk of breast cancer from radiation exposure is higher in women who received radiation before age 30 and at high doses. For women older than 40 years, the benefits of an annual screening mammogram may be greater than the risks from radiation exposure.

There may be pain or discomfort during a mammogram.

During a mammogram, the breast is placed between 2 plates that are pressed together. Pressing the breast helps to get a better

X-ray of the breast. Some women have pain or discomfort during a mammogram.

The risks and benefits of screening for breast cancer may be different in different age groups.

The benefits of breast cancer screening may vary among age groups:

- In women who are expected to live 5 years or fewer, finding and treating early stage breast cancer may reduce their quality of life without helping them live longer.

- As with other women, in women older than 65 years, the results of a screening test may lead to more diagnostic tests and anxiety while waiting for the test results. Also, the breast cancers found are usually not life-threatening.

- It has not been shown that women with an average risk of developing breast cancer benefit from starting screening mammography before age 40.

Women who have had radiation treatment to the chest, especially at a young age, are advised to have routine breast cancer screening. Yearly MRI screening may begin 8 years after treatment or by age 25 years, whichever is later. The benefits and risks of mammograms and MRIs for these women have not been studied.

There is no information on the benefits or risks of breast cancer screening in men.

No matter how old you are, if you have risk factors for breast cancer you should ask for medical advice about when to begin having breast cancer screening tests and how often to have them.

Section 38.2

Screening for Cervical Cancer

Text in this section is excerpted from "Cervical Cancer Screening (PDQ®)," National Cancer Institute (NCI), January 21, 2015.

General Information about Cervical Cancer

Cervical cancer is a disease in which malignant (cancer) cells form in the cervix.

The cervix is the lower, narrow end of the uterus (the hollow, pear-shaped organ where a fetus grows). The cervix leads from the uterus to the vagina (birth canal).

Cervical cancer usually develops slowly over time. Before cancer appears in the cervix, the cells of the cervix go through changes known as dysplasia, in which cells that are not normal begin to appear in the cervical tissue. Later, cancer cells start to grow and spread more deeply into the cervix and to surrounding areas.

Screening for cervical cancer using the Pap test has decreased the number of new cases of cervical cancer and the number of deaths due to cervical cancer since 1950.

Cervical dysplasia occurs more often in women who are in their 20s and 30s. Death from cervical cancer is rare in women younger than 30 years and in women of any age who have regular screenings with the Pap test. The Pap test is used to detect cancer and changes that may lead to cancer. The chance of death from cervical cancer increases with age. Deaths from cervical cancer occur more often in Black women than in White women.

Human papillomavirus (HPV) infection is the major risk factor for cervical cancer.

Although most women with cervical cancer have the human papillomavirus (HPV) infection, not all women with an HPV infection will develop cervical cancer. Many different types of HPV can affect the cervix and only some of them cause abnormal cells that may become cancer. Some HPV infections go away without treatment.

HPV infections are spread mainly through sexual contact. Women who become sexually active at a young age and have many sexual partners are at increased risk for HPV infections.

Other risk factors for cervical cancer include:

- Giving birth to many children.

- Smoking cigarettes.

- Using oral contraceptives ("the Pill").

- Having a weakened immune system.

Cervical Cancer Screening

Tests are used to screen for different types of cancer.

Some screening tests are used because they have been shown to be helpful both in finding cancers early and in decreasing the chance of dying from these cancers. Other tests are used because they have been shown to find cancer in some people; however, it has not been proven in clinical trials that use of these tests will decrease the risk of dying from cancer.

Scientists study screening tests to find those with the fewest risks and most benefits. Cancer screening trials also are meant to show whether early detection (finding cancer before it causes symptoms) decreases a person's chance of dying from the disease. For some types of cancer, the chance of recovery is better if the disease is found and treated at an early stage.

Clinical trials that study cancer screening methods are taking place in many parts of the country.

Studies show that screening for cervical cancer helps decrease the number of deaths from the disease.

Regular screening of women between the ages of 21 and 65 years with the Pap test decreases their chance of dying from cervical cancer.

A Pap test is commonly used to screen for cervical cancer.

A Pap test is a procedure to collect cells from the surface of the cervix and vagina. A piece of cotton, a brush, or a small wooden stick is used to gently scrape cells from the cervix and vagina. The cells are viewed under a microscope to find out if they are abnormal. This procedure is also called a Pap smear. A new method of collecting and viewing cells has been developed, in which the cells are placed into a liquid before being placed on a slide. It is not known if the new method will work better than the standard method to reduce the number of deaths from cervical cancer.

After certain positive Pap test results, an HPV test may be done.

An HPV test is a laboratory test that is used to check DNA or RNA for certain types of HPV infection. Cells are collected from the cervix and DNA or RNA from the cells is checked to find out if there is an infection caused by a type of human papillomavirus that is linked to cervical cancer. This test may be done using the sample of cells removed during a Pap test. This test may also be done if the results of a Pap test show certain abnormal cervical cells. When both the HPV test and Pap test are done using cells from the sample removed during a Pap test, it is called a Pap/HPV cotest.

An HPV test may be done with or without a Pap test to screen for cervical cancer.

Screening women aged 30 and older with both the Pap test and the HPV test every 5 years finds more cervical changes that can lead to cancer than screening with the Pap test alone. Screening with both the Pap test and the HPV test lowers the number of cases of cervical cancer.

An HPV DNA test may be used without a Pap test for cervical cancer screening in women aged 25 years and older.

Other screening tests are being studied in clinical trials.

Screening clinical trials are taking place in many parts of the country.

Risks of Cervical Cancer Screening

Screening tests have risks.

Decisions about screening tests can be difficult. Not all screening tests are helpful and most have risks. Before having any screening test, you may want to discuss the test with your doctor. It is important to know the risks of the test and whether it has been proven to reduce the risk of dying from cancer.

511

The risks of cervical cancer screening include the following:

Unnecessary follow-up tests may be done.

In women younger than 21 years, screening with the Pap test may show changes in the cells of the cervix that are not cancer. This may lead to unnecessary follow-up tests and possibly treatment. Women in this age group have a very low risk of cervical cancer and it is likely that any abnormal cells will go away on their own.

False-negative test results can occur.

Screening test results may appear to be normal even though cervical cancer is present. A woman who receives a false-negative test result (one that shows there is no cancer when there really is) may delay seeking medical care even if she has symptoms.

False-positive test results can occur.

Screening test results may appear to be abnormal even though no cancer is present. Also, some abnormal cells in the cervix never become cancer. When a Pap test shows a false-positive result (one that shows there is cancer when there really isn't), it can cause anxiety and is usually followed by more tests and procedures (such as colposcopy, cryotherapy, or LEEP), which also have risks. The long-term effects of these procedures on fertility and pregnancy are not known.

The HPV test finds many infections that will not lead to cervical dysplasia or cervical cancer, especially in women younger than 30 years.

When both the Pap test and the HPV test are done, false-positive test results are more common.

Your doctor can advise you about your risk for cervical cancer and your need for screening tests.

Studies show that the number of cases of cervical cancer and deaths from cervical cancer are greatly reduced by screening with Pap tests. Many doctors recommend a Pap test be done every year. New studies have shown that after a woman has a Pap test and the results show no sign of abnormal cells, the Pap test can be repeated every 2 to 3 years.

The Pap test is not a helpful screening test for cervical cancer in the following groups of women:

- Women who are younger than 21 years.

- Women who have had a total hysterectomy (surgery to remove the uterus and cervix) for a condition that is not cancer.

- Women who are aged 65 years or older and have a Pap test result that shows no abnormal cells. These women are very unlikely to have abnormal Pap test results in the future.

The decision about how often to have a Pap test is best made by you and your doctor.

Section 38.3

Screening for Endometrial Cancer

Text in this section is excerpted from "Endometrial Cancer Screening (PDQ®)," National Cancer Institute (NCI), July 23, 2015.

General Information about Endometrial Cancer

Endometrial cancer is a disease in which malignant (cancer) cells form in the tissues of the endometrium.

The endometrium is the innermost lining of the uterus. The uterus is a hollow, muscular organ in a woman's pelvis. The uterus is where a fetus grows. In most nonpregnant women, the uterus is about 3 inches long.

Cancer of the endometrium is different from cancer of the muscle of the uterus, which is called uterine sarcoma.

In the United States, endometrial cancer is the most common invasive cancer of the female reproductive system.

Endometrial cancer is diagnosed most often in postmenopausal women at an average age of 60 years.

Since 1992, the number of White women diagnosed with endometrial cancer has remained stable, but the number of new cases in Black women has increased slightly. Endometrial cancer occurs more often in White women than in Black women. When endometrial cancer is diagnosed in Black women, it is usually more advanced and less likely to be cured. The number of deaths from endometrial cancer has stayed about the same in White women but has increased slightly in Black women each year since 1998.

Health history and certain medicines can affect the risk of developing endometrial cancer.

Anything that increases your chance of getting a disease is called a risk factor. Having a risk factor does not mean that you will get cancer; not having risk factors doesn't mean that you will not get cancer. People who think they may be at risk should discuss this with their doctor. Risk factors for endometrial cancer include the following:

- Taking tamoxifen for treatment or prevention of breast cancer.

- Taking estrogen alone. (Taking estrogen in combination with progestin does not appear to increase the risk of endometrial cancer.)

- Being overweight.

- Eating a high-fat diet.

- Never giving birth.

- Beginning menstruation at an early age.

- Reaching menopause at an older age.

- Having the gene for hereditary non-polyposis colon cancer (HNPCC).

- Being White.

Endometrial Cancer Screening

Tests are used to screen for different types of cancer.

Some screening tests are used because they have been shown to be helpful both in finding cancers early and decreasing the chance of dying from these cancers. Other tests are used because they have been shown to find cancer in some people; however, it has not been proven in clinical trials that use of these tests will decrease the risk of dying from cancer.

Scientists study screening tests to find those with the fewest risks and most benefits. Cancer screening trials also are meant to show whether early detection (finding cancer before it causes symptoms) decreases a person's chance of dying from the disease. For some types of cancer, finding and treating the disease at an early stage may result in a better chance of recovery.

Endometrial cancer is usually found early.

Endometrial cancer usually causes symptoms (such as vaginal bleeding) and is found at an early stage, when there is a good chance of recovery.

There is no standard or routine screening test for endometrial cancer.

Screening for endometrial cancer is under study and there are screening clinical trials taking place in many parts of the country.

Tests that may detect (find) endometrial cancer are being studied:

Pap test

A Pap test is a procedure to collect cells from the surface of the cervix and vagina. A piece of cotton, a brush, or a small wooden stick is used to gently scrape cells from the cervix and vagina. The cells are viewed under a microscope to find out if they are abnormal. This procedure is also called a Pap smear.

Pap tests are not used to screen for endometrial cancer; however, Pap test results sometimes show signs of an abnormal endometrium (lining of the uterus). Follow-up tests may detect endometrial cancer.

Transvaginal ultrasound

No studies have shown that screening by transvaginal ultrasound (TVU) lowers the number of deaths caused by endometrial cancer.

Transvaginal ultrasound (TVU) is a procedure used to examine the vagina, uterus, fallopian tubes, and bladder. It is also called endovaginal ultrasound. An ultrasound transducer (probe) is inserted into the vagina and used to bounce high-energy sound waves (ultrasound) off internal tissues or organs and make echoes. The echoes form a picture of body tissues called a sonogram. The doctor can identify tumors by looking at the sonogram.

TVU is commonly used to examine women who have abnormal vaginal bleeding. For women who have or are at risk for hereditary non-polyposis colon cancer, experts suggest yearly screening with transvaginal ultrasound, beginning as early as age 25.

The use of tamoxifen to treat or prevent breast cancer increases the risk of endometrial cancer. TVU is not useful in screening for endometrial cancer in women who take tamoxifen but do not have any symptoms of endometrial cancer. In women taking tamoxifen, TVU should be used in those who have vaginal bleeding.

Endometrial sampling

It has not been proven that screening by endometrial sampling (biopsy) lowers the number of deaths caused by endometrial cancer.

Endometrial sampling is the removal of tissue from the endometrium by inserting a brush, curette, or thin, flexible tube through the cervix and into the uterus. The tool is used to gently scrape a small amount of tissue from the endometrium and then remove the tissue samples. A pathologist views the tissue under a microscope to look for cancer cells.

Endometrial sampling is commonly used to examine women who have abnormal vaginal bleeding. If you have abnormal vaginal bleeding, check with your doctor.

Risks of Endometrial Cancer Screening

Screening tests have risks.

Decisions about screening tests can be difficult. Not all screening tests are helpful and most have risks. Before having any screening test, you may want to discuss the test with your doctor. It is important to know the risks of the test and whether it has been proven to reduce the risk of dying from cancer.

The risks of endometrial cancer screening tests include the following:

Finding endometrial cancer may not improve health or help a woman live longer.

Screening may not improve your health or help you live longer if you have advanced endometrial cancer or if it has already spread to other places in your body.

Some cancers never cause symptoms or become life-threatening, but if found by a screening test, the cancer may be treated. It is not known if treatment of these cancers would help you live longer than if no treatment were given, and treatments for cancer may have serious side effects.

False-negative test results can occur.

Screening test results may appear to be normal even though endometrial cancer is present. A woman who receives a false-negative test result (one that shows there is no cancer when there really is) may delay seeking medical care even if she has symptoms.

False-positive test results can occur.

Screening test results may appear to be abnormal even though no cancer is present. A false-positive test result (one that shows there is cancer when there really isn't) can cause anxiety and is usually followed by more tests (such as biopsy), which also have risks.

Side effects may be caused by the test itself.

Side effects that may be caused by screening tests for endometrial cancer include:

- Discomfort.

- Bleeding.

- Infection.

- Puncture of the uterus (rare).

If you have any questions about your risk for endometrial cancer or the need for screening tests, check with your doctor.

Section 38.4

Screening for Ovarian, Fallopian Tube, and Primary Peritoneal Cancer

Text in this section is excerpted from "Ovarian, Fallopian Tube, and Primary Peritoneal Cancer Screening (PDQ®)," National Cancer Institute (NCI), July 2, 2015.

General Information about Ovarian, Fallopian Tube, and Primary Peritoneal Cancer

Ovarian, fallopian tube, and primary peritoneal cancers are diseases in which malignant (cancer) cells form in the ovaries, fallopian tubes, or peritoneum.

The ovaries are a pair of organs in the female reproductive system. They are located in the pelvis, one on each side of the uterus

517

(the hollow, pear-shaped organ where a fetus grows). Each ovary is about the size and shape of an almond. The ovaries produce eggs and female hormones (chemicals that control the way certain cells or organs function).

The fallopian tubes are a pair of long, slender tubes, one on each side of the uterus. Eggs pass from the ovaries, through the fallopian tubes, to the uterus. Cancer sometimes begins at the end of the fallopian tube near the ovary and spreads to the ovary.

The peritoneum is the tissue that lines the abdominal wall and covers organs in the abdomen. Primary peritoneal cancer is cancer that forms in the peritoneum and has not spread there from another part of the body. Cancer sometimes begins in the peritoneum and spreads to the ovary.

In the United States, ovarian cancer is the fifth leading cause of cancer death in women.

Ovarian cancer is also the leading cause of death from cancer of the female reproductive system. Since 1992, the number of new cases of ovarian cancer has gone down slightly. The number of deaths from ovarian cancer has slightly decreased since 2002.

Different factors increase or decrease the risk of ovarian, fallopian tube, and primary peritoneal cancer.

Anything that increases your chance of getting a disease is called a risk factor. Anything that decreases your chance of getting a disease is called a protective factor

Ovarian, Fallopian Tube, and Primary Peritoneal Cancer Screening

Tests are used to screen for different types of cancer.

Some screening tests are used because they have been shown to be helpful both in finding cancers early and in decreasing the chance of dying from these cancers. Other tests are used because they have been shown to find cancer in some people; however, it has not been proven in clinical trials that use of these tests will decrease the risk of dying from cancer.

Scientists study screening tests to find those with the fewest risks and most benefits. Cancer screening trials also are meant to show whether early detection (finding cancer before it causes symptoms)

decreases a person's chance of dying from the disease. For some types of cancer, finding and treating the disease at an early stage may result in a better chance of recovery.

There is no standard or routine screening test for ovarian, fallopian tube, and primary peritoneal cancer.

Screening for ovarian cancer has not been proven to decrease the death rate from the disease.

Screening for ovarian cancer is under study and there are screening clinical trials taking place in many parts of the country.

Tests that may detect (find) ovarian, fallopian tube, and primary peritoneal cancer are being studied:

Pelvic exam

A pelvic exam is an exam of the vagina, cervix, uterus, fallopian tubes, ovaries, and rectum. A speculum is inserted into the vagina and the doctor or nurse looks at the vagina and cervix for signs of disease. The doctor or nurse also inserts one or two lubricated, gloved fingers of one hand into the vagina and places the other hand over the lower abdomen to feel the size, shape, and position of the uterus and ovaries. The doctor or nurse also inserts a lubricated, gloved finger into the rectum to feel for lumps or abnormal areas.

Ovarian cancer is usually advanced when first found by a pelvic exam.

Transvaginal ultrasound

Transvaginal ultrasound (TVU) is a procedure used to examine the vagina, uterus, fallopian tubes, and bladder. An ultrasound transducer (probe) is inserted into the vagina and used to bounce high-energy sound waves (ultrasound) off internal tissues or organs and make echoes. The echoes form a picture of body tissues called a sonogram.

CA-125 assay

A CA 125 assay is a test that measures the level of CA 125 in the blood. CA 125 is a substance released by cells into the bloodstream. An increased CA-125 level is sometimes a sign of certain types of cancer, including ovarian cancer, or other conditions.

Scientists at the National Cancer Institute studied the combination of using TVU and CA-125 levels as a way to screen for and prevent deaths from ovarian cancer. The results of this study showed no decrease in deaths from ovarian cancer.

Risks of Ovarian, Fallopian Tube, and Primary Peritoneal Cancer Screening

Screening tests have risks.

Decisions about screening tests can be difficult. Not all screening tests are helpful and most have risks. Before having any screening test, you may want to talk about the test with your doctor. It is important to know the risks of the test and whether it has been proven to reduce the risk of dying from cancer.

The risks of ovarian, fallopian tube, and primary peritoneal cancer screening tests include the following:

Finding ovarian, fallopian tube, and primary peritoneal cancer may not improve health or help a woman live longer.

Screening may not improve your health or help you live longer if you have advanced ovarian cancer or if it has already spread to other places in your body.

Some cancers never cause symptoms or become life-threatening, but if found by a screening test, the cancer may be treated. It is not known if treatment of these cancers would help you live longer than if no treatment were given, and treatments for cancer may have serious side effects.

False-negative test results can occur.

Screening test results may appear to be normal even though ovarian cancer is present. A woman who receives a false-negative test result (one that shows there is no cancer when there really is) may delay seeking medical care even if she has symptoms.

False-positive test results can occur.

Screening test results may appear to be abnormal even though no cancer is present. A false-positive test result (one that shows there is cancer when there really isn't) can cause anxiety and is usually followed by more tests (such as a laparoscopy or a laparotomy to see if cancer is present), which also have risks. Complications from tests to diagnose ovarian cancer include infection, blood loss, bowel injury, and heart and blood vessel problems. An unnecessary oophorectomy (removal of one or both ovaries) may also result.

Your doctor can advise you about your risk for ovarian cancer and your need for screening tests.

Chapter 39

Cancer Screening Tests for Men

Chapter Contents

Section 39.1

Screening for Prostate Cancer

Text in this section is excerpted from "Prostate Cancer Screening
(PDQ®)," National Cancer Institute (NCI), July 31, 2015.

General Information about Prostate Cancer

*Prostate cancer is a disease in which malignant (cancer) cells form in
the tissues of the prostate.*

The prostate is a gland in the male reproductive system located just
below the bladder (the organ that collects and empties urine) and in
front of the rectum (the lower part of the intestine). It is about the size
of a walnut and surrounds part of the urethra (the tube that empties
urine from the bladder). The prostate gland produces fluid that makes
up part of semen.

As men age, the prostate may get bigger. A bigger prostate may
block the flow of urine from the bladder and cause problems with
sexual function. This condition is called benign prostatic hyperplasia
(BPH), and although it is not cancer, surgery may be needed to correct
it. The symptoms of benign prostatic hyperplasia or of other problems
in the prostate may be similar to symptoms of prostate cancer.

*Prostate cancer is the most common nonskin cancer among men in the
United States.*

Prostate cancer is found mainly in older men. Although the number
of men with prostate cancer is large, most men diagnosed with this
disease do not die from it. Prostate cancer occurs more often in African-American men than in White men. African-American men with
prostate cancer are more likely to die from the disease than White
men with prostate cancer.

*Age, race, and family history of prostate cancer can affect the risk of
developing prostate cancer.*

Anything that increases a person's chance of developing a disease is
called a risk factor. Risk factors for prostate cancer include the following:

- Being 50 years of age or older.

- Being Black.

- Having a brother, son, or father who had prostate cancer.

- Eating a diet high in fat or drinking alcoholic beverages.

Prostate Cancer Screening

Tests are used to screen for different types of cancer.

Some screening tests are used because they have been shown to be helpful both in finding cancers early and decreasing the chance of dying from these cancers. Other tests are used because they have been shown to find cancer in some people; however, it has not been proven in clinical trials that use of these tests will decrease the risk of dying from cancer.

Scientists study screening tests to find those with the fewest risks and most benefits. Cancer screening trials also are meant to show whether early detection (finding cancer before it causes symptoms) decreases a person's chance of dying from the disease. For some types of cancer, finding and treating the disease at an early stage may result in a better chance of recovery.

There is no standard or routine screening test for prostate cancer.

Screening tests for prostate cancer are under study, and there are screening clinical trials taking place in many parts of the country.

Tests to detect (find) prostate cancer that are being studied include the following:

Digital rectal exam

Digital rectal exam (DRE) is an exam of the rectum. The doctor or nurse inserts a lubricated, gloved finger into the lower part of the rectum to feel the prostate for lumps or anything else that seems unusual.

Prostate-specific antigen test

A prostate-specific antigen (PSA) test is a test that measures the level of PSA in the blood. PSA is a substance made mostly by the prostate that may be found in an increased amount in the blood of men who have prostate cancer. The level of PSA may also be high in men who have an infection or inflammation of the prostate or benign prostatic hyperplasia (BPH; an enlarged, but noncancerous, prostate).

If a man has a high PSA level and a biopsy of the prostate does not show cancer, a prostate cancer gene 3 (PCA3) test may be done. This test measures the amount of PCA3 in the urine. If the PCA3 level is high, another biopsy may help diagnose prostate cancer.

Scientists are studying the combination of PSA testing and digital rectal exam as a way to get more accurate results from the screening tests.

Risks of Prostate Cancer Screening

Screening tests have risks.

Decisions about screening tests can be difficult. Not all screening tests are helpful and most have risks. Before having any screening test, you may want to discuss the test with your doctor. It is important to know the risks of the test and whether it has been proven to reduce the risk of dying from cancer.

The risks of prostate screening include the following:

Finding prostate cancer may not improve health or help a man live longer.

Screening may not improve your health or help you live longer if you have cancer that has already spread to the area outside of the prostate or to other places in your body.

Some cancers never cause symptoms or become life-threatening, but if found by a screening test, the cancer may be treated. Finding these cancers is called overdiagnosis. It is not known if treatment of these cancers would help you live longer than if no treatment were given, and treatments for cancer, such as surgery and radiation therapy, may have serious side effects.

Some studies of patients with prostate cancer showed these patients had a higher risk of death from cardiovascular (heart and blood vessel) disease or suicide. The risk was greatest the first year after diagnosis.

Follow-up tests, such as a biopsy, may be done to diagnose cancer.

If a PSA test is higher than normal, a biopsy of the prostate may be done. Complications from a biopsy of the prostate may include fever, pain, blood in the urine or semen, and urinary tract infection. Even if a biopsy shows that a patient does not have prostate cancer, he may worry more about developing prostate cancer in the future.

False-negative test results can occur.

Screening test results may appear to be normal even though prostate cancer is present. A man who receives a false-negative test result (one that shows there is no cancer when there really is) may delay seeking medical care even if he has symptoms.

False-positive test results can occur.

Screening test results may appear to be abnormal even though no cancer is present. A false-positive test result (one that shows there is cancer when there really isn't) can cause anxiety and is usually followed by more tests, (such as biopsy) which also have risks.

Your doctor can advise you about your risk for prostate cancer and your need for screening tests.

Section 39.2

Screening for Testicular Cancer

Text in this section is excerpted from "Testicular Cancer Screening (PDQ®)," National Cancer Institute (NCI), July 19, 2012.

General Information about Testicular Cancer

Testicular cancer is a disease in which malignant (cancer) cells form in the tissues of one or both testicles.

The testicles are 2 egg-shaped glands inside the scrotum (a sac of loose skin that lies directly below the penis). The testicles are held within the scrotum by the spermatic cord. The spermatic cord also contains the vas deferens and vessels and nerves of the testicles.

The testicles are the male sex glands and make testosterone and sperm. Germ cells in the testicles make immature sperm. These sperm travel through a network of tubules (tiny tubes) and larger tubes into the epididymis (a long coiled tube next to the testicles). This is where the sperm mature and are stored.

Almost all testicular cancers start in the germ cells. The two main types of testicular germ cell tumors are seminomas and nonseminomas.

Testicular cancer is the most common cancer in men aged 15 to 34 years.

Testicular cancer is very rare, but it is the most common cancer found in men between the ages of 15 and 34. White men are four times more likely than Black men to have testicular cancer

Testicular cancer can usually be cured.

Although the number of new cases of testicular cancer has doubled in the last 40 years, the number of deaths caused by testicular cancer has decreased greatly because of better treatments. Testicular cancer can usually be cured, even in late stages of the disease.

A condition called cryptorchidism (an undescended testicle) is a risk factor for testicular cancer.

Anything that increases the chance of getting a disease is called a risk factor. Having a risk factor does not mean that you will get cancer; not having risk factors doesn't mean that you will not get cancer. Talk to your doctor if you think you may be at risk. Risk factors for testicular cancer include the following:

- Having cryptorchidism (an undescended testicle).

- Having a testicle that is not normal, such as a small testicle that does not work the way it should.

- Having testicular carcinoma in situ.

- Being White.

- Having a personal or family history of testicular cancer.

- Having Klinefelter syndrome.

Men who have cryptorchidism, a testicle that is not normal, or testicular carcinoma in situ have an increased risk of testicular cancer in one or both testicles, and need to be followed closely.

Testicular Cancer Screening

Tests are used to screen for different types of cancer.

Some screening tests are used because they have been shown to be helpful both in finding cancers early and in decreasing the chance of dying from these cancers. Other tests are used because they have been shown to find cancer in some people; however, it has not been proven in clinical trials that use of these tests will decrease the risk of dying from cancer.

Scientists study screening tests to find those with the fewest risks and most benefits. Cancer screening trials also are meant to show whether early detection (finding cancer before it causes symptoms) decreases a person's chance of dying from the disease. For some types of cancer, the chance of recovery is better if the disease is found and treated at an early stage.

There is no standard or routine screening test for testicular cancer.

There is no standard or routine screening test used for early detection of testicular cancer. Most often, testicular cancer is first found by men themselves, either by chance or during self-exam. Sometimes the cancer is found by a doctor during a routine physical exam.

No studies have been done to find out if testicular self-exams, regular exams by a doctor, or other screening tests in men with no symptoms would decrease the risk of dying from this disease. However, routine screening probably would not decrease the risk of dying from testicular cancer. This is partly because testicular cancer can usually be cured at any stage. Finding testicular cancer early may make it easier to treat. Patients who are diagnosed with testicular cancer that has not spread to other parts of the body may need less chemotherapy and surgery, resulting in fewer side effects.

If a lump is found in the testicle by the patient or during a routine physical exam, tests may be done to check for cancer. Some tests have risks, and may cause anxiety.

Chapter 40

Celiac Disease Tests

What is celiac disease?

Celiac disease is an immune disease in which people can't eat gluten because it will damage their small intestine. Gluten is a protein found in wheat, rye, and barley. Gluten may also be used in products such as vitamin and nutrient supplements, lip balms, and some medicines. Other names for celiac disease are celiac sprue and gluten intolerance.

Your body's natural defense system, called the immune system, keeps you healthy by fighting against things that can make you sick, such as bacteria and viruses. When people with celiac disease eat gluten, their body's immune system reacts to the gluten by attacking the lining of the small intestine. The immune system's reaction to gluten damages small, fingerlike growths called villi. When the villi are damaged, the body cannot get the nutrients it needs.

Celiac disease is hereditary, meaning it runs in families. Adults and children can have celiac disease. As many as 2 million Americans may have celiac disease, but most don't know it.

This chapter includes excerpts from "What I need to know about Celiac Disease," National Institute of Diabetes and Digestive and Kidney Diseases (NIDDK), September 11, 2013; and text from "Testing for Celiac Disease (For Healthcare Providers)," National Institute of Diabetes and Digestive and Kidney Diseases (NIDDK), September 11, 2013.

Is celiac disease serious?

Yes. Celiac disease can be very serious. It often causes long-lasting digestive problems and keeps your body from getting all the nutrition it needs. Over time, celiac disease can cause anemia, infertility, weak and brittle bones, an itchy skin rash, and other health problems.

What are the symptoms of celiac disease?

Symptoms of celiac disease include

- stomach pain
- gas
- diarrhea
- extreme tiredness
- change in mood
- weight loss
- a very itchy skin rash with blisters
- slowed growth

Some people with celiac disease may not feel sick or have symptoms. Or if they feel sick, they don't know celiac disease is the cause. Most people with celiac disease have one or more symptoms. Not all people with celiac disease have digestive problems. Having one or more of these symptoms does not always mean a person has celiac disease because other disorders can cause these symptoms.

How is celiac disease diagnosed?

Celiac disease can be hard to diagnose because some of its symptoms are like the symptoms of other diseases. People with celiac disease may go undiagnosed and untreated for many years. If your doctor thinks you have celiac disease, you will need a blood test. You must be on your regular diet before the test. If not, the results could be wrong.

If your blood test results show you might have celiac disease, your doctor will perform a biopsy, which involves taking a tiny piece of tissue from your small intestine. A biopsy may be performed at a hospital or outpatient center.

Your doctor will provide you instructions about how to prepare for a biopsy. Generally, no eating or drinking is allowed 8 hours before a biopsy. Smoking and chewing gum are also prohibited during this time. Tell your doctor about any health conditions you may have, especially heart and lung problems, diabetes, and allergies. Also tell your doctor about any medicines you take. You may be asked to stop taking them for a short time before and after the test.

To perform the biopsy, the doctor inserts a long, narrow tube into your mouth, down through your stomach, and into your small intestine. At the end of the tube are small tools that the doctor uses to snip out a bit of tissue. The tissue will then be viewed with a microscope to look for signs of celiac disease damage. You will take medicine before the biopsy that makes you sleepy and keeps you from feeling any pain. Many people sleep through the procedure.

How is celiac disease treated?

The only treatment for celiac disease is a gluten-free diet. If you avoid gluten, your small intestine will heal. If you eat gluten or use items that contain gluten, celiac disease will continue to harm your small intestine.

Have regular checkups so your doctor can diagnose and treat problems from celiac disease. Celiac disease can cause problems, such as weak or brittle bones, even if you are on a gluten-free diet.

Eating, Diet, and Nutrition

A dietitian can help you select gluten-free foods. A dietitian is an expert in food and healthy eating. You will learn how to check labels of foods and other items for gluten.

Serologic Tests

Serologic tests for celiac disease provide an effective first step in identifying candidates for intestinal biopsy.

If serologic or genetic tests indicate the possibility of celiac disease, a biopsy should be done promptly and before initiating any dietary changes. Genetic tests that confirm the presence or absence of specific genes associated with celiac disease may be beneficial in some cases.

Serologic tests look for three antibodies common in celiac disease:

- anti-tissue transglutaminase (tTG) antibodies

- endomysial antibodies (EMA)

- deamidated gliadin peptide (DGP) antibodies

The most sensitive antibody tests are of the immunoglobulin A (IgA) class; however, immunoglobulin G (IgG) tests may be used in people with IgA deficiency. Panels are often used because no one serologic test is ideal. However, the tests included in a celiac panel vary by lab, and one or more may be unwarranted. Some reference labs—labs used for specialized tests—have developed cascades of tests in an attempt to minimize the use of less accurate tests whose automatic inclusion in a panel would add little or no sensitivity and/or detract from specificity. For accurate diagnostic test results, patients must be on a gluten-containing diet.

tTG

The tTG-IgA test is an enzyme-linked immunosorbent assay (ELISA) test. The tTG-IgA test is the preferred screening method and has a sensitivity of 93 percent, yielding few false negative results. The tTG test also has a specificity of more than 98 percent.

The performance of the tTG-IgA test may depend on the degree of intestinal damage, making the test less sensitive among people with milder celiac disease. In addition to screening, the tTG test may be used to assess initiation and maintenance of a gluten-free diet.

Point-of-care tTG tests have been developed commercially; however, because of lower sensitivity and specificity, assay results may differ from those in the lab.

The tTG-IgG test is only useful in those subjects who have IgA deficiency, which is 1/400 of the general population or 2 to 3 percent of people with celiac disease.

EMA

The test for EMA-IgA is highly specific for celiac disease, with 99 percent accuracy. The reason the test has a variable sensitivity of 70 to 100 percent may be due in part to the high technical difficulty in performing this test. EMA are measured by indirect immunofluorescent assay, a more expensive and time-consuming process than ELISA testing. In addition, the EMA test is qualitative, making the results more subjective than those for tTG. EMA is often used as an adjunctive test to the routine tTG-IgA test when EMA make celiac disease more certain.

A jejunal biopsy may help diagnose patients who are EMA or tTG negative and suspected of having celiac disease.

DGP

A new generation of tests that use DGP antibodies has sensitivity and specificity that is substantially better than the older gliadin tests. However, based on a meta-analysis of 11 studies, insufficient evidence exists to support the use of DGP over tTG or EMA tests. The tTG test is less expensive than the DGP test and offers better diagnostic performance.

IgA Deficiency

If tTG-IgA or EMA-IgA is negative and celiac disease is still suspected, total IgA should be measured to identify selective IgA deficiency. In cases of IgA deficiency, tTG-IgG or DGP-IgG should be measured. DGP-IgG may be sensitive for celiac disease, and it is preferable to tTG-IgG if used in a cascade. DGP-IgG has reasonable sensitivity for celiac disease in IgA-sufficient as well as IgA-deficient patients.

Genetic Screening Tests

Most people with celiac disease have gene pairs that encode for at least one of the human leukocyte antigen (HLA) gene variants, or alleles, designated HLA-DQ2—found in 95 percent of people with the disease—and HLA-DQ8. However, these alleles are found in about 30 to 35 percent of Caucasians, and most people with the variants do not develop celiac disease. Negative findings for HLA-DQ2 and HLA-DQ8 make current or future celiac disease very unlikely in patients for whom other tests, including biopsy, do not provide a clear diagnostic result. An increased risk of developing celiac disease has recently been described in individuals who carry a new HLA-G I allele in addition to HLA-DQ2.

Chapter 41

Cystic Fibrosis (CF) Tests

What Is Cystic Fibrosis?

Cystic fibrosis, or CF, is an inherited disease of the secretory glands. Secretory glands include glands that make mucus and sweat.

"Inherited" means the disease is passed from parents to children through genes. People who have CF inherit two faulty genes for the disease—one from each parent. The parents likely don't have the disease themselves.

CF mainly affects the lungs, pancreas, liver, intestines, sinuses, and sex organs.

Overview

Mucus is a substance made by tissues that line some organs and body cavities, such as the lungs and nose. Normally, mucus is a slippery, watery substance. It keeps the linings of certain organs moist and prevents them from drying out or getting infected.

If you have CF, your mucus becomes thick and sticky. It builds up in your lungs and blocks your airways. (Airways are tubes that carry air in and out of your lungs.)

Text in this chapter is excerpted from "Cystic Fibrosis," National Heart, Lung, and Blood Institute (NHLBI), December 26, 2013.

The buildup of mucus makes it easy for bacteria to grow. This leads to repeated, serious lung infections. Over time, these infections can severely damage your lungs.

The thick, sticky mucus also can block tubes, or ducts, in your pancreas (an organ in your abdomen). As a result, the digestive enzymes that your pancreas makes can't reach your small intestine.

These enzymes help break down food. Without them, your intestines can't fully absorb fats and proteins. This can cause vitamin deficiency and malnutrition because nutrients pass through your body without being used. You also may have bulky stools, intestinal gas, a swollen belly from severe constipation, and pain or discomfort.

CF also causes your sweat to become very salty. Thus, when you sweat, you lose large amounts of salt. This can upset the balance of minerals in your blood and cause many health problems. Examples of these problems include dehydration (a lack of fluid in your body), increased heart rate, fatigue (tiredness), weakness, decreased blood pressure, heat stroke, and, rarely, death.

If you or your child has CF, you're also at higher risk for diabetes or two bone-thinning conditions called osteoporosis and osteopenia.

CF also causes infertility in men, and the disease can make it harder for women to get pregnant. (The term "infertility" refers to the inability to have children.)

Outlook

The symptoms and severity of CF vary. If you or your child has the disease, you may have serious lung and digestive problems. If the disease is mild, symptoms may not show up until the teen or adult years.

The symptoms and severity of CF also vary over time. Sometimes you'll have few symptoms. Other times, your symptoms may become more severe. As the disease gets worse, you'll have more severe symptoms more often.

Lung function often starts to decline in early childhood in people who have CF. Over time, damage to the lungs can cause severe breathing problems. Respiratory failure is the most common cause of death in people who have CF.

As treatments for CF continue to improve, so does life expectancy for those who have the disease. Today, some people who have CF are living into their forties or fifties, or longer.

Early treatment for CF can improve your quality of life and increase your lifespan. Treatments may include nutritional and respiratory therapies, medicines, exercise, and other treatments.

Your doctor also may recommend pulmonary rehabilitation (PR). PR is a broad program that helps improve the well-being of people who have chronic (ongoing) breathing problems.

Other Names for Cystic Fibrosis

- Cystic fibrosis of the pancreas

- Fibrocystic disease of the pancreas

- Mucoviscidosis

- Mucoviscidosis of the pancreas

- Pancreas fibrocystic disease

- Pancreatic cystic fibrosis

What Causes Cystic Fibrosis?

A defect in the CFTR gene causes cystic fibrosis (CF). This gene makes a protein that controls the movement of salt and water in and out of your body's cells. In people who have CF, the gene makes a protein that doesn't work well. This causes thick, sticky mucus and very salty sweat.

Research suggests that the CFTR protein also affects the body in other ways. This may help explain other symptoms and complications of CF.

More than a thousand known defects can affect the CFTR gene. The type of defect you or your child has may affect the severity of CF. Other genes also may play a role in the severity of the disease.

How Is Cystic Fibrosis Inherited?

Every person inherits two CFTR genes—one from each parent. Children who inherit a faulty CFTR gene from each parent will have CF.

Children who inherit one faulty CFTR gene and one normal CFTR gene are "CF carriers." CF carriers usually have no symptoms of CF and live normal lives. However, they can pass the faulty CFTR gene to their children.

The image below shows how two parents who are both CF carriers can pass the faulty CFTR gene to their children.

Example of an Inheritance Pattern for Cystic Fibrosis

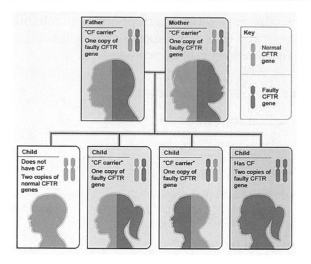

Figure 41.1. *Inheritance Pattern for Cystic Fibrosis: The image shows how CFTR genes are inherited. A person inherits two copies of the CFTR gene—one from each parent. If each parent has a normal CFTR gene and a faulty CFTR gene, each child has a 25 percent chance of inheriting two normal genes; a 50 percent chance of inheriting one normal gene and one faulty gene; and a 25 percent chance of inheriting two faulty genes.*

Who Is at Risk for Cystic Fibrosis?

Cystic fibrosis (CF) affects both males and females and people from all racial and ethnic groups. However, the disease is most common among Caucasians of Northern European descent.

CF also is common among Latinos and American Indians, especially the Pueblo and Zuni. The disease is less common among African Americans and Asian Americans.

More than 10 million Americans are carriers of a faulty CF gene. Many of them don't know that they're CF carriers.

What Are the Signs and Symptoms of Cystic Fibrosis?

The signs and symptoms of cystic fibrosis (CF) vary from person to person and over time. Sometimes you'll have few symptoms. Other times, your symptoms may become more severe.

One of the first signs of CF that parents may notice is that their baby's skin tastes salty when kissed, or the baby doesn't pass stool when first born.

Most of the other signs and symptoms of CF happen later. They're related to how CF affects the respiratory, digestive, or reproductive systems of the body.

Respiratory System Signs and Symptoms

People who have CF have thick, sticky mucus that builds up in their airways. This buildup of mucus makes it easier for bacteria to grow and cause infections. Infections can block the airways and cause frequent coughing that brings up thick sputum (spit) or mucus that's sometimes bloody.

People who have CF tend to have lung infections caused by unusual germs that don't respond to standard antibiotics. For example, lung infections caused by bacteria called mucoid Pseudomonas are much more common in people who have CF than in those who don't. An infection caused by these bacteria may be a sign of CF.

People who have CF have frequent bouts of sinusitis, an infection of the sinuses. The sinuses are hollow air spaces around the eyes, nose, and forehead. Frequent bouts of bronchitis and pneumonia also can occur. These infections can cause long-term lung damage.

As CF gets worse, you may have more serious problems, such as pneumothorax or bronchiectasis.

Some people who have CF also develop nasal polyps (growths in the nose) that may require surgery.

Digestive System Signs and Symptoms

In CF, mucus can block tubes, or ducts, in your pancreas (an organ in your abdomen). These blockages prevent enzymes from reaching your intestines.

As a result, your intestines can't fully absorb fats and proteins. This can cause ongoing diarrhea or bulky, foul-smelling, greasy stools. Intestinal blockages also may occur, especially in newborns. Too much gas or severe constipation in the intestines may cause stomach pain and discomfort.

A hallmark of CF in children is poor weight gain and growth. These children are unable to get enough nutrients from their food because of the lack of enzymes to help absorb fats and proteins.

As CF gets worse, other problems may occur, such as:

- Pancreatitis. This is a condition in which the pancreas become inflamed, which causes pain.

- Rectal prolapse. Frequent coughing or problems passing stools may cause rectal tissue from inside you to move out of your rectum.

- Liver disease due to inflamed or blocked bile ducts.

- Diabetes.

- Gallstones.

Reproductive System Signs and Symptoms

Men who have CF are infertile because they're born without a vas deferens. The vas deferens is a tube that delivers sperm from the testes to the penis.

Women who have CF may have a hard time getting pregnant because of mucus blocking the cervix or other CF complications.

Other Signs, Symptoms, and Complications

Other signs and symptoms of CF are related to an upset of the balance of minerals in your blood.

CF causes your sweat to become very salty. As a result, your body loses large amounts of salt when you sweat. This can cause dehydration (a lack of fluid in your body), increased heart rate, fatigue (tiredness), weakness, decreased blood pressure, heat stroke, and, rarely, death.

CF also can cause clubbing and low bone density. Clubbing is the widening and rounding of the tips of your fingers and toes. This sign develops late in CF because your lungs aren't moving enough oxygen into your bloodstream.

Low bone density also tends to occur late in CF. It can lead to bone-thinning disorders called osteoporosis and osteopenia.

How Is Cystic Fibrosis Diagnosed?

Doctors diagnose cystic fibrosis (CF) based on the results from various tests.

Newborn Screening

All States screen newborns for CF using a genetic test or a blood test. The genetic test shows whether a newborn has faulty CFTR genes. The blood test shows whether a newborn's pancreas is working properly.

Sweat Test

If a genetic test or blood test suggests CF, a doctor will confirm the diagnosis using a sweat test. This test is the most useful test for diagnosing CF. A sweat test measures the amount of salt in sweat.

For this test, the doctor triggers sweating on a small patch of skin on an arm or leg. He or she rubs the skin with a sweat-producing chemical and then uses an electrode to provide a mild electrical current. This may cause a tingling or warm feeling.

Sweat is collected on a pad or paper and then analyzed. The sweat test usually is done twice. High salt levels confirm a diagnosis of CF.

Other Tests

If you or your child has CF, your doctor may recommend other tests, such as:

- Genetic tests to find out what type of CFTR defect is causing your CF.

- A chest X-ray. This test creates pictures of the structures in your chest, such as your heart, lungs, and blood vessels. A chest X-ray can show whether your lungs are inflamed or scarred, or whether they trap air.

- A sinus X-ray. This test may show signs of sinusitis, a complication of CF.

- Lung function tests. These tests measure how much air you can breathe in and out, how fast you can breathe air out, and how well your lungs deliver oxygen to your blood.

- A sputum culture. For this test, your doctor will take a sample of your sputum (spit) to see whether bacteria are growing in it. If you have bacteria called mucoid *Pseudomonas*, you may have more advanced CF that needs aggressive treatment.

Prenatal Screening

If you're pregnant, prenatal genetic tests can show whether your fetus has CF. These tests include amniocentesis and chorionic villus sampling (CVS).

In amniocentesis, your doctor inserts a hollow needle through your abdominal wall into your uterus. He or she removes a small amount of fluid from the sac around the baby. The fluid is tested to see whether both of the baby's CFTR genes are normal.

541

In CVS, your doctor threads a thin tube through the vagina and cervix to the placenta. The doctor removes a tissue sample from the placenta using gentle suction. The sample is tested to see whether the baby has CF.

Cystic Fibrosis Carrier Testing

People who have one normal CFTR gene and one faulty CFTR gene are CF carriers. CF carriers usually have no symptoms of CF and live normal lives. However, carriers can pass faulty CFTR genes on to their children.

If you have a family history of CF or a partner who has CF (or a family history of it) and you're planning a pregnancy, you may want to find out whether you're a CF carrier.

A genetics counselor can test a blood or saliva sample to find out whether you have a faulty CF gene. This type of testing can detect faulty CF genes in 9 out of 10 cases.

Chapter 42

Diagnostic Tests for Diabetes and Prediabetes

Chapter Contents

Section 42.1

Overview of Diagnostic Tests for Diabetes and Prediabetes

Text in this section is excerpted from "Diagnosis of Diabetes and
Prediabetes," National Institute of Diabetes and Digestive and
Kidney Diseases (NIDDK), June 2014.

What is diabetes?

Diabetes is a complex group of diseases with a variety of causes.
People with diabetes have high blood glucose, also called high blood
sugar or hyperglycemia.

Diabetes is a disorder of metabolism—the way the body uses
digested food for energy. The digestive tract breaks down carbohydrates—sugars and starches found in many foods—into glucose, a form
of sugar that enters the bloodstream. With the help of the hormone
insulin, cells throughout the body absorb glucose and use it for energy.
Insulin is made in the pancreas, an organ located behind the stomach.
As the blood glucose level rises after a meal, the pancreas is triggered
to release insulin. Within the pancreas, clusters of cells called islets
contain beta cells, which make the insulin and release it into the blood.

Diabetes develops when the body doesn't make enough insulin or is
not able to use insulin effectively, or both. As a result, glucose builds up
in the blood instead of being absorbed by cells in the body. The body's
cells are then starved of energy despite high blood glucose levels.

Over time, high blood glucose damages nerves and blood vessels,
leading to complications such as heart disease, stroke, kidney disease,
blindness, dental disease, and amputations. Other complications of
diabetes may include increased susceptibility to other diseases, loss
of mobility with aging, depression, and pregnancy problems.

Main Types of Diabetes

The three main types of diabetes are type 1, type 2, and gestational
diabetes:

- **Type 1 diabetes**, formerly called juvenile diabetes, is usually
  first diagnosed in children, teenagers, and young adults. In this

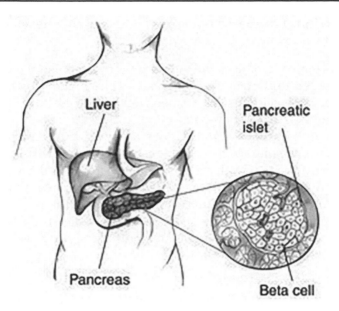

Figure 42.1. *Islets within the pancreas contain beta cells, which make insulin and release it into the blood.*

type of diabetes, the beta cells of the pancreas no longer make insulin because the body's immune system has attacked and destroyed them.

- **Type 2 diabetes**, formerly called adult-onset diabetes, is the most common type of diabetes. About 90 to 95 percent of people with diabetes have type 2.1 People can develop type 2 diabetes at any age, even during childhood, but this type of diabetes is most often associated with older age. Type 2 diabetes is also associated with excess weight, physical inactivity, family history of diabetes, previous history of gestational diabetes, and certain ethnicities.

Type 2 diabetes usually begins with insulin resistance, a condition linked to excess weight in which muscle, liver, and fat cells do not use insulin properly. As a result, the body needs more insulin to help glucose enter cells to be used for energy. At first, the pancreas keeps up with the added demand by producing more insulin. But in time, the pancreas loses its ability to produce enough insulin in response to meals, and blood glucose levels rise.

- **Gestational diabetes** is a type of diabetes that develops only during pregnancy.

The hormones produced during pregnancy increase the amount of insulin needed to control blood glucose levels. If the body can't meet this increased need for insulin, women can develop gestational diabetes during the late stages of pregnancy.

Gestational diabetes usually goes away after the baby is born. Shortly after pregnancy, 5 to 10 percent of women with gestational diabetes continue to have high blood glucose levels and are diagnosed as having diabetes, usually type 2. Research has shown that lifestyle changes and the diabetes medication, metformin, can reduce or delay the risk of type 2 diabetes in these women. Babies born to mothers who had gestational diabetes are also more likely to develop obesity and type 2 diabetes as they grow up.

Other Types of Diabetes

Many other types of diabetes exist, and a person can exhibit characteristics of more than one type. For example, in latent autoimmune diabetes in adults, people show signs of both type 1 and type 2 diabetes. Other types of diabetes include those caused by genetic defects, diseases of the pancreas, excess amounts of certain hormones resulting from some medical conditions, medications that reduce insulin action, chemicals that destroy beta cells, infections, rare autoimmune disorders, and genetic syndromes associated with diabetes.

What is prediabetes?

Prediabetes is when blood glucose levels are higher than normal but not high enough for a diagnosis of diabetes. Prediabetes means a person is at increased risk for developing type 2 diabetes, as well as for heart disease and stroke. Many people with prediabetes develop type 2 diabetes within 10 years.

However, modest weight loss and moderate physical activity can help people with prediabetes delay or prevent type 2 diabetes.

How are diabetes and prediabetes diagnosed?

Blood tests are used to diagnosis diabetes and prediabetes because early in the disease type 2 diabetes may have no symptoms. All diabetes blood tests involve drawing blood at a health care provider's office or commercial facility and sending the sample to a lab for analysis. Lab analysis of blood is needed to ensure test results are accurate.

Glucose measuring devices used in a health care provider's office, such as finger-stick devices, are not accurate enough for diagnosis but may be used as a quick indicator of high blood glucose.

Testing enables health care providers to find and treat diabetes before complications occur and to find and treat prediabetes, which can delay or prevent type 2 diabetes from developing.

Any one of the following tests can be used for diagnosis:

- an A1C test, also called the hemoglobin A1c, HbA1c, or glycohemoglobin test

- a fasting plasma glucose (FPG) test

- an oral glucose tolerance test (OGTT)

Another blood test, the random plasma glucose (RPG) test, is sometimes used to diagnose diabetes during a regular health checkup. If the RPG measures 200 micrograms per deciliter or above, and the individual also shows symptoms of diabetes, then a health care provider may diagnose diabetes.

Symptoms of diabetes include

- increased urination

- increased thirst

- unexplained weight loss

Other symptoms can include fatigue, blurred vision, increased hunger, and sores that do not heal.

Any test used to diagnose diabetes requires confirmation with a second measurement unless clear symptoms of diabetes exist.

A1C Test

The A1C test is used to detect type 2 diabetes and prediabetes but is not recommended for diagnosis of type 1 diabetes or gestational diabetes. The A1C test is a blood test that reflects the average of a person's blood glucose levels over the past 3 months and does not show daily fluctuations. The A1C test is more convenient for patients than the traditional glucose tests because it does not require fasting and can be performed at any time of the day.

The A1C test result is reported as a percentage. The higher the percentage, the higher a person's blood glucose levels have been. A normal A1C level is below 5.7 percent.

An A1C of 5.7 to 6.4 percent indicates prediabetes. People diagnosed with prediabetes may be retested in 1 year. People with an A1C below

5.7 percent maystill be at risk for diabetes, depending on the presence of other characteristics that put them at risk, also known as risk factors. People with an A1C above 6.0 percent should be considered at very high risk of developing diabetes. A level of 6.5 percent or above means a person has diabetes.

Laboratory analysis. When the A1C test is used for diagnosis, the blood sample must be sent to a laboratory using a method that is certified by the NGSP to ensure the results are standardized. Blood samples analyzed in a health care provider's office, known as point-of-care tests, are not standardized for diagnosing diabetes.

Abnormal results. The A1C test can be unreliable for diagnosing or monitoring diabetes in people with certain conditions known to interfere with the results. Interference should be suspected when A1C results seem very different from the results of a blood glucose test. People of African, Mediterranean, or Southeast Asian descent or people with family members with sickle cell anemia or a thalassemia are particularly at risk of interference.

However, not all of the A1C tests are unreliable for people with these diseases.

False A1C test results may also occur in people with other problems that affect their blood or hemoglobin such as chronic kidney disease, liver disease, or anemia.

Changes in Diagnostic Testing

In the past, the A1C test was used to monitor blood glucose levels but not for diagnosis. The A1C test has now been standardized, and in 2009, an international expert committee recommended it be used for diagnosis of type 2 diabetes and prediabetes.

Fasting Plasma Glucose Test

The FPG test is used to detect diabetes and prediabetes. The FPG test has been the most common test used for diagnosing diabetes because it is more convenient than the OGTT and less expensive. The FPG test measures blood glucose in a person who has fasted for at least 8 hours and is most reliable when given in the morning.

People with a fasting glucose level of 100 to 125 mg/dL have impaired fasting glucose (IFG), or prediabetes. A level of 126 mg/dL or above, confirmed by repeating the test on another day, means a person has diabetes.

Oral Glucose Tolerance Test

The OGTT can be used to diagnose diabetes, prediabetes, and gestational diabetes. Research has shown that the OGTT is more sensitive than the FPG test, but it is less convenient to administer. When used to test for diabetes or prediabetes, the OGTT measures blood glucose after a person fasts for at least 8 hours and 2 hours after the person drinks a liquid containing 75 grams of glucose dissolved in water.

If the 2-hour blood glucose level is between 140 and 199 mg/dL, the person has a type of prediabetes called impaired glucose tolerance (IGT). If confirmed by a second test, a 2-hour glucose level of 200 mg/dL or above means a person has diabetes.

Are diabetes blood test results always accurate?

All laboratory test results can vary from day to day and from test to test. Results can vary

- **within the person being tested.** A person's blood glucose levels normally move up and down depending on meals, exercise, sickness, and stress.

- **between different tests.** Each test measures blood glucose levels in a different way.

- **within the same test.** Even when the same blood sample is repeatedly measured in the same laboratory, the results may vary due to small changes in temperature, equipment, or sample handling.

Although all these tests can be used to indicate diabetes, in some people one test will indicate a diagnosis of diabetes when another test does not. People with differing test results may be in an early stage of the disease, where blood glucose levels have not risen high enough to show on every test.

Health care providers take all these variations into account when considering test results and repeat laboratory tests for confirmation. Diabetes develops over time, so even with variations in test results, health care providers can tell when overall blood glucose levels are becoming too high.

Diagnosis of Gestational Diabetes

Health care providers test for gestational diabetes using the OGTT. Women may be tested during their first visit to the health care provider after becoming pregnant or between 24 to 28 weeks of pregnancy depending on their risk factors and symptoms. Women found to have diabetes at the first visit to the health care provider after becoming pregnant may be diagnosed with type 2 diabetes.

Defining Safe Blood Glucose Levels for Pregnancy

Many studies have shown that gestational diabetes can cause complications for the mother and baby. An international, multicenter study, the Hyperglycemia and Adverse Pregnancy Outcome (HAPO) study, showed that the higher a pregnant woman's blood glucose is, the higher her risk of pregnancy complications. The HAPO researchers found that pregnancy complications can occur at blood glucose levels that were once considered to be normal.

Based on the results of the HAPO study, new guidelines for diagnosis of gestational diabetes were recommended by the International Association of the Diabetes and Pregnancy Study Groups in 2011. So far, the new guidelines have been adopted by the American Diabetes Association (ADA) but not by the American College of Obstetricians and Gynecologists (ACOG) or other medical organizations. Researchers estimate these new guidelines, if widely adopted, will increase the proportion of pregnant women diagnosed with gestational diabetes to nearly 18 percent.

Both ADA and ACOG guidelines for using the OGTT in diagnosing gestational diabetes are shown in the following tables.

Table 42.1. Recommendations for Testing Pregnant Women for Diabetes

Time of testing	ACOG	ADA
At first visit during pregnancy	No recommendation	Test women with risk factors for diabetes using standard testing for diagnosis of type 2 diabetes. Women found to have diabetes at this time should be diagnosed with type 2 diabetes, not gestational diabetes.
At 24 to 28 weeks of pregnancy	Test women for diabetes based on their history, risk factors, or a 50-gram, 1-hour, nonfasting, glucose challenge test—a modified OGTT. If score is 130–140 mg/dL, test again with fasting, 100-gram, 3-hour OGTT.*	Test all women for diabetes who are not already diagnosed, using a fasting, 75-gram, 2-hour OGTT.*

*See the next table "OGTT Levels for Diagnosis of Gestational Diabetes" for blood glucose levels.

Table 42.2. OGTT Levels for Diagnosis of Gestational Diabetes

Time of Sample Collection	ACOG Levels**,4 (mg/dL)	ADA Levels3(mg/dL)
	100-gram Glucose Drink	75-gram Glucose Drink
Fasting, before drinking glucose	95 or above	92 or above
1 hour after drinking glucose	180 or above	180 or above
2 hours after drinking glucose	155 or above	153 or above
3 hours after drinking glucose	140 or above	Not used
Requirements for Diagnosis	TWO or more of the above levels must be met	ONE or more of the above levels must be met

*Carpenter and Coustan Conversion, some labs use different numbers.

Who should be tested for diabetes and prediabetes?

Adults, pregnant women, children, and teens should be tested for diabetes and prediabetes according to their risk factors.

Adults

Anyone age 45 or older should consider getting tested for diabetes or prediabetes. Testing is strongly recommended for people older than age 45 who are overweight or obese. People younger than 45 should consider testing if they are overweight or obese and have one or more of the following risk factors:

- physical inactivity
- parent, brother, or sister with diabetes
- family background that is African American, Alaska Native, American Indian, Asian American, Hispanic/Latino, or Pacific Islander American
- history of giving birth to at least one baby weighing more than 9 pounds
- history of gestational diabetes
- high blood pressure—140/90 mmHg or higher—or being diagnosed with high blood pressure

- high-density lipoprotein, or HDL, cholesterol—"good" cholesterol—level below 35 mg/dL or a triglyceride level above 250 mg/dL

- polycystic ovary syndrome, also called PCOS

- prediabetes—an A1C level of 5.7 to 6.4 percent; an FPG test result of 100–125 mg/dL, indicating IFG; or a 2-hour OGTT result of 140–199 mg/dL, indicating IGT

- acanthosis nigricans, a condition associated with insulin resistance and characterized by a dark, velvety rash around the neck or armpits

- history of cardiovascular disease—disease affecting the heart and blood vessels

In addition to weight, the location of excess fat on the body can be important. A waist measurement of 40 inches or more for men and 35 inches or more for women is linked to insulin resistance and increases a person's risk for type 2 diabetes. This is true even if a person's body mass index (BMI) falls within the normal range.

How to Measure the Waist

To measure the waist, a person should

- place a tape measure around the bare abdomen just above the hip bone

- make sure the tape is snug but isn't digging into the skin and is parallel to the floor

- relax, exhale, and measure

If results of testing are normal, testing should be repeated at least every 3 years. Health care providers may recommend more frequent testing depending on initial results and risk status. People whose test results indicate they have prediabetes may be tested again in 1 year and should take steps to prevent or delay type 2 diabetes.

Pregnant Women

All pregnant women with risk factors for type 2 diabetes should be tested using standard diabetes blood tests during their first visit to the health care provider during pregnancy to see if they had undiagnosed diabetes before becoming pregnant. After that, pregnant women should be tested for gestational diabetes between 24 and 28 weeks of their pregnancy using the OGTT.

Women who develop gestational diabetes should also have follow-up testing 6 to 12 weeks after the baby is born to find out if they have type 2 diabetes or prediabetes. If results of testing are normal, testing should be repeated at least every 3 years. Blood glucose tests, rather than the A1C test, should be used for testing within 12 weeks of delivery.

Children and Teens

Type 2 diabetes has become increasingly common in children and teens. Children are at high risk for developing type 2 diabetes and should be tested if they are

- overweight or obese and have other risk factors, such as a family history of diabetes

- older than age 10 or have already gone through puberty

Body Mass Index (BMI)

Body mass index is a measurement of body weight relative to height for adults age 20 or older. To use the chart

- find the person's height in the left-hand column

- move across the row to find the number closest to the person's weight

- find the number at the top of that column

The number at the top of the column is the person's BMI. The words above the BMI number indicate whether the person is normal weight, overweight, or obese. People who are overweight or obese should consider talking with a health care provider about ways to lose weight and reduce the risk of diabetes.

The BMI has certain limitations. The BMI may overestimate body fat in athletes and others who have a muscular build and underestimate body fat in older adults and others who have lost muscle.

The BMI for children and teens must be determined based on age, height, weight, and sex.

What steps can delay or prevent type 2 diabetes?

A major research study, the Diabetes Prevention Program (DPP), proved that people with prediabetes were able to sharply reduce their

Table 42.3. Body Mass Index Table – A

BMI	Normal						Overweight					Obese					
	19	20	21	22	23	24	25	26	27	28	29	30	31	32	33	34	35
Height (inches)	Body Weight (pounds)																
58	91	96	100	105	110	115	119	124	129	134	138	143	148	153	158	162	167
59	94	99	104	109	114	119	124	128	133	138	143	148	153	158	163	168	173
60	97	102	107	112	118	123	128	133	138	143	148	153	158	163	168	174	179
61	100	106	111	116	122	127	132	137	143	148	153	158	164	169	174	180	185
62	104	109	115	120	126	131	136	142	147	153	158	164	169	175	180	186	191
63	107	113	118	124	130	135	141	146	152	158	163	169	175	180	186	191	197
64	110	116	122	128	134	140	145	151	157	163	169	174	180	186	192	197	204
65	114	120	126	132	138	144	150	156	162	168	174	180	186	192	198	204	210
66	118	124	130	136	142	148	155	161	167	173	179	186	192	198	204	210	216
67	121	127	134	140	146	153	159	166	172	178	185	191	198	204	211	217	223
68	125	131	138	144	151	158	164	171	177	184	190	197	203	210	216	223	230
69	128	135	142	149	155	162	169	176	182	189	196	203	209	216	223	230	236
70	132	139	146	153	160	167	174	181	188	195	202	209	216	222	229	236	243
71	136	143	150	157	165	172	179	186	193	200	208	215	222	229	236	243	250
72	140	147	154	162	169	177	184	191	199	206	213	221	228	235	242	250	258
73	144	151	159	166	174	182	189	197	204	212	219	227	235	242	250	257	265
74	148	155	163	171	179	186	194	202	210	218	225	233	241	249	256	264	272
75	152	160	168	176	184	192	200	208	216	224	232	240	248	256	264	272	279
76	156	164	172	180	189	197	205	213	221	230	238	246	254	263	271	279	287

Table 42.4. Body Mass Index Table – B

BMI	Obese				Extreme Obesity														
	36	37	38	39	40	41	42	43	44	45	46	47	48	49	50	51	52	53	54
"Height (inches)"	Body Weight (pounds)																		
58	172	177	181	186	191	196	201	205	210	215	220	224	229	234	239	244	248	253	258
59	178	183	188	193	198	203	208	212	217	222	227	232	237	242	247	252	257	262	267
60	184	189	194	199	204	209	215	220	225	230	235	240	245	250	255	261	266	271	276
61	190	195	201	206	211	217	222	227	232	238	243	248	254	259	264	269	275	280	285
62	196	202	207	213	218	224	229	235	240	246	251	256	262	267	273	278	284	289	295
63	203	208	214	220	225	231	237	242	248	254	259	265	270	278	282	287	293	299	304
64	209	215	221	227	232	238	244	250	256	262	267	273	279	285	291	296	302	308	314
65	216	222	228	234	240	246	252	258	264	270	276	282	288	294	300	306	312	318	324
66	223	229	235	241	247	253	260	266	272	278	284	291	297	303	309	315	322	328	334
67	230	236	242	249	255	261	268	274	280	287	293	299	306	312	319	325	331	338	344
68	236	243	249	256	262	269	276	282	289	295	302	308	315	322	328	335	341	348	354
69	243	250	257	263	270	277	284	291	297	304	311	318	324	331	338	345	351	358	365
70	250	257	264	271	278	285	292	299	306	313	320	327	334	341	348	355	362	369	376
71	257	265	272	279	286	293	301	308	315	322	329	338	343	351	358	365	372	379	386
72	265	272	279	287	294	302	309	316	324	331	338	346	353	361	368	375	383	390	397
73	272	280	288	295	302	310	318	325	333	340	348	355	363	371	378	386	393	401	408
74	280	287	295	303	311	319	326	334	342	350	358	365	373	381	389	396	404	412	420
75	287	295	303	311	319	327	335	343	351	359	367	375	383	391	399	407	415	423	431
76	295	304	312	320	328	336	344	353	361	369	377	385	394	402	410	418	426	435	443

risk of developing diabetes during the study by losing 5 to 7 percent of their body weight through dietary changes and increased physical activity.

Study participants followed a low-fat, low-calorie diet and engaged in regular physical activity, such as walking briskly five times a week for 30 minutes. These strategies worked well for both men and women in all racial and ethnic groups, but were especially effective for participants age 60 and older. A follow-up study, the Diabetes Prevention Program Outcomes Study (DPPOS), showed losing weight and being physically active provide lasting results. Ten years after the DPP, modest weight loss delayed onset of type 2 diabetes by an average of 4 years.

The diabetes medication metformin also lowers the risk of type 2 diabetes in people with prediabetes, especially those who are younger and heavier and women who have had gestational diabetes. The DPPOS showed that metformin delayed type 2 diabetes by 2 years. People at high risk should ask their health care provider if they should take metformin to prevent type 2 diabetes. Metformin is a medication that makes insulin work better and can reduce the risk of type 2 diabetes.

How is diabetes managed?

People can manage their diabetes with meal planning, physical activity, and if needed, medications.

Section 42.2

Blood Glucose Meter

Text in this section is excerpted from "Tips and Articles on Device Safety," U.S. Food and Drug Administration (FDA), August 5, 2015.

Home Healthcare Medical Devices: Blood Glucose Meters

Getting the Most Out of Your Meter
Testing Your Blood Glucose Accurately

It is important to test your blood glucose (sugar) accurately so you can manage your blood glucose levels. Keeping your blood glucose under control helps you feel better and lowers the risk of blindness, kidney disease, and nerve damage.

Tips for Using Your Blood Glucose Meter

Although blood glucose meters are simple to operate, many things can go wrong. Follow the tips below to get the most accurate results from your blood glucose meter.

Preparing to Test

- Read and save all instructions for your meter and test strips.

- Watch and practice with an experienced blood glucose meter user, a diabetes educator, or a healthcare professional. Don't be afraid to ask questions!

- Wash your hands. Even small amounts of food or sugar on your fingers can affect your results.

- Read the test strip packaging to make sure the strips will work with your meter.

- Do not use test strips from a cracked or damaged bottle.

- Do not use test strips that have passed their expiration dates.

- Make sure you have entered the correct calibration code (if your meter requires one).

- Test strips may look alike, but they are not all the same. Strips often have very specific chemical coatings or sizes.

- Even if an incorrect test strip fits in your meter, it could give you wrong results.

Testing Your Blood Glucose

- Use the correct blood drop size. If there is not enough blood on the test strip, the meter may not read the blood glucose level accurately. Repeat the test if you have any doubts.

- Let the blood flow freely from your fingertip; do not squeeze your finger. Squeezing your finger can affect the results.

- Use a whole test strip each time you use your meter.

- Insert the test strip into the meter until you feel it stop against the end of the meter guide.

Even if your meter is supposed to give an error message when the blood drop is too small, the message may appear only when the drop is much too small. If the blood drop is too small, your meter can be wrong without giving an error message!

- **Maintaining Your Blood Glucose Meter**

- Keep your meter clean.

- Test your meter regularly with control solution.

- Keep extra batteries charged and ready.

- Store your meter and supplies properly. Heat and humidity can damage test strips.

- Replace the bottle cap promptly after removing a test strip.

- **Following Up**

- Take your meter with you when you visit your doctor so you can compare it with your laboratory results.

- Talk with your doctor or call the manufacturer's toll-free phone number if you are having problems with your meter.

- **Note on Alternative Site Testing**

- **Some** blood glucose meters can use blood samples from the upper arm, forearm, base of the thumb, or thigh.

- Using alternative sites gives you more options. But be aware that blood glucose levels from these sites may not always be as accurate as readings from the fingertips. Alternative site results differ from fingertip results when glucose levels are changing rapidly such as after a meal, after taking insulin, during exercise, or when you are ill or under stress.

- Use blood from a fingertip rather than an alternative site if:

- you think your blood glucose is low,

- you don't regularly have symptoms when your blood glucose is low, or

- how you feel doesn't match the results from the alternative site.

  Caution: Not all meters can use blood from alternative sites, and not all alternative sites are the same. Only test from sites that are identified in the instructions. Alternative site testing is not for everyone. Talk with your doctor before you test from a site other than your fingertip.

Recognizing Low and High Blood Glucose

Some people have recognizable symptoms of low or high blood glucose and some do not. The only reliable way to know when you have low or high blood glucose is to test it.

When your blood glucose is low, you may feel faint, shaky, dizzy, or confused. You may begin to sweat. You may have a headache, sudden behavior change, or seizure.

When your blood glucose is high, your symptoms may be similar to when your blood glucose is low. You may feel dizzy or have a headache. You may also feel thirsty or have an urgent need to urinate.

But many people have no symptoms with low or high blood sugar levels. Other people have symptoms that change over time, so they no longer recognize them. Often, older patients or people who have had diabetes for many years stop having symptoms.

Blood Glucose Meters Are Not Perfect

Although blood glucose meters are generally reliable and help to manage diabetes, they are not perfect. The technology used in blood glucose meters is not as accurate as testing done in a hospital or a doctor's office.

Your blood glucose meter may give a wrong reading if you are dehydrated, are going into shock, or have a high red blood cell count (hematocrit). Even a very low blood glucose level can cause an incorrect reading.

If you suspect your blood glucose is too low or too high, call your doctor or go to an emergency room immediately... even if your meter shows that everything is fine.

Reporting Problems with Your Glucose Meter

FDA encourages you to report any serious injuries, deaths or malfunctions you experience with medical products. FDA will take action when needed to protect the public's health.

Report the events to FDA at 1-800-332-1088 and to the product manufacturer.

Chapter 43

Heart and Vascular Disease Screening and Diagnostic Tests

How Is Heart Disease Diagnosed?

Your doctor will diagnose coronary heart disease (CHD) based on your medical and family histories, your risk factors, a physical exam, and the results from tests and procedures.

No single test can diagnose CHD. If your doctor thinks you have CHD, he or she may recommend one or more of the following tests.

EKG (Electrocardiogram)

An EKG is a simple, painless test that detects and records the heart's electrical activity. The test shows how fast the heart is beating and its rhythm (steady or irregular). An EKG also records the strength and timing of electrical signals as they pass through the heart.

An EKG can show signs of heart damage due to CHD and signs of a previous or current heart attack.

Text in this chapter is excerpted from "Heart Disease in Women," National Heart, Lung, and Blood Institute (NHLBI), April 21, 2014.

Stress Testing

During stress testing, you exercise to make your heart work hard and beat fast while heart tests are done. If you can't exercise, you may be given medicines to increase your heart rate.

When your heart is working hard and beating fast, it needs more blood and oxygen. Plaque-narrowed coronary (heart) arteries can't supply enough oxygen-rich blood to meet your heart's needs.

A stress test can show possible signs and symptoms of CHD, such as:

- Abnormal changes in your heart rate or blood pressure

- Shortness of breath or chest pain

- Abnormal changes in your heart rhythm or your heart's electrical activity

If you can't exercise for as long as what is considered normal for someone your age, your heart may not be getting enough oxygen-rich blood. However, other factors also can prevent you from exercising long enough (for example, lung diseases, anemia, or poor general fitness).

As part of some stress tests, pictures are taken of your heart while you exercise and while you rest. These imaging stress tests can show how well blood is flowing in your heart and how well your heart pumps blood when it beats.

Echocardiography

Echocardiography (echo) uses sound waves to create a moving picture of your heart. The test provides information about the size and shape of your heart and how well your heart chambers and valves are working.

Echo also can show areas of poor blood flow to the heart, areas of heart muscle that aren't contracting normally, and previous injury to the heart muscle caused by poor blood flow.

Chest X-Ray

A chest X-ray creates pictures of the organs and structures inside your chest, such as your heart, lungs, and blood vessels.

A chest X-ray can reveal signs of heart failure, as well as lung disorders and other causes of symptoms not related to CHD.

Blood Tests

Blood tests check the levels of certain fats, cholesterol, sugar, and proteins in your blood. Abnormal levels may be a sign that you're at risk for CHD. Blood tests also help detect anemia, a risk factor for CHD.

During a heart attack, heart muscle cells die and release proteins into the bloodstream. Blood tests can measure the amount of these proteins in the bloodstream. High levels of these proteins are a sign of a recent heart attack.

Coronary Angiography and Cardiac Catheterization

Your doctor may recommend coronary angiography if other tests or factors suggest you have CHD. This test uses dye and special X-rays to look inside your coronary arteries.

To get the dye into your coronary arteries, your doctor will use a procedure called cardiac catheterization.

A thin, flexible tube called a catheter is put into a blood vessel in your arm, groin (upper thigh), or neck. The tube is threaded into your coronary arteries, and the dye is released into your bloodstream.

Special X-rays are taken while the dye is flowing through your coronary arteries. The dye lets your doctor study the flow of blood through your heart and blood vessels.

Coronary angiography detects blockages in the large coronary arteries. However, the test doesn't detect coronary microvascular disease (MVD). This is because coronary MVD doesn't cause blockages in the large coronary arteries.

Even if the results of your coronary angiography are normal, you may still have chest pain or other CHD symptoms. If so, talk with your doctor about whether you might have coronary MVD.

Your doctor may ask you to fill out a questionnaire called the Duke Activity Status Index. This questionnaire measures how easily you can do routine tasks. It gives your doctor information about how well blood is flowing through your coronary arteries.

Your doctor also may recommend other tests that measure blood flow in the heart, such as a cardiac MRI (magnetic resonance imaging) stress test.

Cardiac MRI uses radio waves, magnets, and a computer to create pictures of your heart as it beats. The test produces both still and moving pictures of your heart and major blood vessels.

Other tests done during cardiac catheterization can check blood flow in the heart's small arteries and the thickness of the artery walls.

Tests Used to Diagnose Broken Heart Syndrome

If your doctor thinks you have broken heart syndrome, he or she may recommend coronary angiography. Other tests are also used to diagnose this disorder, including blood tests, EKG, echo, and cardiac MRI.

Chapter 44

Infectious Disease Testing

Chapter Contents

Section 44.1

Tests for HIV / AIDS

Text in this section begins with excerpts from "HIV Basics," Centers for Disease Control and Prevention (CDC), January 16, 2015;

and text from "Getting an HIV test" is excerpted from"Testing," Centers for Disease Control and Prevention (CDC), June 30, 2015.

About HIV/AIDS

HIV is a virus spread through body fluids that affects specific cells of the immune system, called CD4 cells, or T cells. Over time, HIV can destroy so many of these cells that the body can't fight off infections and disease. When this happens, HIV infection leads to AIDS. Learn more about the stages of HIV and how to tell whether you're infected.

What is HIV?

HIV stands for human immunodeficiency virus. It is the virus that can lead to acquired immunodeficiency syndrome, or AIDS. Unlike some other viruses, the human body cannot get rid of HIV. That means that once you have HIV, you have it for life.

No safe and effective cure currently exists, but scientists are working hard to find one, and remain hopeful. Meanwhile, with proper medical care, HIV can be controlled. Treatment for HIV is often called antiretroviral therapy or ART. It can dramatically prolong the lives of many people infected with HIV and lower their chance of infecting others. Before the introduction of ART in the mid-1990s, people with HIV could progress to AIDS in just a few years. Today, someone diagnosed with HIV and treated before the disease is far advanced can have a nearly normal life expectancy.

HIV affects specific cells of the immune system, called CD4 cells, or T cells. Over time, HIV can destroy so many of these cells that the body can't fight off infections and disease. When this happens, HIV infection leads to AIDS.

What are the stages of HIV?

HIV disease has a well-documented progression. Untreated, HIV is almost universally fatal because it eventually overwhelms the immune system—resulting in acquired immunodeficiency syndrome (AIDS). HIV treatment helps people at all stages of the disease, and treatment can slow or prevent progression from one stage to the next.

A person can transmit HIV to others during any of these stages:

Acute infection: Within **2 to 4 weeks** after infection with HIV, you may feel sick with flu-like symptoms. This is called acute retroviral syndrome (ARS) or primary HIV infection, and it's the body's natural response to the HIV infection. (Not everyone develops ARS, however—and some people may have no symptoms.)

During this period of infection, large amounts of HIV are being produced in your body. The virus uses important immune system cells called CD4 cells to make copies of itself and destroys these cells in the process. Because of this, the CD4 count can fall quickly.

Your ability to spread HIV is highest during this stage because the amount of virus in the blood is very high.

Eventually, your immune response will begin to bring the amount of virus in your body back down to a stable level. At this point, your CD4 count will then begin to increase, but it may not return to pre-infection levels.

Clinical latency (inactivity or dormancy): This period is sometimes called asymptomatic HIV infection or chronic HIV infection. During this phase, HIV is still active, but reproduces at very low levels. You may not have any symptoms or get sick during this time. People who are on antiretroviral therapy (ART) may live with clinical latency for several decades. For people who are not on ART, this period can last up to a decade, but some may progress through this phase faster. It is important to remember that you are still able to transmit HIV to others during this phase even if you are treated with ART, although ART greatly reduces the risk. Toward the middle and end of this period, your viral load begins to rise and your CD4 cell count begins to drop. As this happens, you may begin to have symptoms of HIV infection as your immune system becomes too weak to protect you.

AIDS (acquired immunodeficiency syndrome): This is the stage of infection that occurs when your immune system is badly damaged and you become vulnerable to infections and infection-related cancers called opportunistic illnesses. When the number of your CD4 cells falls below 200 cells per cubic millimeter of blood (200 cells/mm3), you are considered to have progressed to AIDS. (Normal CD4 counts are between 500 and 1,600 cells/mm3.) You can also be diagnosed with AIDS if you develop one or more opportunistic illnesses, regardless of your CD4 count. Without treatment, people who are diagnosed with AIDS typically survive about 3 years. Once someone has a dangerous opportunistic illness, life expectancy without treatment falls to about 1 year. People with AIDS need medical treatment to prevent death.

How can I tell if I'm infected with HIV?

The only way to know if you are infected with HIV is to be tested. You cannot rely on symptoms to know whether you have HIV. Many people who are infected with HIV **do not have any symptoms at all** for 10 years or more. Some people who are infected with HIV report having flu-like symptoms (often described as "the worst flu ever") 2 to 4 weeks after exposure. Symptoms can include:

• Fever

• Enlarged lymph nodes

• Sore throat

• Rash

These symptoms can last anywhere from a few days to several weeks. During this time, HIV infection may not show up on an HIV test, but people who have it are highly infectious and can spread the infection to others.

However, you should not assume you have HIV if you have any of these symptoms. Each of these symptoms can be caused by other illnesses. Again, the only way to determine whether you are infected is to be tested for HIV infection.

You can also ask your health care provider to give you an HIV test.

Two types of home testing kits are available in most drugstores or pharmacies: one involves pricking your finger for a blood sample, sending the sample to a laboratory, then phoning in for results. The other involves getting a swab of fluid from your mouth, using the kit to test it, and reading the results in 20 minutes. Confidential counseling and referrals for treatment are available with both kinds of home tests.

If you test positive for HIV, you should see your doctor as soon as possible to begin treatment.

Is there a cure for HIV?

For most people, the answer is no. Most reports of a cure involve HIV-infected people who needed treatment for a cancer that would have killed them otherwise. But these treatments are very risky, even life-threatening, and are used only when the HIV-infected people would have died without them. Antiretroviral therapy (ART), however, can dramatically prolong the lives of many people infected with HIV and lower their chance of infecting others. It is important that people get tested for HIV and know that they are infected early so that medical care and treatment have the greatest effect.

Testing

Getting an HIV test is the only way to know if you have HIV. This section answers some of the most common questions related to HIV testing, including the types of tests available, where to get one, and what to expect when you go to get tested.

Should I get tested for HIV?

CDC recommends that health care providers test everyone between the ages of 13 and 64 at least once as part of routine health care. One in eight people in the United States who have HIV do not know they are infected.

Behaviors that put you at risk for HIV include having vaginal or anal sex without a condom or without being on medicines that prevent or treat HIV, or sharing injection drug equipment with someone who has HIV. If you answer yes to any of the following questions, you should definitely get an HIV test:

- Have you had sex with someone who is HIV-positive or whose status you didn't know since your last HIV test?

- Have you injected drugs (including steroids, hormones, or silicone) and shared equipment (or works, such as needles and syringes) with others?

- Have you exchanged sex for drugs or money?

- Have you been diagnosed with or sought treatment for a sexually transmitted disease, like syphilis?

- Have you been diagnosed with or sought treatment for hepatitis or tuberculosis (TB)?

- Have you had sex with someone who could answer yes to any of the above questions or someone whose history you don't know?

If you continue having unsafe sex or sharing injection drug equipment, you should get tested at least once a year. Sexually active gay and bisexual men may benefit from more frequent testing (e.g., every 3 to 6 months).

You should also get tested if

- You have been sexually assaulted.

- You are a woman who is planning to get pregnant or who is pregnant.

How can testing help me?

Getting tested can give you some important information and can help keep you—and others—safe. For example,

- Knowing your HIV status can give you peace of mind—and testing is the **only way** you can know your HIV status for sure.

- When you and your partner know each other's HIV status, you can make informed decisions about your sexual behaviors and how to stay safe.

- If you are pregnant, or planning to get pregnant, knowing your status can help protect your baby from becoming infected.

- If you find out you are HIV-positive, you can start taking medicine for your HIV. Getting treated for HIV improves your health, prolongs your life, and greatly lowers your chance of spreading HIV to others.

- If you know you are HIV-positive, you can take steps to protect your sex partners from becoming infected.

I don't believe I am at high risk. Why should I get tested?

Some people who test positive for HIV were not aware of their risk. That's why CDC recommends that providers in all health care settings make HIV testing a routine part of medical care for patients aged 13 to 64, unless the patient declines (opts out). This practice would get more people tested and help reduce the stigma around testing.

Even if you have been in a long-term relationship with one person, you should find out for sure whether you or your partner has HIV. If you are both HIV-negative and you both stay faithful (monogamous) and do not have other risks for HIV infection, then you probably won't need another HIV test unless your situation changes.

I am pregnant. Why should I get tested?

HIV testing during each pregnancy is important because, if your result is positive, treatment can improve your health and greatly lower the chance that you will pass HIV to your infant before, during, or after birth. The treatment is most effective for preventing HIV transmission to babies when started as early as possible during pregnancy. However, there are still great health benefits to beginning preventive treatment even during labor or shortly after the baby is born.

CDC recommends that health care providers screen all pregnant women for HIV, talk to them about HIV or give them written materials, and, for women with risk factors, provide referrals to prevention counseling.

Screening all pregnant women for HIV, and giving them the right medical care, helped decrease the number of babies born with HIV from a high of 1,650 in 1991 to 127 in 2011.

When should I get tested?

The immune system usually takes 3 to 8 weeks to make antibodies against HIV, but tests differ in how early they are able to detect antibodies. Although most HIV tests look for these antibodies, some look for the virus itself. The period after infection but before the test becomes positive is called the window period.

Deciding when to get tested therefore depends on when you may have been exposed and which test is used. You can ask your health care provider about the window period for the HIV test you are taking. If you are using a home test, you can get that information from the materials included in the packaging of the test.

A few people will have a longer window period, so if you get a negative antibody test result in the first 3 months after possible exposure, you should get a repeat test after 3 months. Ninety-seven percent of people will develop antibodies in the first 3 months after they are infected. In very rare cases, it can take up to 6 months to develop antibodies to HIV.

Where can I get tested?

You can ask your health care provider for an HIV test. Many medical clinics, substance abuse programs, community health centers, and hospitals offer them, too. You can also

Visit National HIV and STD Testing Resources (https://gettested.cdc.gov/) and enter your ZIP code.

- Text your ZIP code to KNOWIT (566948), and you will receive a text back with a testing site near you.

- Call 800-CDC-INFO (800-232-4636) to ask for free testing sites in your area.

- Contact your local health department.

- Get a home testing kit (the Home Access HIV-1 Test System or the OraQuick In-Home HIV Test) from a drugstore.

- What kinds of tests are available, and how do they work?

The most common HIV test is the **antibody screening test (immunoassay),** which tests for the antibodies that your body makes against HIV. The immunoassay may be conducted in a lab or as a rapid test at the testing site. It may be performed on blood or oral fluid (not saliva). Because the level of antibody in oral fluid is lower than it is in blood, blood tests tend to find infection sooner after exposure than do oral fluid tests. In addition, most blood-based lab tests find infection sooner after exposure than rapid HIV tests.

Several tests are being used more commonly that can detect both **antibodies and antigen (part of the virus itself).** These tests can find recent infection earlier than tests that detect only antibodies. These antigen/antibody combination tests can find HIV as soon as 3 weeks after exposure to the virus, but they are only available for testing blood, not oral fluid.

The **rapid test** is an immunoassay used for screening, and it produces quick results, in 30 minutes or less. Rapid tests use blood or oral fluid to look for antibodies to HIV. If an immunoassay (lab test or rapid test) is conducted during the window period (i.e., the period after exposure but before the test can find antibodies), the test may not find antibodies and may give a false-negative result. All immunoassays that are positive need a follow-up test to confirm the result.

Follow-up diagnostic testing is performed if the first immunoassay result is positive. Follow-up tests include: an antibody differentiation test, which distinguishes HIV-1 from HIV-2; an HIV-1 nucleic acid test, which looks for virus directly, or the Western blot or indirect immunofluorescence assay, which detect antibodies.

Immunoassays are generally very accurate, but follow-up testing allows you and your health care provider to be sure the diagnosis is right. If your first test is a rapid test, and it is positive, you will be directed to a medical setting to get follow-up testing. If your first test is a lab test, and it is positive, the lab will conduct follow-up testing, usually on the same blood specimen as the first test.

Currently there are only two home HIV tests: the Home Access HIV-1 Test System and the OraQuick In-home HIV test. If you buy your home test online make sure the HIV test is FDA-approved.

The **Home Access HIV-1 Test System** is a home collection kit, which involves pricking your finger to collect a blood sample, sending the sample to a licensed laboratory, and then calling in for results as early as the next business day. This test is anonymous. If the test is positive, a follow-up test is performed right away, and the results include the follow-up test. The manufacturer provides confidential counseling and referral to treatment. The tests conducted on the blood sample collected at home find infection later after infection than most lab-based tests using blood from a vein, but earlier than tests conducted with oral fluid.

The **OraQuick In-Home HIV Test** provides rapid results in the home. The testing procedure involves swabbing your mouth for an oral fluid sample and using a kit to test it. Results are available in 20 minutes. If you test positive, you will need a follow-up test. The manufacturer provides confidential counseling and referral to follow-up testing sites. Because the level of antibody in oral fluid is lower than it is in blood, oral fluid tests find infection later after exposure than do blood tests. Up to 1 in 12 people may test false-negative with this test.

RNA tests detect the virus directly (instead of the antibodies to HIV) and thus can detect HIV at about 10 days after infection—as soon as it appears in the bloodstream, before antibodies develop. These tests cost more than antibody tests and are generally not used as a screening test, although your doctor may order one as a follow-up test, after a positive antibody test, or as part of a clinical workup.

What should I expect when I go in for an HIV test?

When it's time to take the test, a health care provider will take your sample (blood or oral fluid) and you may be able to wait for the results (if it's a rapid HIV test). If the test comes back negative, and you haven't had an exposure for 3 months, you can be confident you're not infected with HIV.

If your test comes back positive, you will need to get a follow-up test, which the testing site will arrange.

Your health care provider or counselor may talk with you about your risk factors, answer questions about your general health, and discuss next steps with you, especially if your result is positive.

What does a negative test result mean?

A negative result does not necessarily mean that you don't have HIV. That's because of the window period—the period after you may have been exposed to HIV but before a test can detect it. The window period depends on the kind of test that was used on your blood or oral fluid. For antibody tests, if you get a negative result within 3 months of your most recent possible exposure, you need to get tested again at the 3-month mark. For RNA tests or antibody/ antigen tests, that timeframe may be shorter. Ask your health care provider if and when you need to be retested with a negative test result. And meanwhile, practice abstinence or mutual monogamy with a trusted partner, use condoms every time you have sex (and for every sex act—anal, oral, or vaginal), and don't share needles and other drug equipment (works).

If I have a negative result, does that mean that my partner is HIV-negative also?

No. Your HIV test result reveals only your HIV status. HIV is not necessarily transmitted every time you have sex. Therefore, taking an HIV test is not a way to find out if your partner is infected. Ask your partner if he or she has been tested for HIV and about his or her risk behaviors, both now and in the past. Consider getting tested together, often referred to as couples testing.

What does a positive result mean?

If you had a rapid screening test, the testing site will arrange a follow-up test to make sure the screening test result was correct. If your blood was tested in a lab, the lab will conduct a follow-up test on the same sample. If the follow-up test is also positive, it means you are HIV-positive.

The sooner you take steps to protect your health, the better. Early treatment with antiretroviral drugs and a healthy lifestyle can help you stay well. Prompt medical care prevents the onset of AIDS and some life-threatening conditions.

Here are some important steps you can take right away to protect your health:

- **See a licensed health care provider, even if you don't feel sick.** Your local health department can help you find a health care provider who has experience treating HIV. There are medicines to treat HIV infection and help you stay healthy. It's never too early to start treatment. Current guidelines recommend treatment with antiretroviral therapy (ART) for all people with HIV, including those with early infection.

- Get screened for other sexually transmitted infections (STIs). STIs can cause serious health problems, even when they don't cause symptoms. Using a condom during all sexual contact (anal, vaginal, or oral) can help prevent many STIs.

- Have a TB (tuberculosis) test. You may be infected with TB and not know it. Undetected TB can cause serious illness, but it can be successfully treated if caught early.

- Get help if you smoke cigarettes, drink too much alcohol, or use illegal drugs (such as methamphetamine), which can weaken your immune system. Find substance abuse treatment facilities near you.

To avoid giving HIV to anyone else,

Tell your partner or partners about your HIV status before you have any type of sexual contact with them (anal, vaginal, or oral).

- Use latex condoms and/or dental dams with every sexual contact. If either partner is allergic to latex, plastic (polyurethane) condoms for either the male or female can be used.

- Don't share needles, syringes, or other drug paraphernalia with anyone.

- Stay on ART to keep your virus under control and greatly reduce your ability to spread HIV to others.

- If your steady partner is HIV-negative, discuss whether he or she should consider pre-exposure prophylaxis (PrEP)—medications to *prevent* HIV.

If I test positive for HIV, does that mean I have AIDS?

No. Being HIV-positive does not mean you have AIDS. AIDS is the most advanced stage of HIV disease. Proper treatment can keep you from developing AIDS.

Will other people know my test result?

Your test results are protected by state and federal privacy laws. They can only be released with your permission. Whether anyone can know about your test results or your HIV status depends on what kind of test you take: confidential or anonymous. Some states only offer confidential testing.

- **Confidential testing** means that your name and other identifying information will be attached to your test results. The results will go in your medical record and may be shared with your health care providers and your health insurance company. Otherwise, the results are protected by state and federal privacy laws.

- **Anonymous testing** means that nothing ties your test results to you. When you take an anonymous HIV test, you get a unique identifier that allows you to get your test results.

With confidential testing, if you test positive for HIV or another STI, the test result and your name will be reported to the state or local health department to help public health officials get better estimates of the rates of HIV in the state. The state health department will then **remove all personal information** about you (name, address, etc.) and share the remaining non-identifying information with CDC. CDC does not share this information with anyone else, including insurance companies.

Should I share my positive test result with others?

Whether you share, or disclose, your status to others is your decision.

Partners

If you test positive for HIV, your sex or drug-using partners may also be infected. It's important that they know they have been exposed so that they can be tested too.

You can tell them yourself—but if you're nervous about disclosing your test result, or you have been threatened or injured by your partner, you can ask your doctor or the local health department to tell them that they might have been exposed to HIV. Health departments do not reveal your name to your partners. They will only tell your partners that they have been exposed to HIV and should get tested.

Most states have laws that require you to tell your sexual partners if you are HIV-positive be**fore** you have sex (anal, vaginal, or oral) or share drugs. You can be charged with a crime in some states if you don't tell—even if your partner doesn't become infected.

Family and friends

In most cases, your family and friends will not know your test results or HIV status unless you tell them yourself. While telling your family that you have HIV may seem hard, you should know that disclosure actually has many benefits—studies have shown that people who disclose their HIV status respond better to treatment than those who don't.

If you are under 18, however, some states allow your health care provider to tell your parent(s) that you received services for sexually transmitted infections, including HIV, if they think doing so is in your best interest.

Employers

In most cases, your employer will not know your HIV status unless you tell. But your employer does have a right to ask if you have any health conditions that would affect your ability to do your job or pose a serious risk to others. (An example might be a health care professional, like a surgeon, who does procedures where there is a risk of blood or other body fluids being exchanged.)

If you have health insurance through your employer, the insurance company cannot **legally** tell your employer that you have HIV. But it is possible that your employer could find out if the insurance company provides detailed information to your employer about the benefits it pays or the costs of insurance.

All people with HIV are covered under the Americans with Disabilities Act. This means that your employer cannot discriminate against you because of your HIV status as long as you can do your job.

Who will pay for my HIV test?

HIV screening is covered by health insurance without a co-pay, as required by the Affordable Care Act. If you do not have medical insurance, there are places where you can get an HIV test at a reduced cost or for free.

Who will pay for my treatment if I am HIV-positive?

If you have insurance, your insurer may pay for treatment. If you do not have insurance, or your insurer will not pay for treatment, government programs, such as Medicaid, Medicare, Ryan White Care Act treatment centers, and community health centers may be able to help if you meet their rules for eligibility (usually low income and/or disability). CDC is working with its federal partners to make sure that all people who need treatment can get it. Your health care provider or local public health department can direct you to HIV treatment programs.

Section 44.2

Flu/Influenza Testing

Text in this section begins with excerpts from "Seasonal Influenza: Flu Basics," Centers for Disease Control and Prevention (CDC), August 25, 2015; and text from "Diagnosing Flu," Centers for Disease Control and Prevention (CDC), August 13, 2015.

Seasonal Influenza: Flu Basics

Influenza (flu) is a contagious respiratory illness caused by influenza viruses. It can cause mild to severe illness. Serious outcomes of flu infection can result in hospitalization or death. Some people, such as older people, young children, and people with certain health conditions, are at high risk for serious flu complications. The best way to prevent the flu is by getting **vaccinated** each year.

Diagnosing Flu

How do I know if I have the flu?

Your respiratory illness might be the flu if you have fever, cough, sore throat, runny or stuffy nose, body aches, headache, chills and fatigue. Some people may have vomiting and diarrhea. People may be infected with the flu and have respiratory symptoms without a fever. Flu viruses usually cause the most illness during the colder months of the year. However, influenza can also occur outside of the typical flu season. In addition, other viruses can also cause respiratory illness similar to the flu. So, it is impossible to tell for sure if you have the flu based on symptoms alone. If your doctor needs to know for sure whether you have the flu, there are laboratory tests that can be done.

What kinds of flu tests are there?

A number of flu tests are available to detect influenza viruses. The most common are called "rapid influenza diagnostic tests." These tests can provide results in 30 minutes or less. Unfortunately, the ability of these tests to detect the flu can vary greatly. Therefore, you could still have the flu, even though your rapid test result is negative. In addition to rapid tests, there are several more accurate and sensitive flu tests available that must be performed in specialized laboratories, such as those found in hospitals or state public health laboratories. All of these tests require that a health care provider swipe the inside of your nose or the back of your throat with a swab and then send the swab for testing. These tests do not require a blood sample.

How well can rapid tests detect the flu?

During an influenza outbreak, a positive rapid flu test is likely to indicate influenza infection. However, rapid tests vary in their ability to detect flu viruses, depending on the type of rapid test used, and on the type of flu viruses circulating. Also, rapid tests appear to be better at detecting flu in children than adults. This variation in ability to detect viruses can result in some people who are infected with the flu having a negative rapid test result. (This situation is called a false negative test result.) Despite a negative rapid test result, your health care provider may diagnose you with flu based on your symptoms and their clinical judgment.

Will my health care provider test me for flu if I have flu-like symptoms?

Not necessarily. Most people with flu symptoms do not require testing because the test results usually do not change how you are treated.

Your health care provider may diagnose you with flu based on your symptoms and their clinical judgment or they may choose to use an influenza diagnostic test. During an outbreak of respiratory illness, testing for flu can help determine if flu viruses are the cause of the outbreak. Flu testing can also be helpful for some people with suspected flu who are pregnant or have a weakened immune system, and for whom a diagnosis of flu can help their doctor make decisions about their care.

Section 44.3

Test for Hepatitis

Text in this section is excerpted from "Testing for the Hepatitis
C Virus," Agency for Healthcare Research and Quality (AHRQ),
September 2013.

What is hepatitis C?

Hepatitis C is a disease caused by a virus that infects your liver. Your liver is an important organ in your body and has many functions. The liver removes harmful chemicals from your body, aids digestion, and processes vitamins and nutrients from food. The liver also makes chemicals that help your blood clot when you have a cut. You cannot live without a liver.

For some people with hepatitis C, the infection lasts only a short time, and their body is able to clear the virus. But, most people infected with hepatitis C develop chronic hepatitis C.

Chronic hepatitis C is a long-term illness that happens when the hepatitis C virus stays in your body. Most people who have chronic hepatitis C do not have symptoms for many years until the infection has started to damage their liver.

How can hepatitis C be harmful?

If hepatitis C is left untreated, over time (up to 20 years or longer in some people), the infection can damage the liver and make it not work properly. It can cause cirrhosis (scarring of the liver that makes the liver not work correctly and causes other problems), liver cancer, liver failure, and death.

- Hepatitis C is a leading cause of liver cancer.

- Hepatitis C is the most common reason for liver transplants in the United States.

- Out of 100 people with chronic hepatitis C who do not receive treatment, up to 20 people will develop cirrhosis within 20 years of being infected. After 20 years, the number of people with chronic hepatitis C who develop cirrhosis can be much higher.

Cirrhosis increases the chance of liver cancer and death.

- Hepatitis C causes about 15,000 deaths in the United States each year.

Who is at risk for hepatitis C?

The hepatitis C virus is spread through infected blood or other bodily fluids. There is no vaccine for hepatitis C.

People at risk for hepatitis C include people who:

- Received a blood product, such as clotting factors for blood clotting problems, before 1987

- Had a blood transfusion or an organ transplant before 1992

- Got a tattoo with unsterilized tools

- Injected drugs (took drugs through a needle) or snorted drugs (inhaled drugs through a tube or straw), even if it was only one time

- Were exposed to the hepatitis C virus at work, such as a health care worker coming in contact with infected blood

- Spent many years on dialysis for kidney failure

- Were born to a mother with hepatitis C

- Have been in jail

You **cannot** catch the hepatitis C virus from simply being around infected people, shaking hands, or hugging.

A mother with hepatitis C can pass the virus to her child during birth. Researchers found that the risk is about the same for both Cesarean section (C-section) and vaginal delivery. Researchers also found that breastfeeding is not associated with an increased risk of passing the hepatitis C virus from mother to child.

How common is hepatitis C?

- About 4 million people in the United States have chronic hepatitis C.

- Around three out of every four Americans infected with the hepatitis C virus were born in the years between 1945 and 1965 (Baby Boomers).

- About 8 out of every 10 people infected with the hepatitis C virus develop chronic hepatitis C.

What are the symptoms of hepatitis C?

Most people do not notice any symptoms of hepatitis C for many years until the virus begins to damage their liver. Other people have symptoms right away.

When symptoms of hepatitis C do appear, they can include those listed below. However, some of these symptoms can be caused by common illnesses as well.

- Fever

- Upset stomach and nausea

- Diarrhea

- Loss of appetite

- Feeling exhausted

- Yellowed eyes and skin, called "jaundice"

- Swelling of the belly

- Easy bruising

- Taking longer for bleeding to stop

How do I know if I have the hepatitis C virus?

A simple blood test can show if you have been infected with the hepatitis C virus in the past. If the blood test comes back positive, your doctor will do a second blood test to see if the virus is still in your blood. These blood tests are very accurate.

Why is testing for hepatitis C important?

Many people who are infected with the hepatitis C virus do not know they have it. Symptoms usually do not show up until the infection begins to damage the liver. For some people, this can happen up to 20 years or longer after being infected. Testing for the hepatitis C virus can help identify infected people early so they can get treatment before their liver becomes damaged. Infected people can also make lifestyle changes to help protect their liver, such as avoiding alcohol. Testing can also help identify infected people so they can take steps to prevent spreading the virus to others. Hepatitis C is spread through blood. An infected person can prevent infecting others by not sharing any items that come into contact with his or her blood.

Who should be tested for hepatitis C?

The Centers for Disease Control and Prevention (CDC) and a national group of doctors, nurses, and others who are experts in prevention reviewed research on testing for hepatitis C and recommend the following:

- Doctors should offer one-time hepatitis C testing to adults born in the years from 1945 through 1965.

- Adults at an increased risk for hepatitis C should be tested.

- Risk factors include having injected drugs (shared drug needles), having received a blood transfusion before 1992.

- People who continue to be at risk (such as those who continue to inject drugs) may need to be tested for hepatitis C more than once.

If you feel you should be tested for hepatitis C, talk with your doctor.

What if I find out that I have hepatitis C?

Hepatitis C can be cured, although not everyone who has hepatitis C needs to be treated right away. Your doctor will talk with you about if and when you may need treatment. You can also make lifestyle changes to help protect your liver, such as avoiding alcohol.

Treatments are available that can help your body clear the virus for good. Before deciding on treatment, your doctor may do blood tests to check your liver for signs of damage. Some doctors may also suggest a liver biopsy. During a liver biopsy, the doctor removes a tiny piece of your liver to look for damage. The results of the biopsy can help the doctor decide if you need treatment right away or if you can wait to be treated. Some people wait years before starting treatment.

Hepatitis C treatments consist of medicines (a weekly shot along with pills taken by mouth) that you take for 6 months to a year. Out of every 10 people who complete treatment, up to 7 are able to clear the hepatitis C virus from their body. The success rate depends on several things, including the specific type of hepatitis C virus a person has, the type of treatment used, and how long the treatment lasted.

The medicines to treat hepatitis C can cause many side effects, including flu- like symptoms, anemia (a low number of red blood cells), a rash, and depression. The side effects can sometimes be severe.

New medicines to treat hepatitis C are currently being developed. These new medicines that are taken by mouth are thought to work better and have fewer side effects than the medicines available right now. Some of these new medicines may be approved by the U.S. Food and Drug Administration (FDA) in the next few years.

What should I think about?

In deciding whether you should be tested for hepatitis C, you may want to think about:

- Whether you were born between 1945 and 1965
- Whether you have any of the risk factors for hepatitis C
- Whether you continue to be at risk for becoming infected with hepatitis C
- The benefits of getting tested for hepatitis C
- What a positive test result would mean

Section 44.4

Tests for Chlamydia

Text in this chapter is excerpted from "Chlamydia - CDC Fact Sheet (Detailed)," Centers for Disease Control and Prevention (CDC), September 24, 2015.

Who should be tested for chlamydia?

Any sexually active person can be infected with chlamydia. Anyone with genital symptoms such as discharge, burning during urination, unusual sores, or rash should refrain from having sex until they are able to see a health care provider about their symptoms.

Also, anyone with an oral, anal, or vaginal sex partner who has been recently diagnosed with an STD should see a health care provider for evaluation.

Because chlamydia is usually asymptomatic, screening is necessary to identify most infections. Screening programs have been demonstrated to reduce rates of adverse sequelae in women. CDC recommends yearly chlamydia screening of all sexually active women younger than 25, as well as older women with risk factors such as new or multiple partners, or a sex partner who has a sexually transmitted infection. Pregnant women should be screened during their first prenatal care visit. Pregnant women under or at increased risk for chlamydia (e.g., women who have a new or more than one sex partner) should be screened again in their third trimester. Any woman who is sexually active should discuss her risk factors with a health care provider who can then determine if more frequent screening is necessary.

Routine screening is not recommended for men. However, the screening of sexually active young men should be considered in clinical settings with a high prevalence of chlamydia (e.g., adolescent clinics, correctional facilities, and STD clinics) when resources permit and do not hinder screening efforts in women.

Men who have sex with men (MSM) who have receptive anal sex should be screened for chlamydia each year. MSM who have multiple and/or anonymous sex partners should be screened more frequently (e.g., at 3-6 month intervals).

HIV-infected sexually active women who are age 25 or younger or have other risk factors, and all HIV-infected patients who report having receptive anal sex should be screened for chlamydia at their first HIV care visit and then at least annually. A patient's health care providermight determine more frequent screening is necessary, based on the patient's risk factors.

How is chlamydia diagnosed?

There are a number of diagnostic tests for chlamydia, including nucleic acid amplification tests (NAATs), cell culture, and others. NAATs are the most sensitive tests, and can be performed on easily obtainable specimens such as vaginal swabs (either clinician- or patient-collected) or urine.

Vaginal swabs, either patient- or clinician-collected, are the optimal specimen to screen for genital chlamydia using NAATs in females; urine is the specimen of choice for males, and is an effective alternative specimen type for females. Self-collected vaginal swab specimens perform at least as well as other approved specimens using NAATs.

In addition, patients may prefer self-collected vaginal swabs or urinebased screening to the more invasive endocervical or urethral swab specimens. Adolescent girls may be particularly good candidates for self-collected vaginal swab- or urine-based screening because pelvic aexams are not indicated if they are asymptomatic.

Section 44.5

Test for Tuberculosis

Text in this section is excerpted from "Tuberculosis (TB)," Center for Disease Control and Prevention (CDC), April 10, 2014.

Testing and Diagnosis

Tuberculosis (TB) is a disease that is spread through the air from one person to another. There are two kinds of tests that are used to determine if a person has been infected with TB bacteria: the tuberculin skin test and TB blood tests.

A positive TB skin test or TB blood test only tells that a person has been infected with TB bacteria. It does not tell whether the person has latent TB infection (LTBI) or has progressed to TB disease. Other tests, such as a chest X-ray and a sample of sputum, are needed to see whether the person has TB disease.

Tuberculin skin test: The TB skin test (also called the Mantoux tuberculin skin test) is performed by injecting a small amount of fluid (called tuberculin) into the skin in the lower part of the arm. A person given the tuberculin skin test must return within 48 to 72 hours to have a trained health care worker look for a reaction on the arm. The health care worker will look for a raised, hard area or swelling, and if present, measure its size using a ruler. Redness by itself is not considered part of the reaction.

The skin test result depends on the size of the raised, hard area or swelling. It also depends on the person's risk of being infected with TB bacteria and the progression to TB disease if infected.

Positive skin test: This means the person's body was infected with TB bacteria. Additional tests are needed to determine if the person has latent TB infection or TB disease. A health care worker will then provide treatment as needed.

Negative skin test: This means the person's body did not react to the test, and that latent TB infection or TB disease is not likely.

TB blood tests: TB blood tests (also called interferon-gamma release assays or IGRAs) measure how the immune system reacts to the bacteria that cause TB. An IGRA measures how strong a person's immune system reacts to TB bacteria by testing the person's blood in a laboratory.

Two IGRAs are approved by the U.S. Food and Drug Administration (FDA) and are available in the United States:

1.   QuantiFERON®–TB Gold In-Tube test (QFT-GIT)

2.   T-SPOT®.TB test (T-Spot)

Positive IGRA: This means that the person has been infected with TB bacteria. Additional tests are needed to determine if the person has latent TB infection or TB disease. A health care worker will then provide treatment as needed.

Negative IGRA: This means that the person's blood did not react to the test and that latent TB infection or TB disease is not likely. IGRAs are the preferred method of TB infection testing for the following:

- People who have received bacille Calmette–Guérin (BCG). BCG is a vaccine for TB disease.

- People who have a difficult time returning for a second appointment to look for a reaction to the TST.

There is no problem with repeated IGRAs.

Who Should Get Tested for TB

TB tests are generally not needed for people with a low risk of infection with TB bacteria.

Certain people should be tested for TB bacteria because they are more likely to get TB disease, including:

- People who have spent time with someone who has TB disease weakens the immune system

- People who have symptoms of TB disease (fever, night sweats, cough, and weight loss)
- People from a country where TB disease is common (most countries in Latin America, the Caribbean, Africa, Asia, Eastern Europe, and Russia)
- People who live or work somewhere in the United States where TB disease is more common (homeless shelters, prison or jails, or some nursing homes)
- People who use illegal drugs

Testing for TB in BCG-Vaccinated Persons

Many people born outside of the United States have been BCG-vaccinated.

People who have had a previous BCG vaccine may receive a TB skin test. In some people, BCG may cause a positive skin test when they are not infected with TB bacteria. If a TB skin test is positive, additional tests are needed.

IGRAs, unlike the TB skin tests, are not affected by prior BCG vaccination and are not expected to give a false-positive result in people who have received BCG.

Choosing a TB Test

The person's health care provider should choose which TB test to use. Factors in selecting which test to use include the reason for testing, test availability, and cost. Generally, it is not recommended to test a person with both a TST and an IGRA.

Diagnosis of Latent TB Infection or TB Disease

If a person is found to be infected with TB bacteria, other tests are needed to see if the person has TB disease. TB disease can be diagnosed by medical history, physical examination, chest X-ray, and other laboratory tests. TB disease is treated by taking several drugs as recommended by a health care provider.

If a person does not have TB disease, but has TB bacteria in the body, then latent TB infection is diagnosed. The decision about treatment for latent TB infection will be based on a person's chances of developing TB disease.

Diagnosis of TB Disease

People suspected of having TB disease should be referred for amedical evaluation, which will include

- Medical history,

- Physical examination,

- Test for TB infection (TB skin test or TB blood test),

- Chest radiograph (X-ray), and

- Appropriate laboratory tests.

Section 44.6

Malaria Testing

Text in this section is excerpted from "Malaria," Centers for Disease Control and Prevention (CDC), November 9, 2012.

About Malaria

Malaria is a serious and sometimes fatal disease caused by a parasite that commonly infects a certain type of mosquito which feeds on humans. People who get malaria are typically very sick with high fevers, shaking chills, and flu-like illness. Although malaria can be a deadly disease, illness and death from malaria can usually be prevented.

About 1,500 cases of malaria are diagnosed in the United States each year. The vast majority of cases in the United States are in travelers and immigrants returning from countries where malaria transmission occurs, many from sub-Saharan Africa and South Asia.

Diagnosis of Malaria (United States)

Malaria must be recognized promptly in order to treat the patient in time and to prevent further spread of infection in the community via local mosquitoes.

Malaria should be considered a potential medical emergency and should be treated accordingly. Delay in diagnosis and treatment is a leading cause of death in malaria patients in the United States.

Malaria can be suspected based on the patient's travel history, symptoms, and the physical findings at examination. However, for a definitive diagnosis to be made, laboratory tests must demonstrate the malaria parasites or their components.

Diagnosis of malaria can be difficult:

- Where malaria is not endemic any more (such as in the United States), health-care providers may not be familiar with the disease. Clinicians seeing a malaria patient may forget to consider malaria among the potential diagnoses and not order the needed diagnostic tests. Laboratorians may lack experience with malaria and fail to detect parasites when examining blood smears under the microscope.

- In some malaria-endemic areas, malaria transmission is so intense that a large proportion of the population is infected but not made ill by the parasites. Such carriers have developed just enough immunity to protect them from malarial illness but not from malarial infection. In that situation, finding malaria parasites in an ill person does not necessarily mean that the illness is caused by the parasites.

Clinical Diagnosis of Malaria

Clinical diagnosis is based on the patient's symptoms and on physical findings at examination.

The first symptoms of malaria (most often fever, chills, sweats, headaches, muscle pains, nausea and vomiting) are often not specific and are also found in other diseases (such as the "flu" and common viral infections). Likewise, the physical findings are often not specific (elevated temperature, perspiration, tiredness).

In severe malaria (caused by Plasmodium falciparum), clinical findings (confusion, coma, neurologic focal signs, severe anemia, respiratory difficulties) are more striking and may increase the index of suspicion for malaria.

If possible, clinical findings should always be confirmed by a laboratory test for malaria.

In addition to ordering the malaria specific diagnostic tests described below, the health-care provider should conduct an initial workup and request a complete blood count and a routine chemistry panel. In the event that the person does have a positive malaria test, these additional tests will be useful in determining whether the patient has uncomplicated or severe manifestations of the malaria infection. Specifically, these tests can detect severe anemia, hypoglycemia, renal failure, hyperbilirubinemia, and acid-base disturbances.

Microscopic Diagnosis

Malaria parasites can be identified by examining under the microscope a drop of the patient's blood, spread out as a "blood smear" on a microscope slide. Prior to examination, the specimen is stained (most often with the Giemsa stain) to give the parasites a distinctive appearance. This technique remains the gold standard for laboratory confirmation of malaria. However, it depends on the quality of the reagents, of the microscope, and on the experience of the laboratorian.

Antigen Detection

Various test kits are available to detect antigens derived from malaria parasites. Such immunologic ("immunochromatographic") tests most often use a dipstick or cassette format, and provide results in 2-15 minutes. These "Rapid Diagnostic Tests" (RDTs) offer a useful alternative to microscopy in situations where reliable microscopic diagnosis is not available. Malaria RDTs are currently used in some clinical settings and programs. However, before malaria RDTs can be widely adopted, several issues remain to be addressed, including improving their accuracy; lowering their cost; and ensuring their adequate performance under adverse field conditions. The World Health Organization is conducting comparative performance evaluations of many of the RDTs which are commercially available worldwide based on a panel of parasites derived from a global network of collection sites.

On June 13, 2007, the U.S. Food and Drug Administration (FDA) approved the first RDT for use in the United States. This RDT is approved for use by hospital and commercial laboratories, not by individual clinicians or by patients themselves. It is recommended that all RDTs are followed-up with microscopy to confirm the results and if positive, to quantify the proportion of red blood cells that are infected. The use of this RDT may decrease the amount of time that it takes to determine that a patient is infected with malaria.

Molecular Diagnosis

Parasite nucleic acids are detected using polymerase chain reaction (PCR). Although this technique may be slightly more sensitive than smear microscopy, it is of limited utility for the diagnosis of acutely ill patients in the standard healthcare setting. PCR results are often not available quickly enough to be of value in establishing the diagnosis of malaria infection.

PCR is most useful for confirming the species of malarial parasite after the diagnosis has been established by either smear microscopy or RDT.

Serology

Serology detects antibodies against malaria parasites, using either indirect immunofluorescence (IFA) or enzyme-linked immunosorbent assay (ELISA). Serology does not detect current infection but rather measures past exposure.

Drug Resistance Tests

Drug resistance tests must be performed in specialized laboratories to assess the susceptibility to antimalarial compounds of parasites collected from a specific patient. Two main laboratory methods are available:

In vitro tests: The parasites are grown in culture in the presence of increasing concentrations of drugs; the drug concentration that inhibits parasite growth is used as endpoint.

Molecular characterization: Molecular markers assessed by PCR or gene sequencing also allow the prediction, to some degree, of resistance to some drugs. CDC recommends that all cases of malaria diagnosed in the United States should be evaluated for evidence of drug resistance.

Chapter 45

Lung Function Tests

What Are Lung Function Tests?

Lung function tests, also called pulmonary function tests, measure how well your lungs work. These tests are used to look for the cause of breathing problems, such as shortness of breath.

Lung function tests measure:

- How much air you can take into your lungs. This amount is compared with that of other people your age, height, and sex. This allows your doctor to see whether you're in the normal range.

- How much air you can blow out of your lungs and how fast you can do it.

- How well your lungs deliver oxygen to your blood.

- The strength of your breathing muscles.

Doctors use lung function tests to help diagnose conditions such as asthma, pulmonary fibrosis (scarring of the lung tissue), and COPD (chronic obstructive pulmonary disease).

Lung function tests also are used to check the extent of damage caused by conditions such as pulmonary fibrosis and sarcoidosis (sar-koy-DOE-sis). Also, these tests might be used to check how well treatments, such as asthma medicines, are working.

Text in this chapter is excerpted from "Lung Function Tests," National Heart, Lung, and Blood Institute (NHLBI), September 17, 2012.

Overview

Lung function tests include breathing tests and tests that measure the oxygen level in your blood. The breathing tests most often used are:

- Spirometry. This test measures how much air you can breathe in and out. It also measures how fast you can blow air out.

- Body plethysmography. This test measures how much air is present in your lungs when you take a deep breath. It also measures how much air remains in your lungs after you breathe out fully.

- Lung diffusion capacity. This test measures how well oxygen passes from your lungs to your bloodstream.

These tests may not show what's causing breathing problems. So, you may have other tests as well, such as an exercise stress test. This test measures how well your lungs and heart work while you exercise on a treadmill or bicycle.

Two tests that measure the oxygen level in your blood are pulse oximetry and arterial blood gas tests. These tests also are called blood oxygen tests.

Pulse oximetry measures your blood oxygen level using a special light. For an arterial blood gas test, your doctor takes a sample of your blood, usually from an artery in your wrist. The sample is sent to a laboratory, where its oxygen level is measured.

Outlook

Lung function tests usually are painless and rarely cause side effects. You may feel some discomfort during an arterial blood gas test when the blood sample is taken.

Types of Lung Function Tests

Breathing Tests

Spirometry

Spirometry measures how much air you breathe in and out and how fast you blow it out. This is measured two ways: peak expiratory flow rate (PEFR) and forced expiratory volume in 1 second (FEV1).

PEFR is the fastest rate at which you can blow air out of your lungs. FEV1 refers to the amount of air you can blow out in 1 second.

During the test, a technician will ask you to take a deep breath in. Then, you'll blow as hard as you can into a tube connected to a small machine. The machine is called a spirometer.

Spirometry

Your doctor may have you inhale a medicine that helps open your airways. He or she will want to see whether the medicine changes or improves the test results.

Spirometry helps check for conditions that affect how much air you can breathe in, such as pulmonary fibrosis (scarring of the lung tissue). The test also helps detect diseases that affect how fast you can breathe air out, like asthma and COPD (chronic obstructive pulmonary disease).

Lung Volume Measurement

Body plethysmography (pleth-iz-MOG-re-fe) is a test that measures how much air is present in your lungs when you take a deep breath. It also measures how much air remains in your lungs after you breathe out fully.

During the test, you sit inside a glass booth and breathe into a tube that's attached to a computer.

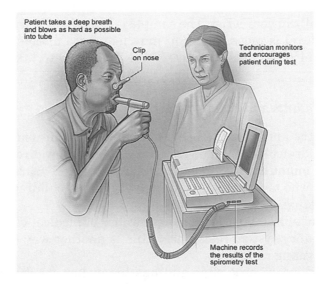

Figure 45.1. Spirometry: *The image shows how spirometry is done. The patient takes a deep breath and blows as hard as possible into a tube connected to a spirometer. The spirometer measures the amount of air breathed out. It also measures how fast the air was blown out.*

For other lung function tests, you might breathe in nitrogen or helium gas and then blow it out. The gas you breathe out is measured to show how much air your lungs can hold.

Lung volume measurement can help diagnose pulmonary fibrosis or a stiff or weak chest wall.

Lung Diffusion Capacity

This test measures how well oxygen passes from your lungs to your bloodstream. During this test, you breathe in a type of gas through a tube. You hold your breath for a brief moment and then blow out the gas.

Abnormal test results may suggest loss of lung tissue, emphysema (a type of COPD), very bad scarring of the lung tissue, or problems with blood flow through the body's arteries.

Tests to Measure Oxygen Level

Pulse oximetry and arterial blood gas tests show how much oxygen is in your blood. During pulse oximetry, a small sensor is attached to your finger or ear. The sensor uses light to estimate how much oxygen is in your blood. This test is painless and no needles are used.

For an arterial blood gas test, a blood sample is taken from an artery, usually in your wrist. The sample is sent to a laboratory, where its oxygen level is measured. You may feel some discomfort during an arterial blood gas test because a needle is used to take the blood sample.

Testing in Infants and Young Children

Spirometry and other measures of lung function usually can be done for children older than 6 years, if they can follow directions well. Spirometry might be tried in children as young as 5 years. However, technicians who have special training with young children may need to do the testing.

Instead of spirometry, a growing number of medical centers measure respiratory system resistance. This is another way to test lung function in young children.

The child wears nose clips and has his or her cheeks supported with an adult's hands. The child breathes in and out quietly on a mouthpiece, while the technician measures changes in pressure at the mouth. During these lung function tests, parents can help comfort their children and encourage them to cooperate.

Very young children (younger than 2 years) may need an infant lung function test. This requires special equipment and medical staff. This type of test is available only at a few medical centers.

The doctor gives the child medicine to help him or her sleep through the test. A technician places a mask over the child's nose and mouth and a vest around the child's chest.

The mask and vest are attached to a lung function machine. The machine gently pushes air into the child's lungs through the mask. As the child exhales, the vest slightly squeezes his or her chest. This helps push more air out of the lungs. The exhaled air is then measured.

In children younger than 5 years, doctors likely will use signs and symptoms, medical history, and a physical exam to diagnose lung problems.

Doctors can use pulse oximetry and arterial blood gas tests for children of all ages.

Who Needs Lung Function Tests?

People who have breathing problems, such as shortness of breath, may need lung function tests. These tests help find the cause of breathing problems.

Doctors use lung function tests to help diagnose conditions such as asthma, pulmonary fibrosis (scarring of the lung tissue), and COPD (chronic obstructive pulmonary disease).

Lung function tests also are used to check the extent of damage caused by conditions such as pulmonary fibrosis and sarcoidosis. Also, these tests might be used to check how well treatments, such as asthma medicines, are working.

Diagnosing Lung Conditions

Your doctor will diagnose a lung condition based on your medical and family histories, a physical exam, and test results.

Medical and Family Histories

Your doctor will ask you questions, such as:

- Do you ever feel like you can't get enough air?

- Does your chest feel tight sometimes?

- Do you have periods of coughing or wheezing (a whistling sound when you breathe)?

- Do you ever have chest pain?

- Can you walk or run as fast as other people your age?

Your doctor also will ask whether you or anyone in your family has ever:

- Had asthma or allergies

- Had heart disease

- Smoked

- Traveled to places where they may have been exposed to tuberculosis

- Had a job that exposed them to dust, fumes, or particles (like asbestos)

Physical Exam

Your doctor will check your heart rate, breathing rate, and blood pressure. He or she also will listen to your heart and lungs with a stethoscope and feel your abdomen and limbs.

Your doctor will look for signs of heart or lung disease, or another disease that might be causing your symptoms.

Lung and Heart Tests

Based on your medical history and physical exam, your doctor will recommend tests. A chest X-ray usually is the first test done to find the cause of a breathing problem. This test takes pictures of the organs and structures inside your chest.

Your doctor may do lung function tests to find out even more about how well your lungs work.

Your doctor also may do tests to check your heart, such as an EKG (electrocardiogram) or an exercise stress test. An EKG detects and records your heart's electrical activity. A stress test shows how well your heart works during physical activity.

What to Expect before Lung Function Tests

If you take breathing medicines, your doctor may ask you to stop them for a short time before spirometry, lung volume measurement, or lung diffusion capacity tests.

No special preparation is needed before pulse oximetry and arterial blood gas tests. If you're getting oxygen therapy, your doctor may ask you to stop using it for a short time before the tests. This allows your doctor to check your blood oxygen level without the added oxygen.

What to Expect during Lung Function Tests

Breathing Tests

Spirometry might be done in your doctor's office or in a special lung function laboratory (lab). Lung volume measurement and lung diffusion capacity tests are done in a special lab or clinic. For these tests, you sit in a chair next to a machine that measures your breathing. For spirometry, you sit or stand next to the machine.

Before the tests, a technician places soft clips on your nose. This allows you to breathe only through a tube that's attached to the testing machine. The technician will tell you how to breathe into the tube. For example, you might be asked to breathe normally, slowly, or rapidly.

Some tests require deep breathing, which might make you feel short of breath, dizzy, or light-headed, or it might make you cough.

Spirometry

For this test, you take a deep breath and then exhale as fast and as hard as you can into the tube. With spirometry, your doctor may give you medicine to help open your airways. Your doctor will want to see whether the medicine changes or improves the test results.

Lung Volume Measurement

For body plethysmography, you sit in a clear glass booth and breathe through the tube attached to the testing machine. The changes in pressure inside the booth are measured to show how much air you can breathe into your lungs.

For other tests, you breathe in nitrogen or helium gas and then exhale. The gas that you breathe out is measured.

Lung Diffusion Capacity

During this test, you breathe in gas through the tube, hold your breath for 10 seconds, and then rapidly blow it out. The gas contains a small amount of carbon monoxide, which won't harm you.

Tests to Measure Oxygen Level

Pulse oximetry is done in a doctor's office or hospital. An arterial blood gas test is done in a lab or hospital.

Pulse Oximetry

For this test, a small sensor is attached to your finger or ear using a clip or flexible tape. The sensor is then attached to a cable that leads to a small machine called an oximeter. The oximeter shows the amount of oxygen in your blood. This test is painless and no needles are used.

Arterial Blood Gas

During this test, your doctor or technician inserts a needle into an artery, usually in your wrist, and takes a sample of blood. You may feel some discomfort when the needle is inserted. The sample is then sent to a lab where its oxygen level is measured.

After the needle is removed, you may feel mild pressure or throbbing at the needle site. Applying pressure to the area for 5 to 10 minutes should stop the bleeding. You'll be given a small bandage to place on the area.

What to Expect after Lung Function Tests

You can return to your normal activities and restart your medicines after lung function tests. Talk with your doctor about when you'll get the test results.

What Do Lung Function Tests Show?

Breathing Tests

Spirometry

Spirometry can show whether you have:

- A blockage (obstruction) in your airways. This may be a sign of asthma, COPD (chronic obstructive pulmonary disease), or another obstructive lung disorder.

- Smaller than normal lungs (restriction). This may be a sign of heart failure, pulmonary fibrosis (scarring of the lung tissue), or another restrictive lung disorder.

Lung Volume Measurement

These tests measure how much air your lungs can hold when you breathe in and how much air is left in your lungs when you breathe out. Abnormal test results may show that you have pulmonary fibrosis or a stiff or weak chest wall.

Lung Diffusion Capacity

This test can show a problem with oxygen moving from your lungs into your bloodstream. This might be a sign of loss of lung tissue, emphysema (a type of COPD), or problems with blood flow through the body's arteries.

Tests to Measure Oxygen Level

Pulse oximetry and **arterial blood gas tests** measure the oxygen level in your blood. These tests show how well your lungs are taking in oxygen and moving it into the bloodstream. A low level of oxygen in the blood might be a sign of a lung or heart disorder.

What Are the Risks of Lung Function Tests?

Spirometry, lung volume measurement, and lung diffusion capacity tests usually are safe. These tests rarely cause problems.

Pulse oximetry has no risks. Side effects from arterial blood gas tests are rare.

Chapter 46

Sleep Disorder Tests

What Are Sleep Studies?

Sleep studies are tests that measure how well you sleep and how your body responds to sleep problems. These tests can help your doctor find out whether you have a sleep disorder and how severe it is.

Sleep studies are important because untreated sleep disorders can raise your risk for heart disease, high blood pressure, stroke, and other medical conditions. Sleep disorders also have been linked to an increased risk of injury, such as falling (in the elderly) and car accidents.

People usually aren't aware of their breathing and movements while sleeping. They may never think to talk to their doctors about issues that might be related to sleep problems.

However, sleep disorders can be treated. Talk with your doctor if you snore regularly or feel very tired while at work or school most days of the week.

You also may want to talk with your doctor if you often have trouble falling or staying asleep, or if you wake up too early and aren't able to go back to sleep. These are common signs of a sleep disorder.

Your doctor might be able to diagnose a sleep disorder based on your sleep schedule and habits. However, he or she also might need the results from sleep studies and other medical tests to diagnose a sleep disorder.

Text in this chapter is excerpted from "Sleep Studies," National Heart, Lung, and Blood Institute (NHLBI), March 29, 2012.

Sleep studies can help diagnose:

- Sleep-related breathing disorders, such as sleep apnea

- Sleep-related seizure disorders

- Sleep-related movement disorders, such as periodic limb movement disorder

- Sleep disorders that cause extreme daytime tiredness, such as narcolepsy

Doctors might use sleep studies to help diagnose or rule out restless legs syndrome (RLS). However, RLS usually is diagnosed based on signs and symptoms, medical history, and a physical exam.

Types of Sleep Studies

To diagnose sleep-related problems, doctors may use one or more of the following sleep studies:

- Polysomnogram (PSG)

- Multiple sleep latency test (MSLT)

- Maintenance of wakefulness test (MWT)

- Home-based portable monitor

Your doctor may use actigraphy if he or she thinks you have a circadian rhythm disorder. This is a disorder that disrupts your body's natural sleep-wake cycle.

Polysomnogram

For a PSG, you usually will stay overnight at a sleep center. This study records brain activity, eye movements, heart rate, and blood pressure.

A PSG also records the amount of oxygen in your blood, air movement through your nose while you breathe, snoring, and chest movements. The chest movements show whether you're making an effort to breathe.

PSG results are used to help diagnose:

- Sleep-related breathing disorders, such as sleep apnea

- Sleep-related seizure disorders

- Sleep-related movement disorders, such as periodic limb movement disorder

- Sleep disorders that cause extreme daytime tiredness, such as narcolepsy (PSG and MSLT results will be reviewed together)

Your doctor also may use a PSG to find the right setting for you on a CPAP (continuous positive airway pressure) machine. CPAP is a treatment for sleep apnea.

Sleep apnea is a common disorder in which you have one or more pauses in breathing or shallow breaths while you sleep. In obstructive sleep apnea, the airway collapses or becomes blocked during sleep. A CPAP machine uses mild air pressure to keep your airway open while you sleep.

If your doctor thinks that you have sleep apnea, he or she might schedule a split-night sleep study. During the first half of the night, your sleep is checked without a CPAP machine. This will show whether you have sleep apnea and how severe it is.

If the PSG shows that you have sleep apnea, you'll use a CPAP machine during the second half of the split-night study. A technician will help you select a CPAP mask that fits and is comfortable.

While you sleep, the technician will check the amount of oxygen in your blood and whether your airway stays open. He or she will adjust the flow of air through the mask to find the setting that's right for you. This process is called CPAP titration.

Sometimes the entire study isn't done during the same night. Some people need to go back to the sleep center for the CPAP titration study.

Also, some people might need more than one PSG. For example, your doctor may recommend a followup PSG to:

- Adjust your CPAP settings after weight loss or weight gain

- Recheck your sleep if symptoms return despite treatment with CPAP

- Find out how well surgery has worked to correct a sleep-related breathing disorder

Multiple Sleep Latency Test

This daytime sleep study measures how sleepy you are. It typically is done the day after a PSG. You relax in a dark, quiet room for about 30 minutes while a technician checks your brain activity.

The MSLT records whether you fall asleep during the test and what types and stages of sleep you're having. Sleep has two basic types: rapid eye movement (REM) and non-REM. Non-REM sleep has three distinct stages. REM sleep and the three stages of non-REM sleep occur in regular cycles throughout the night.

The types and stages of sleep you have can help your doctor diagnose sleep disorders such as narcolepsy, idiopathic hypersomnia, and other sleep disorders that cause daytime tiredness.

An MSLT takes place over the course of a full day. This is because your ability to fall asleep changes throughout the day.

Maintenance of Wakefulness Test

This daytime sleep study measures your ability to stay awake and alert. It's usually done the day after a PSG and takes most of the day.

Results can show whether your inability to stay awake is a public or personal safety concern. Results also can show how you're responding to treatment.

Home-Based Portable Monitor

Your doctor may recommend a home-based sleep test with a portable monitor. The portable monitor will record some of the same information as a PSG. For example, it may record:

- The amount of oxygen in your blood

- Air movement through your nose while you breathe

- Your heart rate

- Chest movements that show whether you're making an effort to breathe

A sleep specialist might use the results from a home-based sleep test to help diagnose sleep apnea. He or she also might use the results to see how well some treatments for sleep apnea are working.

Home-based testing is appropriate only for some people. Talk with your doctor to find out whether a portable monitor is an option for you. If your doctor recommends this test, you'll need to visit a sleep center or your doctor's office to pick up the equipment and learn how to use it.

If you're diagnosed with sleep apnea, your doctor may prescribe treatment with CPAP. If so, he or she will need to find the correct airflow setting for your CPAP machine. To do this, you may need to go to a sleep center to have a PSG. Or, you may be able to find the correct setting at home with an autotitrating CPAP machine.

An autotitrating CPAP machine automatically finds the right airflow setting for you. These machines work well for some people who have sleep apnea. A technician or a doctor will teach you how to use the machine.

Actigraphy

Actigraphy is a test that's done while you do your normal daily routine. This test is useful for all age groups and doesn't require an overnight stay at a sleep center.

An actigraph is a simple device that's usually worn like a wristwatch. Your doctor may ask you to wear the device for several days and nights, except when bathing or swimming.

Actigraphy gives your doctor a better idea about your sleep schedule, such as when you sleep or nap and whether the lights are on while you sleep.

Doctors can use actigraphy to help diagnose many sleep disorders, including circadian rhythm disorders (such as jet lag and shift work disorder). Doctors also may use the test to check how well sleep treatments are working.

Actigraphy might be used with a PSG or alone.

Who Needs a Sleep Study?

Your doctor might not detect a sleep problem during a routine office visit because you're awake. Thus, you should let your doctor know if you or a family member/sleep partner thinks you might have a sleep problem.

For example, talk with your doctor if you:

- Have chronic (ongoing) snoring

- Often feel sleepy during the day, even though you've spent enough time in bed to be well rested

- Don't wake up feeling refreshed and alert

- Have trouble adapting to shift work

Your doctor might be able to diagnose a sleep disorder based on your sleep schedule and habits. However, he or she also might need the results from sleep studies and other medical tests to diagnose a sleep disorder.

Sleep studies often are used to diagnose sleep-related breathing disorders, such as sleep apnea. Signs of these disorders include loud snoring, gasping, or choking sounds while you sleep or pauses in breathing during sleep.

Other common signs and symptoms of sleep disorders include the following:

- It takes you more than 30 minutes to fall asleep at night.

- You often wake up during the night and then have trouble falling asleep again, or you wake up too early and aren't able to go back to sleep.

- You feel sleepy during the day and fall asleep within 5 minutes if you have a chance to nap, or you fall asleep at inappropriate times during the day.

- You have creeping, tingling, or crawling feelings in your legs that you can relieve by moving or massaging them, especially in the evening and when you try to fall asleep.

- You have vivid, dreamlike experiences while falling asleep or dozing.

- You have episodes of sudden muscle weakness when you're angry, fearful, or when you laugh.

- You feel as though you can't move when you first wake up.

- Your bed partner notes that your legs or arms jerk often during sleep.

- You regularly feel the need to use stimulants, such as caffeine, to stay awake during the day.

Many of the same signs and symptoms of sleep disorders can occur in infants and children. If your child snores or has other signs or symptoms of sleep problems, talk with his or her doctor.

If you've had a sleep disorder for a long time, you may not notice how it affects your daily routine.

Your doctor will work with you to decide whether you need a sleep study. A sleep study allows your doctor to observe sleep patterns and diagnose a sleep disorder, which can then be treated.

Certain medical conditions have been linked to sleep disorders, such as heart failure, kidney disease, high blood pressure, diabetes, stroke, obesity, and depression.

If you have or have had one of these conditions, ask your doctor whether it would be helpful to have a sleep study.

What to Expect before a Sleep Study

Before a sleep study, your doctor may ask you about your sleep habits and whether you feel well rested and alert during the day.

Your doctor also may ask you to keep a sleep diary. You'll record information such as when you went to bed, when you woke up, how many times you woke up during the night, and more.

What to Bring with You

Depending on what type of sleep study you're having, you may need to bring:

- Notes from your sleep diary. These notes may help your doctor.

- Pajamas and a toothbrush for overnight sleep studies.

- A book or something to do between testing periods if you're having a maintenance of wakefulness test (MWT) or multiple sleep latency test (MSLT).

How to Prepare

Your doctor may advise you to stop or limit the use of tobacco, caffeine, and other stimulants before having a sleep study.

Your doctor also may ask whether you're taking any medicines. Make sure you tell your doctor about all of the medicines you're taking, including over-the-counter products. Some medicines can affect the sleep study results.

Your doctor also may ask about any allergies you have.

You should try to sleep well for 2 nights before having a sleep study. If you're being tested as a requirement for a transportation- or safety-related job, you might be asked to take a drug-screening test.

If you're going to have a home-based sleep test with a portable monitor, you'll need to visit a sleep center or your doctor's office to pick up the equipment. Your doctor or a technician will show you how to use the equipment.

What to Expect during a Sleep Study

Sleep studies are painless. The polysomnogram (PSG), multiple sleep latency test (MSLT), and maintenance of wakefulness test (MWT) usually are done at a sleep center.

The room the sleep study is done in may look like a hotel room. A technician makes the room comfortable for you and sets the temperature to your liking.

Most of your contact at the sleep center will be with nurses or technicians. They can answer questions about the test itself, but they usually can't give you the test results.

During a Polysomnogram

Sticky patches with sensors called electrodes are placed on your scalp, face, chest, limbs, and a finger. While you sleep, these sensors record your brain activity, eye movements, heart rate and rhythm, blood pressure, and the amount of oxygen in your blood.

Elastic belts are placed around your chest and belly. They measure chest movements and the strength and duration of inhaled and exhaled breaths.

Wires attached to the sensors transmit the data to a computer in the next room. The wires are very thin and flexible. They are bundled together so they don't restrict movement, disrupt your sleep, or cause other discomfort.

Polysomnogram

If you have signs of sleep apnea, you may have a split-night sleep study. During the first half of the night, the technician records your sleep patterns. At the start of the second half of the night, he or she wakes you to fit a CPAP (continuous positive airway pressure) mask over your nose and/or mouth.

A small machine gently blows air through the mask. This creates mild pressure that keeps your airway open while you sleep.

The technician checks how you sleep with the CPAP machine. He or she adjusts the flow of air through the mask to find the setting that's right for you.

At the end of the PSG, the technician removes the sensors. If you're having a daytime sleep study, such as an MSLT, some of the sensors might be left on for that test.

Parents usually are required to spend the night with their child during the child's PSG.

During a Multiple Sleep Latency Test

The MSLT is a daytime sleep study that's usually done after a PSG. This test often involves sensors placed on your scalp, face, and chin. These sensors record brain activity and eye movements. They show various stages of sleep and how long it takes you to fall asleep. Sometimes your breathing is checked during an MSLT.

A technician in another room watches these recordings as you sleep. He or she fixes any problems that occur with the recordings.

About 2 hours after you wake from the PSG, you're asked to relax and try to fall asleep in a dark, quiet room. The test is repeated four or five times throughout the day. This is because your ability to fall asleep changes throughout the day.

You get 2-hour breaks between tests. You need to stay awake during the breaks.

The MSLT records whether you fall asleep during the test and what types and stages of sleep you have. Sleep has two basic types: rapid eye movement (REM) and non-REM. Non-REM sleep has three distinct stages. REM sleep and the three stages of non-REM sleep occur in regular cycles throughout the night.

The types and stages of sleep you have during the day can help your doctor diagnose sleep disorders such as narcolepsy, idiopathic hypersomnia, and other sleep disorders that cause daytime tiredness.

During a Maintenance of Wakefulness Test

This sleep study usually is done the day after a PSG, and it takes most of the day. Sensors on your scalp, face, and chin are used to measure when you're awake and asleep.

You sit quietly on a chair in a comfortable position and look straight ahead. Then you simply try to stay awake for a period of time.

An MWT typically includes four trials lasting about 40 minutes each. If you fall asleep, the technician will wake you after about 90 seconds. There usually are 2-hour breaks between trials. During these breaks, you can read, watch television, etc.

If you're being tested as a requirement for a transportation- or safety-related job, you may need a drug-screening test before an MWT.

During a Home-Based Portable Monitor Test

If you're having a home-based portable monitor test, you'll need to set up the equipment at home before you go to sleep.

When you pick up the equipment at the sleep center or your doctor's office, someone will show you how to use it. In some cases, a technician will come to your home to help you prepare for the study.

During Actigraphy

You don't have to go to a sleep center for this test. An actigraph is a small device that's usually worn like a wristwatch. You can do your normal daily routine while you wear it. You remove it while bathing or swimming.

The actigraph measures your sleep-wake behavior over 3 to 14 days and nights. Results give your doctor a better idea about your sleep habits, such as when you sleep or nap and whether the lights are on while you sleep.

Your doctor may ask you to keep a sleep diary while you wear an actigraph.

About 1.5 to 3 hours after you wake from the PSG, you're asked to relax in a quiet room for about 30 minutes. The test is repeated four or five times throughout the day. This is because your ability to fall asleep changes throughout the day.

You get 2-hour breaks between tests. You need to stay awake during the breaks.

The MSLT records whether you fall asleep during the test and what types and stages of sleep you have. Sleep has two basic types: rapid eye movement (REM) and non-REM. Non-REM sleep has three distinct stages. REM sleep and the three stages of non-REM sleep occur in patterns throughout the night.

The types and stages of sleep you have during the day can help your doctor diagnose sleep disorders such as narcolepsy and idiopathic hypersomnia.

What to Expect after a Sleep Study

Once the sensors are removed after a polysomnogram (PSG), multiple sleep latency test, or maintenance of wakefulness test, you can go home. If you used an actigraph or a home-based portable monitor, you'll return the equipment to a sleep center or your doctor's office.

You won't receive a diagnosis right away. A sleep specialist and your primary care doctor will review the results of your sleep study. They will use your medical history, your sleep history, and the test results to make a diagnosis.

You may not get the sleep study results for a couple of weeks. Usually, your doctor, nurse, or sleep specialist will explain the test results and work with you to develop a treatment plan.

What Do Sleep Studies Show?

Sleep studies allow doctors to look at sleep patterns and note sleep-related problems that patients don't know about or can't describe during routine office visits. Sleep studies are needed to diagnose certain sleep disorders, such as sleep apnea and narcolepsy.

Your sleep study results might include information about sleep and wake times, sleep stages, abnormal breathing, the amount of oxygen in your blood, and any movement during sleep.

Your doctor will use your sleep study results and your medical history to make a diagnosis and create a treatment plan.

Results from a Polysomnogram

Polysomnogram (PSG) results are used to help diagnose:

- Sleep-related breathing disorders, such as sleep apnea

- Sleep-related seizure disorders

- Sleep-related movement disorders, such as periodic limb movement disorder

- Sleep disorders that cause extreme daytime tiredness, such as narcolepsy (PSG and MSLT results will be reviewed together)

If you have sleep apnea, your doctor also may use a PSG to find the correct setting for you on a CPAP (continuous positive airway pressure) machine.

A CPAP machine supplies air to your nose and/or mouth through a special mask. Finding the right setting involves adding just enough extra air to create mild pressure that keeps your airway open while you sleep.

Your doctor may recommend a followup PSG to:

- Adjust your CPAP settings after weight loss or weight gain

- Recheck your sleep if symptoms return despite treatment with CPAP

- Find out how well surgery has worked to correct a sleep-related breathing disorder

Technicians also use PSGs to record the number of abnormal breathing events that occur with sleep-related breathing disorders, such as sleep apnea. These events include pauses in breathing or dips in the level of oxygen in your blood.

Results from a Multiple Sleep Latency Test

MSLT results are used to help diagnose narcolepsy, idiopathic hypersomnia, and other sleep disorders that cause daytime sleepiness.

For narcolepsy, technicians study how quickly you fall asleep. The MSLT also shows how long it takes you to reach different types and stages of sleep.

Sleep has two basic types: rapid eye movement (REM) and non-REM. Non-REM sleep has three distinct stages. REM sleep and the three stages of non-REM sleep occur in regular cycles throughout the night.

People who fall asleep in less than 5 minutes or quickly reach REM sleep may need treatment for a sleep disorder.

Results from a Maintenance of Wakefulness Test

Maintenance of wakefulness test (MWT) results can show whether your inability to stay awake is a public or personal safety concern. This study also is used to show how well treatment for a sleep disorder is working.

Results from a Home-Based Portable Monitor Test

Home-based portable monitors might be used to help diagnose sleep apnea. Portable monitors also can show how well some treatments for sleep apnea are working.

Sometimes, home-based monitors don't record enough information. If this happens, you might have to take the monitor home again and repeat the test, or your sleep specialist may ask you to have a PSG.

Results from Actigraphy

Actigraphy results give your doctor a better idea about your sleep habits, such as when you sleep or nap and whether the lights are on while you sleep. This test also is used to help diagnose circadian rhythm disorders.

What Are the Risks of Sleep Studies?

Sleep studies are painless. There's a small risk of skin irritation from the sensors. The irritation will go away once the sensors are removed.

Although the risks of sleep studies are minimal, these studies take time (at least several hours). If you're having a daytime sleep study, bring a book or something to do during the test.

Chapter 47

Thyroid and Other Endocrine Tests

Chapter Contents

Section 47.1

Thyroid Tests

Text in this section is excerpted from "Thyroid Tests," National
Institute of Diabetes and Digestive and Kidney Diseases (NIDDK),
May 14, 2014.

What is the thyroid?

The thyroid is a 2-inch-long, butterfly-shaped gland weighing less
than 1 ounce. Located in the front of the neck below the larynx, or voice
box, it has two lobes, one on either side of the windpipe.

The thyroid is one of the glands that make up the endocrine system.
The glands of the endocrine system produce and store hormones and
release them into the bloodstream. The hormones then travel through
the body and direct the activity of the body's cells.

What is the role of thyroid hormones?

Thyroid hormones regulate metabolism—the way the body uses
energy—and affect nearly every organ in the body. Thyroid hormones
also affect brain development, breathing, heart and nervous system
functions, body temperature, muscle strength, skin dryness, menstrual
cycles, weight, and cholesterol levels.

The thyroid makes two thyroid hormones:

- thyroxine (T_4)

- triiodothyronine (T_3)

Only a small amount of T_3 in the blood comes from the thyroid.
Most T_3 comes from cells all over the body, where it is made from T_4.
Thyroid-stimulating hormone (TSH), which is made by the pituitary
gland in the brain, regulates thyroid hormone production. When thyroid
hormone levels in the blood are low, the pituitary releases more TSH.
When thyroid hormone levels are high, the pituitary decreases TSH
production.

Why do health care providers perform thyroid tests?

Health care providers perform thyroid tests to assess how well the thyroid is working. The tests are also used to diagnose and help find the cause of thyroid disorders such as hyperthyroidism and hypothyroidism:

- Hyperthyroidism is a disorder caused by too much thyroid hormone in the bloodstream, which increases the speed of bodily functions and leads to weight loss, sweating, rapid heart rate, and high blood pressure, among other symptoms.

- Hypothyroidism is a disorder that occurs when the thyroid doesn't make enough thyroid hormone for the body's needs. Without enough thyroid hormone, many of the body's functions slow down. People may have symptoms such as fatigue, weight gain, and cold intolerance.

What blood tests do health care providers use to check a person's thyroid function?

A health care provider may order several blood tests to check thyroid function, including the following:

- TSH test
- T_4 tests
- T_3 test
- thyroid-stimulating immunoglobulin (TSI) test
- antithyroid antibody test, also called the thyroid peroxidase antibody test (TPOab)

A blood test involves drawing blood at a health care provider's office or a commercial facility and sending the sample to a lab for analysis. Blood tests assess thyroid function by measuring TSH and thyroid hormone levels, and by detecting certain autoantibodies present in autoimmune thyroid disease. Autoantibodies are molecules produced by a person's body that mistakenly attack the body's own tissues.

Many complex factors affect thyroid function and hormone levels. Health care providers take a patient's full medical history into account when interpreting thyroid function tests.

TSH Test

A health care provider usually performs the TSH blood test first to check how well the thyroid is working. The TSH test measures the amount of TSH a person's pituitary is secreting. The TSH test is the most accurate test for diagnosing both hyperthyroidism and hypothyroidism. Generally, a below-normal level of TSH suggests hyperthyroidism. An abnormally high TSH level suggests hypothyroidism.

The TSH test detects even tiny amounts of TSH in the blood. Normally, the pituitary boosts TSH production when thyroid hormone levels in the blood are low. The thyroid responds by making more hormone. Then, when the body has enough thyroid hormone circulating in the blood, TSH output drops. The cycle repeats continuously to maintain a healthy level of thyroid hormone in the body. In people whose thyroid produces too much thyroid hormone, the pituitary shuts down TSH production, leading to low or even undetectable TSH levels in the blood.

In people whose thyroid is not functioning normally and produces too little thyroid hormone, the thyroid cannot respond normally to TSH by producing thyroid hormone. As a result, the pituitary keeps making TSH, trying to get the thyroid to respond.

If results of the TSH test are abnormal, a person will need one or more additional tests to help find the cause of the problem.

T_4 Tests

The thyroid primarily secretes T_4 and only a small amount of T_3. T_4 exists in two forms:

- T_4 that is bound to proteins in the blood and is kept in reserve until needed

- a small amount of unbound or "free" T_4 (FT_4), which is the active form of the hormone and is available to enter body tissues when needed

A high level of total T_4—bound and FT_4 together—or FT_4 suggests hyperthyroidism, and a low level of total T_4 or FT_4 suggests hypothyroidism.

Both pregnancy and taking oral contraceptives increase levels of binding protein in the blood. In either of these cases, although a woman may have a high total T_4 level, she may not have hyperthyroidism. Severe illness or the use of corticosteroids—a class of medications that treat asthma, arthritis, and skin conditions, among other health problems—can decrease binding protein levels. Therefore, in these cases, the total T_4 level may be low, yet the person does not have hypothyroidism.

T_3 Test

If a health care provider suspects hyperthyroidism in a person who has a normal FT_4 level, a T_3 test can be useful to confirm the condition. In some cases of hyperthyroidism, FT_4 is normal yet free T_3 (FT_3) is elevated, so measuring both T_4 and T_3 can be useful if a health care provider suspects hyperthyroidism. The T_3 test is not useful in diagnosing hypothyroidism because levels are not reduced until the hypothyroidism is severe.

TSI Test

Thyroid-stimulating immunoglobulin is an autoantibody present in Graves' disease. TSI mimics TSH by stimulating the thyroid cells, causing the thyroid to secrete extra hormone. The TSI test detects TSI circulating in the blood and is usually measured

- in people with Graves' disease when the diagnosis is obscure

- during pregnancy

- to find out if a person is in remission, or no longer has hyperthyroidism and its symptoms

Antithyroid Antibody Test

Antithyroid antibodies are markers in the blood that are extremely helpful in diagnosing Hashimoto's disease. Two principal types of antithyroid antibodies are

- anti-TG antibodies, which attack a protein in the thyroid called thyroglobulin

- anti-thyroperoxidase, or anti-TPO, antibodies, which attack an enzyme in thyroid cells called thyroperoxidase

What do thyroid test results tell health care providers?

Health care providers look at thyroid test results in people with hyperthyroidism or hypothyroidism to find the underlying cause of their thyroid disorder. The following tables illustrate what test results may show based on the type of thyroid problem.

619

Table 47.1. Typical thyroid function test results: Hyperthyroidism

Cause	Test			
	TSH	**T3/T4**	**TSI**	**Radioactive Iodine Uptake Test**
Graves' disease	↓	↑	+	↑
Thyroiditis (with hyperthyroidism)	↓	↑	−	↓
Thyroid nodules (hot, or toxic)	↓	↑	−	↑ or Normal

Key: ↑ *= Above Normal* ↓ *= Below Normal + = Positive − = Negative*

Table 47.2. Typical thyroid function test results: Hypothyroidism

Cause	Test		
	TSH	**T3/T4**	**Antithyroid Antibody**
Hashimoto's disease (thyroiditis, early stage)	↑	↓ or Normal	+
Hashimoto's disease (thyroiditis, later stage)	↑	↓	+
Pituitary abnormality	↓	↓	-

Key: ↑ *= Above Normal* ↓ *= Below Normal + = Positive − = Negative*

What imaging tests do health care providers use to diagnose and find the cause of thyroid disorders?

A health care provider may use one or a combination of imaging tests, such as an ultrasound of the thyroid, a computerized tomography (CT) scan, or nuclear medicine tests, to diagnose and find the cause of thyroid disorders.

- **Ultrasound.** Ultrasound uses a device, called a transducer that bounces safe, painless sound waves off organs to create an image of their structure. A specially trained technician performs the procedure in a health care provider's office, an outpatient center, or a hospital, and a radiologist—a doctor who specializes in medical imaging—interprets the images; a patient does not need anesthesia. The images can show the size and texture of the thyroid, as well as a pattern of typical autoimmune inflammation.

The images can also show nodules or growths within the gland that suggest a malignant tumor.

- **CT scan.** CT scans use a combination of X-rays and computer technology to create images. For a CT scan, a health care provider may give the patient a solution to drink and an injection of a special dye, called contrast medium. CT scans require the patient to lie on a table that slides into a tunnel-shaped device where the X-rays are taken. An X-ray technician performs the procedure in an outpatient center or a hospital, and a radiologist interprets the images. The patient does not need anesthesia. CT scans are usually not needed to diagnose thyroid disease; however, health care providers will use them to view a large goiter. Also, a CT scan will often show a thyroid nodule when a person is having the scan for other health problems.

- **Nuclear medicine tests.** Nuclear medicine tests of the thyroid include a thyroid scan and a radioactive iodine uptake test. People often have to follow a low iodine diet prior to having the tests.

- **Thyroid scan.** A thyroid scan is a type of nuclear medicine imaging. Nuclear medicine uses small amounts of radioactive material to create a picture of an organ and give information about the organ's structure and function. A thyroid scan is used to look at the size, shape, and position of the gland. This test can help find the cause of hyperthyroidism and check for thyroid nodules. The scan also can help a health care provider evaluate thyroid nodules; however, it does not confirm whether the nodules are cancerous or benign.

A specially trained technician performs the procedure in an outpatient center or a hospital, and a radiologist interprets the images; a patient does not need anesthesia. For the scan, radioactive iodine or radioactive technetium is injected into the patient's vein or swallowed in liquid or capsule form. The scan takes place 30 minutes after an injection or 6 to 24 hours after the radioactive substance is swallowed. The patient lies on an exam table for the scan, which takes about 30 minutes.

A device called a gamma camera is suspended over the table or may be located within a large, tunnel-shaped device that resembles a CT scanner. The gamma camera detects the radioactive material and sends images to a computer that show how and where the radioactive substance has been distributed in the thyroid. Nodules that produce too much thyroid hormone—called "hot," or toxic, nodules—show up clearly because they absorb more radioactive material than normal thyroid tissue. Graves' disease shows up as a spread-out, overall increase in radioactivity rather than an increase in a localized spot.

Even though the amount of radiation used in this test is small, women who are pregnant or breastfeeding should not have this test because of the risks of exposing the fetus or the baby to radiation.

- **Radioactive iodine uptake test.** The radioactive iodine uptake test, also known as a thyroid uptake, is a nuclear medicine test used to evaluate the function of the thyroid and find the cause of a patient's hyperthyroidism. A whole-body thyroid scan is used for people who have had thyroid cancer. The test measures the amount of iodine the thyroid collects from the bloodstream in a given time period. The thyroid uptake is not used to assess hypothyroidism.

A specially trained technician performs the test in an outpatient center or a hospital, and a radiologist interprets the images; a patient does not need anesthesia. For this test, the patient swallows a small amount of radioactive iodine in liquid or capsule form. After 4 to 6 hours and again at 24 hours, the patient returns to the testing center, where the technician measures the amount of radioactive iodine taken up by the thyroid. The measurement is taken with a small device called a gamma probe, which resembles a microphone. The gamma probe is positioned near the patient's neck over the thyroid. Measurement takes only a few minutes and is painless.

In the diagnosis of hyperthyroidism, a high thyroid uptake reading usually indicates an overactive thyroid that produces too much thyroid hormone, as seen in Graves' disease or a condition called toxic nodular goiter, an enlargement of the thyroid. A low thyroid uptake reading suggests the thyroid is not overactive.

Several thyroid disorders that cause inflammation of the thyroid, or thyroiditis, may cause leakage of thyroid hormone and iodine out of the thyroid into the bloodstream, which can lead to high T4 levels. When the thyroid is inflamed, it does not take up the radioactive iodine given as part of the thyroid uptake test. For example, hyperthyroidism seen in Graves' disease would be marked by high blood T4 and a high thyroid uptake reading. In thyroiditis, temporary hyperthyroidism may exist because of the release of T4 into the blood; however, the thyroid uptake reading is low because of the inflammation. Temporary hyperthyroidism in thyroiditis is often followed by a period of hypo-thyroidism before the thyroid heals.

Even though the amount of radiation used in this test is small, women who are pregnant or breastfeeding should not have this test because of the risks of exposing the fetus or infant to radiation.

What tests do health care providers use if a thyroid nodule is found?

If a health care provider feels a nodule in a patient's neck during a physical exam or detects one during imaging tests of the thyroid, a fine needle aspiration biopsy may be done to confirm whether the nodule is cancerous or benign.

A fine needle aspiration biopsy of the thyroid involves taking cells from the thyroid for examination with a microscope. The health care provider with experience in needle aspirations performs the biopsy in his or her office, an outpatient center, or a hospital; he or she may use medication to numb the area. The patient may feel mild discomfort during the test and the biopsy site may be tender for 1 to 2 days.

For this test, the patient lies back with support under the shoulders so the neck can be extended and bent back slightly. The health care provider inserts a small, thin needle attached to a syringe into the thy-roid nodule and uses ultrasound to guide its insertion. Samples of the cells in the nodule are drawn through the needle and sent to a lab to be examined by a pathologist—a doctor who specializes in diagnosing diseases. The health care provider may need to take several samples. Once the biopsy is complete, a bandage is placed on the area to lower the chance of bleeding.

Section 47.2

Graves' Disease Testing

Text in this section is excerpted from "Graves' Disease," National
Institute of Diabetes and Digestive and Kidney Diseases (NIDDK),
August 10, 2012.

What is Graves' disease?

Graves' disease, also known as toxic diffuse goiter, is the most common cause of hyperthyroidism in the United States. Hyperthyroidism is a disorder that occurs when the thyroid gland makes more thyroid hormone than the body needs.

Autoimmune Disorder

Graves' disease is an autoimmune disorder. Normally, the immune system protects the body from infection by identifying and destroying bacteria, viruses, and other potentially harmful foreign substances. But in autoimmune diseases, the immune system attacks the body's own cells and organs.

With Graves' disease, the immune system makes an antibody called thyroid-stimulating immunoglobulin (TSI)—sometimes called TSH receptor antibody—that attaches to thyroid cells. TSI mimics TSH and stimulates the thyroid to make too much thyroid hormone. Sometimes the TSI antibody instead blocks thyroid hormone production, leading to conflicting symptoms that may make correct diagnosis more difficult.

What are the symptoms of Graves' disease?

People with Graves' disease may have common symptoms of hyperthyroidism such as

- nervousness or irritability
- fatigue or muscle weakness
- heat intolerance
- trouble sleeping

- hand tremors

- rapid and irregular heartbeat

- frequent bowel movements or diarrhea

- weight loss

- goiter, which is an enlarged thyroid that may cause the neck to look swollen and can interfere with normal breathing and swallowing

A small number of people with Graves' disease also experience thickening and reddening of the skin on their shins. This usually painless problem is called pretibial myxedema or Graves' dermopathy.

In addition, the eyes of people with Graves' disease may appear enlarged because their eyelids are retracted—seem pulled back into the eye sockets—and their eyes bulge out from the eye sockets. This condition is called Graves' ophthalmopathy (GO).

What is Graves' ophthalmopathy?

Graves' ophthalmopathy is a condition associated with Graves' disease that occurs when cells from the immune system attack the muscles and other tissues around the eyes.

The result is inflammation and a buildup of tissue and fat behind the eye socket, causing the eyeballs to bulge out. Rarely, inflammation is severe enough to compress the optic nerve that leads to the eye, causing vision loss.

Other GO symptoms are

- dry, gritty, and irritated eyes

- puffy eyelids

- double vision

- light sensitivity

- pressure or pain in the eyes

- trouble moving the eyes

About 25 to 30 percent of people with Graves' disease develop mild GO, and 2 to 5 percent develop severe GO. This eye condition usually lasts 1 to 2 years and often improves on its own.

GO can occur before, at the same time as, or after other symptoms of hyperthyroidism develop and may even occur in people whose thyroid function is normal. Smoking makes GO worse.

Who is likely to develop Graves' disease?

Scientists cannot predict who will develop Graves' disease. However, factors such as age, sex, heredity, and emotional and environmental stress are likely involved.

Graves' disease usually occurs in people younger than age 40 and is seven to eight times more common in women than men. Women are most often affected between ages 30 and 60. And a person's chance of developing Graves' disease increases if other family members have the disease.

Researchers have not been able to find a specific gene that causes the disease to be passed from parent to child. While scientists know some people inherit an immune system that can make antibodies against healthy cells, predicting who will be affected is difficult.

People with other autoimmune diseases have an increased chance of developing Graves' disease. Conditions associated with Graves' disease include type 1 diabetes, rheumatoid arthritis, and vitiligo—a disorder in which some parts of the skin are not pigmented.

How is Graves' disease diagnosed?

Health care providers can sometimes diagnose Graves' disease based only on a physical examination and a medical history. Blood tests and other diagnostic tests, such as the following, then confirm the diagnosis.

TSH test. The ultrasensitive TSH test is usually the first test performed. This test detects even tiny amounts of TSH in the blood and is the most accurate measure of thyroid activity available.

T_3 and T_4 test. Another blood test used to diagnose Graves' disease measures T_3 and T_4 levels. In making a diagnosis, health care providers look for below-normal levels of TSH, normal to elevated levels of T_4, and elevated levels of T_3.

Because the combination of low TSH and high T_3 and T_4 can occur with other thyroid problems, health care providers may order other tests to finalize the diagnosis. The following two tests use small, safe doses of radioactive iodine because the thyroid uses iodine to make thyroid hormone.

Radioactive iodine uptake test. This test measures the amount of iodine the thyroid collects from the bloodstream. High levels of iodine uptake can indicate Graves' disease.

Thyroid scan. This scan shows how and where iodine is distributed in the thyroid. With Graves' disease the entire thyroid is involved, so the iodine shows up throughout the gland. Other causes of hyperthyroidism such as nodules—small lumps in the gland—show a different pattern of iodine distribution.

TSI test. Health care providers may also recommend the TSI test, although this test usually isn't necessary to diagnose Graves' disease. This test, also called a TSH antibody test, measures the level of TSI in the blood. Most people with Graves' disease have this antibody, but people whose hyperthyroidism is caused by other conditions do not.

Section 47.3

Hashimoto's Disease Testing

Text in this section is excerpted from "Hashimoto's Disease,"
National Institute of Diabetes and Digestive and Kidney Diseases
(NIDDK), May 14, 2014.

What is Hashimoto's disease?

Hashimoto's disease, also called chronic lymphocytic thyroiditis or autoimmune thyroiditis, is an autoimmune disease. An autoimmune disease is a disorder in which the body's immune system attacks the body's own cells and organs. Normally, the immune system protects the body from infection by identifying and destroying bacteria, viruses, and other potentially harmful foreign substances.

In Hashimoto's disease, the immune system attacks the thyroid gland, causing inflammation and interfering with its ability to produce thyroid hormones. Large numbers of White blood cells called lymphocytes accumulate in the thyroid. Lymphocytes make the antibodies that start the autoimmune process.

Hashimoto's disease often leads to reduced thyroid function, or hypothyroidism. Hypothyroidism is a disorder that occurs when the thyroid doesn't make enough thyroid hormone for the body's needs. Thyroid hormones regulate metabolism—the way the body uses energy—and affect nearly every organ in the body. Without enough thyroid hormone, many of the body's functions slow down. Hashimoto's disease is the most common cause of hypothyroidism in the United States.

What are the symptoms of Hashimoto's disease?

Many people with Hashimoto's disease have no symptoms at first. As the disease slowly progresses, the thyroid usually enlarges and may cause the front of the neck to look swollen. The enlarged thyroid, called a goiter, may create a feeling of fullness in the throat, though it is usually not painful. After many years, or even decades, damage to the thyroid causes it to shrink and the goiter to disappear.

Not everyone with Hashimoto's disease develops hypothyroidism. For those who do, the hypothyroidism may be subclinical—mild and without symptoms, especially early in its course. With progression to hypothyroidism, people may have one or more of the following symptoms:

- fatigue

- weight gain

- cold intolerance

- joint and muscle pain

- constipation, or fewer than three bowel movements a week

- dry, thinning hair

- heavy or irregular menstrual periods and problems becoming pregnant

- depression

- memory problems

- a slowed heart rate

Who is more likely to develop Hashimoto's disease?

Hashimoto's disease is much more common in women than men. Although the disease often occurs in adolescent or young women, it more commonly appears between 30 and 50 years of age.

Hashimoto's disease tends to run in families. Researchers are working to identify the gene or genes that cause the disease to be passed from one generation to the next.

Possible environmental factors are also being studied. For example, researchers have found that consuming too much iodine may inhibit thyroid hormone production in susceptible individuals. Chemicals released into the environment, such as pesticides, along with certain medications or viral infections may also contribute to autoimmune thyroid diseases.

People with other autoimmune diseases are more likely to develop Hashimoto's disease. The opposite is also true—people with Hashimoto's disease are more likely to develop other autoimmune diseases. These diseases include

- vitiligo, a condition in which some areas of the skin lose their natural color.

- rheumatoid arthritis, a disease that causes pain, swelling, stiffness, and loss of function in the joints when the immune system attacks the membrane lining the joints.

- Addison's disease, in which the adrenal glands are damaged and cannot produce enough of certain critical hormones.

- type 1 diabetes, in which the pancreas is damaged and can no longer produce insulin, causing high blood glucose, also called blood sugar.

- pernicious anemia, a type of anemia caused by not having enough vitamin B12 in the body. In anemia, the number of red blood cells is less than normal, resulting in less oxygen carried to the body's cells and extreme fatigue.

- celiac disease, a form of gastrointestinal gluten sensitivity, an autoimmune disorder in which people cannot tolerate gluten because it will damage the lining of the small intestine and prevent adsorption of nutrients. Gluten is a protein found in wheat, rye, and barley and in some products.

- autoimmune hepatitis, or nonviral liver inflammation, a disease in which the immune system attacks liver cells.

How is Hashimoto's disease diagnosed?

Diagnosis begins with a physical exam and medical history. A goiter, nodules, or growths may be found during a physical exam, and symptoms may suggest hypothyroidism. Health care providers will then perform blood tests to confirm the diagnosis. A blood test involves drawing blood at a health care provider's office or a commercial facility and sending the sample to a lab for analysis. Diagnostic blood tests may include the

- **TSH test.** The ultrasensitive TSH test is usually the first test performed. This test detects even tiny amounts of TSH in the blood and is the most accurate measure of thyroid activity available. Generally, a TSH reading above normal means a person has hypothyroidism.

- **T_4 test.** The T_4 test measures the actual amount of thyroid hormone circulating in the blood. In hypothyroidism, the level of T_4 in the blood is lower than normal.

- **antithyroid antibody test.** This test looks for the presence of thyroid autoantibodies, or molecules produced by a person's body that mistakenly attack the body's own tissues. Two principal types of antithyroid antibodies are

- anti-TG antibodies, which attack a protein in the thyroid called thyroglobulin

- anti-thyroperoxidase (TPO) antibodies, which attack an enzyme called thyroperoxidase in thyroid cells that helps convert T_4 to T_3. Having TPO autoantibodies in the blood means the body's immune system attacked the thyroid tissue in the past. Most people with Hashimoto's disease have these antibodies, although people whose hypothyroidism is caused by other conditions do not.

A health care provider may also order imaging tests, including an ultrasound or a computerized tomography (CT) scan.

- **Ultrasound.** Ultrasound uses a device, called a transducer, that bounces safe, painless sound waves off organs to create an image of their structure. A specially trained technician performs the procedure in a health care provider's office, an outpatient center, or a hospital, and a radiologist—a doctor who specializes in medical imaging—interprets the images; a patient does not need anesthesia.

The images can show the size and texture of the thyroid, as well as a pattern of typical autoimmune inflammation, helping the health care provider confirm Hashimoto's disease. The images can also show nodules or growths within the gland that suggest a malignant tumor.

- **CT scan.** CT scans use a combination of X-rays and computer technology to create images. For a CT scan, a health care provider may give the patient a solution to drink and an injection of a special dye, called contrast medium. CT scans require the patient to lie on a table that slides into a tunnel-shaped device where the X-rays are taken. An X-ray technician performs the procedure in an outpatient center or a hospital, and a radiologist interprets the images. The patient does not need anesthesia. In some cases of Hashimoto's disease, a CT scan is used to examine the placement and extent of a large goiter, and to show a goiter's effect on nearby structures.

Chapter 48

Vision Tests

Chapter Contents

Section 48.1

Color Blindness Testing

Text in this section is excerpted from "Facts About Color Blindness,"
National Eye Institute (NEI), February 2015.

How is color blindness diagnosed?

Eye care professionals use a variety of tests to diagnose color blindness. These tests can quickly diagnose specific types of color blindness.

The Ishihara Color Test is the most common test for red-green color blindness. The test consists of a series of colored circles, called Ishihara plates, each of which contains a collection of dots in different colors and sizes. Within the circle are dots that form a shape clearly visible to those with normal color vision, but invisible or difficult to see for those with red-green color blindness.

The newer Cambridge Color Test uses a visual array similar to the Ishihara plates, except displayed on a computer monitor. The goal is to identify a C shape that is different in color from the background. The "C" is presented randomly in one of four orientations. When test-takers see the "C," they are asked to press one of four keys that correspond to the orientation.

The anomaloscope uses a test in which two different light sources have to be matched in color. Looking through the eyepiece, the viewer sees a circle. The upper half is a yellow light that can be adjusted in brightness. The lower half is a combination of red and green lights that can be mixed in variable proportions. The viewer uses one knob to adjust the brightness of the top half, and another to adjust the color of the lower half. The goal is to make the upper and lower halves the same brightness and color.

The HRR Pseudoisochromatic Color Test is another red-green color blindness test that uses color plates to test for color blindness.

The Farnsworth-Munsell 100 Hue Test uses a set of blocks or pegs that are roughly the same color but in different hues (shades of the color). The goal is to arrange them in a line in order of hue. This test measures the ability to discriminate subtle color changes. It is used by industries that depend on the accurate color perception of its employees, such as graphic design, photography, and food quality inspection.

The Farnsworth Lantern Test is used by the U.S. military to determine the severity of color blindness. Those with mild forms pass the test and are allowed to serve in the armed forces.

Section 48.2

Cataract Testing

Text in this section is excerpted from "Cataract What You Should Know," National Eye Institute (NEI), September 2014.

What is a cataract?

A cataract is a clouding of the lens in the eye that affects vision. Most cataracts are related to aging. Cataracts are very common in older people. By age 80, more than half of all Americans have either a cataract or have had cataract surgery.

A cataract can occur in either or both eyes. It cannot spread from one eye to the other.

What is the lens?

The lens is a clear part of the eye that helps to focus light, or an image, on the retina. The retina is the light-sensitive tissue at the back of the eye.

In a normal eye, light passes through the transparent lens to the retina. Once it reaches the retina, light is changed into nerve signals that are sent to the brain. The lens must be clear for the retina to receive a sharp image. If the lens is cloudy from a cataract, the image you see will be blurred.

In a normal eye, light passes through the transparent lens to the retina. Once it reaches the retina, light is changed into nerve signals that are sent to the brain.

The lens must be clear for the retina to receive a sharp image. If the lens is cloudy from a cataract, the image you see will be blurred.

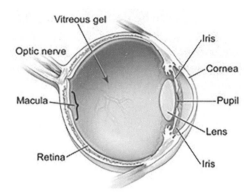

Figure 48.1. *Structure of the eye*

What causes cataracts?

The lens lies behind the iris and the pupil. It works much like a camera lens. It focuses light onto the retina at the back of the eye, where an image is recorded. The lens also adjusts the eye's focus, letting us see things clearly both up close and far away. The lens is made of mostly water and protein. The protein is arranged in a precise way that keeps the lens clear and lets light pass through it.

But as we age, some of the protein may clump together and start to cloud a small area of the lens. This is a cataract. Over time, the cataract may grow larger and cloud more of the lens, making it harder to see.

Smoking and diabetes contribute to the development of cataract. Or, it may be that the protein in the lens just changes from the wear and tear it takes over the years.

How do cataracts affect vision?

Age-related cataracts can affect vision in two ways:

Clumps of protein reduce the sharpness of the image reaching the retina.

The lens consists mostly of water and protein. When the protein clumps up, it clouds the lens and reduces the light that reaches the retina. The clouding may become severe enough to cause blurred vision. Most age-related cataracts develop from protein clumpings.

When a cataract is small, the cloudiness affects only a small part of the lens. You may not notice any changes in your vision. Cataracts tend to "grow" slowly, so vision gets worse gradually. Over time, the cloudy area in the lens may get larger, and the cataract may increase in size. Seeing may become more difficult. Your vision may get duller or blurrier.

The clear lens slowly changes to a yellowish/brownish color, adding a brownish tint to vision.

As the clear lens slowly colors with age, your vision gradually may acquire a brownish shade. At first, the amount of tinting may be small and may not cause a vision problem. Over time, the cataract usually increases in size. This gradual change in the amount of tinting does not affect the sharpness of the image transmitted to the retina.If you have advanced lens discoloration, you may not be able to identify blues and purples. You may be wearing what you believe to be a pair of Black socks, only to find out from friends that you are wearing purple socks.

When are you most likely to have a cataract?

The term "age-related" is a little misleading. You don't have to be a senior citizen to get this type of cataract. In fact, people can have an age-related cataract in their 40s and 50s. But during middle age, most cataracts are small and do not affect vision. It is after age 60 that most cataracts cause problems with a person's vision.

Who is at risk for cataract?

The risk of cataract increases as you get older. Other risk factors for cataract include:

- Certain diseases (for example, diabetes).
- Personal behavior (smoking, alcohol use).
- The environment (prolonged exposure to ultraviolet sunlight).

What are the symptoms of a cataract?

The most common symptoms of a cataract are:

- Cloudy or blurry vision.
- Colors seem faded.
- Glare. Headlights, lamps, or sunlight may appear too bright. A halo may appear around lights.
- Poor night vision.

- Double vision or multiple images in one eye. (This symptom may clear as the cataract gets larger.)

- Frequent prescription changes in your eyeglasses or contact lenses.

These symptoms also can be a sign of other eye problems. If you have any of these symptoms, check with your eye care professional.

How is a cataract detected?

Cataract is detected through a comprehensive eye exam that includes:

- **Visual acuity test.** This eye chart test measures how well you see at various distances.

- **Dilated eye exam.** Drops are placed in your eyes to widen, or dilate, the pupils. Your eye care professional uses a special magnifying lens to examine your retina and optic nerve for signs of damage and other eye problems. After the exam, your close-up vision may remain blurred for several hours.

- **Tonometry.** An instrument measures the pressure inside the eye. Numbing drops may be applied to your eye for this test.

Your eye care professional also may do other tests to learn more about the structure and health of your eye.

Section 48.3

Tests for Diabetic Eye Disease

Text in this section is excerpted from "Facts About Diabetic Eye Disease," National Eye Institute (NEI), September 2015.

What is diabetic eye disease?

Diabetic eye disease is a group of eye conditions that can affect people with diabetes.

- **Diabetic retinopathy** affects blood vessels in the light-sensitive tissue called the retina that lines the back of the eye. It is the most common cause of vision loss among people with diabetes and the leading cause of vision impairment and blindness among working-age adults.

- **Diabetic macular edema (DME).** A consequence of diabetic retinopathy, DME is swelling in an area of the retina called the macula.

Diabetic eye disease also includes cataract and glaucoma:

- **Cataract** is a clouding of the eye's lens. Adults with diabetes are 2-5 times more likely than those without diabetes to develop cataract. Cataract also tends to develop at an earlier age in people with diabetes.

- **Glaucoma** is a group of diseases that damage the eye's optic nerve—the bundle of nerve fibers that connects the eye to the brain. Some types of glaucoma are associated with elevated pressure inside the eye. In adults, diabetes nearly doubles the risk of glaucoma.

All forms of diabetic eye disease have the potential to cause severe vision loss and blindness.

Diabetic Retinopathy

What causes diabetic retinopathy?

Chronically high blood sugar from diabetes is associated with damage to the tiny blood vessels in the retina, leading to diabetic retinopathy. The retina detects light and converts it to signals sent through the optic nerve to the brain. Diabetic retinopathy can cause blood vessels in the retina to leak fluid or hemorrhage (bleed), distorting vision. In its most advanced stage, new abnormal blood vessels proliferate (increase in number) on the surface of the retina, which can lead to scarring and cell loss in the retina.

Diabetic retinopathy may progress through four stages:

1. **Mild nonproliferative retinopathy.** Small areas of balloon-like swelling in the retina's tiny blood vessels, called microaneurysms, occur at this earliest stage of the disease. These microaneurysms may leak fluid into the retina.

2. **Moderate nonproliferative retinopathy.** As the disease progresses, blood vessels that nourish the retina may swell and distort. They may also lose their ability to transport blood. Both conditions cause characteristic changes to the appearance of the retina and may contribute to DME.

3. **Severe nonproliferative retinopathy.** Many more blood vessels are blocked, depriving blood supply to areas of the retina. These areas secrete growth factors that signal the retina to grow new blood vessels.

4. **Proliferative diabetic retinopathy (PDR).** At this advanced stage, growth factors secreted by the retina trigger the proliferation of new blood vessels, which grow along the inside surface of the retina and into the vitreous gel, the fluid that fills the eye. The new blood vessels are fragile, which makes them more likely to leak and bleed. Accompanying scar tissue can contract and cause retinal detachment—the pulling away of the retina from underlying tissue, like wallpaper peeling away from a wall. Retinal detachment can lead to permanent vision loss.

What is diabetic macular edema (DME)?

DME is the build-up of fluid (edema) in a region of the retina called the macula. The macula is important for the sharp, straight-ahead vision that is used for reading, recognizing faces, and driving. DME is the most common cause of vision loss among people with diabetic retinopathy. About half of all people with diabetic retinopathy will develop DME. Although it is more likely to occur as diabetic retinopathy worsens, DME can happen at any stage of the disease.

Who is at risk for diabetic retinopathy?

People with all types of diabetes (type 1, type 2, and gestational) are at risk for diabetic retinopathy. Risk increases the longer a person has diabetes. Between 40 and 45 percent of Americans diagnosed with diabetes have some stage of diabetic retinopathy, although only about half are aware of it. Women who develop or have diabetes during pregnancy may have rapid onset or worsening of diabetic retinopathy.

Symptoms and Detection

What are the symptoms of diabetic retinopathy and DME?

The early stages of diabetic retinopathy usually have no symptoms. The disease often progresses unnoticed until it affects vision.

Bleeding from abnormal retinal blood vessels can cause the appearance of "floating" spots. These spots sometimes clear on their own. But without prompt treatment, bleeding often recurs, increasing the risk of permanent vision loss. If DME occurs, it can cause blurred vision.

How are diabetic retinopathy and DME detected?

Diabetic retinopathy and DME are detected during a comprehensive dilated eye exam that includes:

- **Visual acuity testing.** This eye chart test measures a person's ability to see at various distances.

- **Tonometry.** This test measures pressure inside the eye.

- **Pupil dilation.** Drops placed on the eye's surface dilate (widen) the pupil, allowing a physician to examine the retina and optic nerve.

- **Optical coherence tomography (OCT).** This technique is similar to ultrasound but uses light waves instead of sound waves to capture images of tissues inside the body. OCT provides detailed images of tissues that can be penetrated by light, such as the eye.

A comprehensive dilated eye exam allows the doctor to check the retina for:

1. Changes to blood vessels

2. Leaking blood vessels or warning signs of leaky blood vessels, such as fatty deposits

3. Swelling of the macula (DME)

4. Changes in the lens

Damage to nerve tissue

If DME or severe diabetic retinopathy is suspected, a **fluorescein angiogram** may be used to look for damaged or leaky blood vessels. In this test, a fluorescent dye is injected into the bloodstream, often into an arm vein. Pictures of the retinal blood vessels are taken as the dye reaches the eye.

Section 48.4

Tests for Glaucoma

Text in this section is excerpted from "Glaucoma What You Should Know," National Eye Institute (NEI), November 2014.

What is glaucoma?

Glaucoma is a group of diseases that damage the eye's optic nerve and can result in vision loss and blindness. However, with early detection and treatment, you can often protect your eyes against serious vision loss.

How does the optic nerve get damaged by open-angle glaucoma?

Several large studies have shown that eye pressure is a major risk factor for optic nerve damage. In the front of the eye is a space called

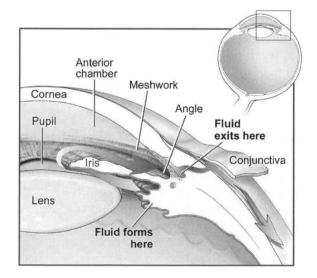

Figure 48.2. *Fluid Pathway*

the anterior chamber. A clear fluid flows continuously in and out of the chamber and nourishes nearby tissues. The fluid leaves the chamber at the open angle where the cornea and iris meet. When the fluid reaches the angle, it flows through a spongy meshwork, like a drain, and leaves the eye.

In open-angle glaucoma, even though the drainage angle is "open," the fluid passes too slowly through the meshwork drain. Since the fluid builds up, the pressure inside the eye rises to a level that may damage the optic nerve. When the optic nerve is damaged from increased pressure, open-angle glaucoma – and vision loss – may result. That's why controlling pressure inside the eye is important.

Another risk factor for optic nerve damage relates to blood pressure. Thus, it is important to also make sure that your blood pressure is at a proper level for your body by working with your medical doctor.

Who is at risk for open-angle glaucoma?

Anyone can develop glaucoma. Some people, listed below, are at higher risk than others:

- African Americans over age 40
- Everyone over age 60, especially Hispanics/ Latinos
- People with a family history of glaucoma

A comprehensive dilated eye exam can reveal more risk factors, such as high eye pressure, thinness of the cornea, and abnormal optic nerve anatomy. In some people with certain combinations of these high-risk factors, medicines in the form of eyedrops reduce the risk of developing glaucoma by about half.

Glaucoma Symptoms

At first, open-angle glaucoma has no symptoms. It causes no pain. Vision stays normal. Glaucoma can develop in one or both eyes.

Without treatment, people with glaucoma will slowly lose their peripheral (side) vision. As glaucoma remains untreated, people may miss objects to the side and out of the corner of their eye. They seem to be looking through a tunnel. Over time, straight-ahead (central) vision may decrease until no vision remains.

How is glaucoma detected

Glaucoma is detected through a comprehensive dilated eye exam that includes the following:

Visual acuity test. This eye chart test measures how well you see at various distances.

Visual field test. This test measures your peripheral (side vision). It helps your eye care professional tell if you have lost peripheral vision, a sign of glaucoma.

Dilated eye exam. In this exam, drops are placed in your eyes to widen, or dilate, the pupils. Your eye care professional uses a special magnifying lens to examine your retina and optic nerve for signs of damage and other eye problems. After the exam, your close-up vision may remain blurred for several hours.

Tonometry is the measurement of pressure inside the eye by using an instrument (right) called a tonometer. Numbing drops may be applied to your eye for this test.

Pachymetry is the measurement of the thickness of your cornea. Your eye care professional applies a numbing drop to your eye and uses an ultrasonic wave instrument to measure the thickness of your cornea.

Can glaucoma be cured?

No. There is no cure for glaucoma. Vision lost from the disease cannot be restored.

Chapter 49

Balance (Vestibular) Disorder Tests

What is a balance disorder?

A balance disorder is a condition that makes you feel unsteady or dizzy. If you are standing, sitting, or lying down, you might feel as if you are moving, spinning, or floating. If you are walking, you might suddenly feel as if you are tipping over.

Everyone has a dizzy spell now and then, but the term "dizziness" can mean different things to different people. For one person, dizziness might mean a fleeting feeling of faintness, while for another it could be an intense sensation of spinning (vertigo) that lasts a long time.

Experts believe that more than four out of 10 Americans, sometime in their lives, will experience an episode of dizziness significant enough to send them to a doctor. Balance disorders can be caused by certain health conditions, medications, or a problem in the inner ear or the brain. A balance disorder can profoundly impact daily activities and cause psychological and emotional hardship.

Text in this chapter is excerpted from "Balance Disorders," National Institute on Deafness and Other Communication Disorders (NIDCD), April 2014.

What are the symptoms of a balance disorder?

If you have a balance disorder, you may stagger when you try to walk, or teeter or fall when you try to stand up. You might experience other symptoms such as:

- Dizziness or vertigo (a spinning sensation)
- Falling or feeling as if you are going to fall
- Lightheadedness, faintness, or a floating sensation
- Blurred vision
- Confusion or disorientation.

Other symptoms might include nausea and vomiting, diarrhea, changes in heart rate and blood pressure, and fear, anxiety, or panic. Symptoms may come and go over short time periods or last for a long time, and can lead to fatigue and depression.

What causes balance disorders?

There are many causes of balance problems, such as medications, ear infections, a head injury, or anything else that affects the inner ear or brain. Low blood pressure can lead to dizziness when you stand up too quickly. Problems that affect the skeletal or visual systems, such as arthritis or eye muscle imbalance, can also cause balance disorders. Your risk of having balance problems increases as you get older.

Unfortunately, many balance disorders start suddenly and with no obvious cause.

How does my body keep its balance?

Your sense of balance relies on a series of signals to the brain from several organs and structures in the body, which together are known as the vestibular system. The vestibular system begins with a maze-like structure in your inner ear called the labyrinth, which is made of bone and soft tissue.

Within the labyrinth are structures known as semicircular canals. The semicircular canals contain three fluid-filled ducts, which form loops arranged roughly at right angles to one another. They tell your brain when your head rotates or moves up or down. Inside each canal is a gel-like structure called the cupula, stretched like a thick drumhead across its duct. The cupula sits on a cluster of sensory hair cells.

Each hair cell has tiny, thin extensions called stereocilia that protrude into the cupula.

When you turn your head, fluid inside the semicircular canal moves, causing the cupula to flex, which bends the stereocilia. This bending creates a nerve signal to the brain to tell it which way your head has turned.

Between the semicircular canals and the cochlea lie two otolithic organs: fluid-filled pouches called the utricle and the saccule. These organs tell your brain the position of your head with respect to gravity, such as whether you are sitting up, leaning back, or lying down, as well as when your head is moving in a straight line, such as up, forward, or sideways.

The utricle and the saccule also have sensory hair cells lining the floor or wall of each organ, with stereocilia extending into an overlying gel-like layer. Here, the gel contains tiny, dense grains of calcium carbonate called otoconia. Whatever the position of your head, gravity pulls on these grains, which then move the stereocilia to signal your head's position to your brain. Any head movement creates a signal that tells your brain about the change in position.

When you move, the vestibular system detects mechanical forces, including gravity, that stimulate the semicircular canals and the otolithic organs. These organs work with other sensory systems in your body, such as your vision and your musculoskeletal sensory system, to control the position of your body at rest or in motion. This helps you maintain stable posture and keep your balance when you're walking or running. It also helps you keep a stable visual focus on objects when your body changes position.

When the signals from any of these sensory systems malfunction, you can have problems with your sense of balance. If you have additional problems with motor control, such as weakness, slowness, tremor, or rigidity, you can lose your ability to recover properly from imbalance. This raises the risk of falling and injury.

What are some types of balance disorders?

There are more than a dozen different balance disorders. Some of the most common are:

- **Benign paroxysmal positional vertigo (BPPV) or positional vertigo:** A brief, intense episode of vertigo triggered by a specific change in the position of the head. You might feel as if you're spinning when you bend down to look under something, tilt your head to look up or over your shoulder, or roll over in bed. BPPV occurs when loose otoconia tumble into one of the semicircular canals and weigh on the cupula. The cupula doesn't flex properly and sends wrong information about your head's position, causing vertigo. BPPV can result from a head injury, or can develop just from getting older.

- **Labyrinthitis:** An infection or inflammation of the inner ear that causes dizziness and loss of balance. It is often associated with an upper respiratory infection such as the flu.

- **Ménière's disease:** Episodes of vertigo, hearing loss, tinnitus a ringing or buzzing in the ear), and a feeling of fullness in the ear. It may be associated with a change in fluid volume within parts of the labyrinth, but the cause or causes are still unknown.

- **Vestibular neuronitis:** An inflammation of the vestibular nerve that can be caused by a virus, and primarily causes vertigo.

- **Perilymph fistula:** A leakage of inner ear fluid into the middle ear. It causes unsteadiness that usually increases with activity, along with dizziness and nausea. Perilymph fistula can occur after a head injury, dramatic changes in air pressure (such as when scuba diving), physical exertion, ear surgery, or chronic ear infections. Some people are born with perilymph fistula.

- **Mal de Debarquement syndrome (MdDS):** A feeling of continuously rocking or bobbing, typically after an ocean cruise or other sea travel. Usually the symptoms go away a few hours or days after you reach land. Severe cases, however, can last months or even years, and the cause remains unknown.

How are balance disorders diagnosed?

Diagnosis of a balance disorder is difficult. To find out if you have a balance problem, your doctor may suggest that you see an otolaryngologist. An otolaryngologist is a physician and surgeon who specializes in diseases and disorders of the ear, nose, neck, and throat.

The otolaryngologist may ask you to have a hearing examination, blood tests, an electronystagmogram (a test that measures eye movements and the muscles that control them), or imaging studies of your head and brain. Another possible test is called posturography. For this test, you stand on a special movable platform in front of a patterned screen. The doctor measures how your body responds to movement of the platform, the patterned screen, or both.

How are balance disorders treated?

The first thing a doctor will do if you have a balance problem is determine if another health condition or a medication is to blame. If so, your doctor will treat the condition, suggest a different medication, or refer you to a specialist if the condition is outside his or her expertise.

If you have BPPV, your doctor might recommend a series of simple movements, such as the Epley maneuver, which can help dislodge the otoconia from the semicircular canal. In many cases, one session works; other people need the procedure several times to relieve their dizziness.

If you are diagnosed with Ménière's disease, your doctor may recommend that you make some changes to your diet and, if you are a smoker, that you stop smoking. Anti-vertigo or anti-nausea medications may relieve your symptoms, but they can also make you drowsy. Other medications, such as gentamicin (an antibiotic) or corticosteroids may be used. Although gentamicin may reduce dizziness better than corticosteroids, it occasionally causes permanent hearing loss. In some severe cases of Ménière's disease, surgery on the vestibular organs may be needed.

Some people with a balance disorder may not be able to fully relieve their dizziness and will need to find ways to cope with it. A vestibular rehabilitation therapist can help you develop an individualized treatment plan.

Talk to your doctor about whether it's safe to drive, as well as ways to lower your risk of falling and getting hurt during daily activities, such as when you walk up or down stairs, use the bathroom, or exercise. To reduce your risk of injury from dizziness, avoid walking in the dark. You should also wear low-heeled shoes or walking shoes outdoors. If necessary, use a cane or walker and modify conditions at your home and workplace, such as by adding handrails.

When should I seek help if I think I have a balance disorder?

To help you decide whether to seek medical help for a dizzy spell, ask yourself the following questions. If you answer "yes" to any of these questions, talk to your doctor:

- Do I feel unsteady?
- Do I feel as if the room is spinning around me?

- Do I feel as if I'm moving when I know I'm sitting or standing still?

- Do I lose my balance and fall?

- Do I feel as if I'm falling?

- Do I feel lightheaded or as if I might faint?

- Do I have blurred vision?

- Do I ever feel disoriented—losing my sense of time or location?

How can I help my doctor make a diagnosis?

You can help your doctor make a diagnosis and determine a treatment plan by answering the questions below. Be prepared to discuss this information during your appointment.

- The best way I can describe my dizziness or balance problem is:

- How often do I feel dizzy or have trouble keeping my balance?

- Have I ever fallen?

- When did I fall?

- Where did I fall?

- Under what conditions did I fall?

- How often have I fallen?

- These are the medicines I take (include prescription medications and over-the-counter medicine, such as aspirin, antihistamines, or sleep aids):

- Name of medicine:

- How much (milligrams) _____and how often (times) _____ per day:

- The condition I take this medicine for is:

Part Seven

Home and Self-Ordered Tests

Chapter 50

Overview of Home and Self-Ordered Tests

Home-use tests allow you to test for some diseases or conditions at home. These tests are cost-effective, quick, and confidential. Home-use tests can help:

- detect possible health conditions when you have no symptoms, so that you can get early treatment and lower your chance of developing later complications (i.e., cholesterol testing, hepatitis testing).

- detect specific conditions when there are no signs so that you can take immediate action (i.e., pregnancy testing).

- monitor conditions to allow frequent changes in treatment (i.e., glucose testing to monitor blood sugar levels in diabetes).

Despite the benefits of home testing, you should take precautions when using home-use tests. Home-use tests are intended to help you with your health care, but they should not replace periodic visits to your doctor. Many times, you should talk to your doctor even if you get normal test results. Most tests are best evaluated together with your medical history, a physical exam, and other testing. Always see your doctor if you are feeling sick, are worried about a possible medical condition, or if the test instructions recommend you do so.

This chapter includes excerpts from "Home Use Tests," U.S. Food and Drug Administration (FDA), June 5, 2014; and text from "How You Can Get the Best Results With Home Use Tests," U.S. Food and Drug Administration (FDA), December 10, 2014.

How You Can Get the Best Results with Home-Use Tests

Follow the tips listed here to use home-use tests as safely and effectively as possible.

- **Read the label and instructions carefully.** Review all instructions and pictures carefully to make sure you understand how to perform the test. Be sure you know:

  - what the test is for and what it is not for

  - how to store the test before you use it

  - how to collect and store the sample

  - when and how to run the test, including timing instructions

  - how to interpret the test

  - what might interfere with the test

  - the manufacturer's phone number if you have questions

- **Use only tests regulated by FDA.**

There are several ways to find out if FDA regulates a home-use test. You can ask your pharmacist or the vendor selling the test. If FDA does not regulate the test, the U.S. government has not determined that the test is reasonably safe or effective, or substantially equivalent to another legally marketed device.

- **Follow all instructions.** You must follow all test instructions to get an accurate result. Most home tests require specific timing, materials, and sample amounts. You should also check the expiration dates and storage conditions before performing a test to make sure the components still work correctly.

- **Keep good records of your testing.**

- **Call the "800" telephone number listed on your home-use test if you have any questions.**

- **When in doubt, contact your doctor.** All tests can give false results. You should see your doctor if you believe your test results are wrong.

- **Don't change medications or dosages based on a home-use test without talking to your doctor.**

Chapter 51

Cholesterol Home Testing

LDL and HDL: "Bad" and "Good" Cholesterol

Molecules called lipoproteins carry cholesterol in the blood. Two important kinds of lipoproteins are low-density lipoprotein (LDL) and high-density lipoprotein (HDL). When checking LDL and HDL, doctors often include another type of fat called triglycerides.

- **Total cholesterol** is a measure of the total amount of cholesterol in your blood and is based on the HDL, LDL, and triglycerides numbers.

- **LDL cholesterol** makes up the majority of the body's cholesterol. LDL is known as "bad" cholesterol because having high levels can lead to plaque buildup in your arteries and result in heart disease and stroke.

- **HDL cholesterol** absorbs cholesterol and carries it back to the liver, which flushes it from the body. HDL is known as "good" cholesterol because having high levels can reduce the risk for heart disease and stroke.

- **Triglycrides** are a type of fat found in your blood that your body uses for energy. The combination of high levels of triglycerides with low HDL cholesterol or high LDL cholesterol can increase your risk for heart attack and stroke.

This chapter includes excerpts from "LDL and HDL: "Bad" and "Good" Cholesterol," Centers for Disease Control and Prevention (CDC), March 16, 2015; and text from "Cholesterol," U.S. Food and Drug Administration (FDA), June 5, 2014.

Know Your Risk

Your health care team can do a simple blood test to check your cholesterol levels. The test is called a lipid profile. The test measures several kinds of total cholesterol and its individual parts including triglycerides. Some doctors do another blood test that just checks total and HDL cholesterol.

Whether your lipid levels require treatment is not solely based on your lipid profile numbers. Your primary care provider will look at these numbers, and your other risk factors, to determine your overall risk for heart disease and help decide if you need treatment.

There are no signs or symptoms of high LDL cholesterol. That is why it's so important to get your cholesterol checked. Talk to your doctor about what your numbers mean for you.

Who needs to get their cholesterol checked?

Cholesterol is something that needs to be monitored just like blood pressure. Talk to your health care team about what's best for you. All adults, aged 20 or older, need to get their cholesterol checked.

If you are 20 years or older and have not been diagnosed with heart disease, it is recommended that your cholesterol be checked every 5 years. Some people need to get their cholesterol checked more often.

All children and adolescents should have their cholesterol monitored at least once between the ages of 9 and 11 years, and again between ages 17 and 21 years.

Lowering Cholesterol

Knowing your cholesterol levels together with other factors, such age, gender, race/ethnicity, smoking status, and blood pressure, will help your health care team decide whether you should take cholesterol-lowering medication to help reduce your risk for heart disease and stroke.

Cholesterol—Home-Use Test

What this test does: This is a home-use test kit to measure total cholesterol.

What cholesterol is: Cholesterol is a fat (lipid) in your blood. High-density lipoprotein (HDL) ("good" cholesterol) helps protect your heart, but low-density lipoprotein (LDL) ("bad" cholesterol) can clog the arteries of your heart. Some cholesterol tests also measure tri-glycerides, another type of fat in the blood.

What type of test this is: This is a quantitative test—you find out the amount of total cholesterol present in your sample.

Why you should do this test: You should do this test to find out if you have high total cholesterol. High cholesterol increases your risk of heart disease. When the blood vessels of your heart become clogged by cholesterol, your heart does not receive enough oxygen. This can cause heart disease.

How often you should do this test: If you are more than 20 years old, you should test your cholesterol about every 5 years. If your doctor has you on a special diet or drugs to control your cholesterol, you may need to check your cholesterol more frequently. Follow your doctor's recommendations about how often you test your cholesterol.

What you cholesterol levels should be: Your total cholesterol level should be 200 mg/dL or less, according to recommendations in the National Cholesterol Education Program (NCEP) Third Adult Treatment Panel (ATP III). You should try to keep your LDL values less than 100 mg/dL, your HDL values greater or equal to 40 mg/dL, and your triglyceride values less than 150 mg/dL.

How accurate this test is: This test is about as accurate as the test your doctor uses, but you must follow the directions carefully.

Total cholesterol tests vary in accuracy from brand to brand. Information about the test's accuracy is printed on its package. Tests that say they are "traceable" to a program of the Centers for Disease Control and Prevention (CDC) may be more accurate than others.

What to do you if your test shows high cholesterol: Talk to your doctor if your test shows that your cholesterol is higher than 200 mg/dL. Many things can cause high cholesterol levels including diet, exercise, and other factors. Your doctor may want you to test your cholesterol again.

How you do this test: You prick your finger with a lancet to get a drop of blood. Then put the drop of blood on a piece paper that contains special chemicals. The paper will change color depending on how much cholesterol is in your blood. Some testing kits use a small machine to tell you how much cholesterol there is in the sample.

Chapter 52

Drugs of Abuse Home-Use Test

What do these tests do?

These tests indicate if one or more prescription or illegal drugs are present in urine. These tests detect the presence of drugs such as marijuana, cocaine, opiates, methamphetamine, amphetamines, phencyclidine (PCP), benzodiazepine, barbiturates, methadone, tricyclic antidepressants, ecstasy, and oxycodone.

The testing is done in two steps. First, you do a quick at-home test. Second, if the test suggests that drugs may be present, you send the sample to a laboratory for additional testing.

What are drugs of abuse?

Drugs of abuse are illegal or prescription medicines (for example, Oxycodone or Valium) that are taken for a non-medical purpose. Non-medical purposes for a prescription drug include taking the medication for longer than your doctor prescribed it for or for a purpose other than what the doctor prescribed it for. Medications are not drugs of abuse if they are taken according to your doctor's instructions.

Text in this chapter is excerpted from "Drugs of Abuse Home Use Test," U.S. Food and Drug Administration (FDA), June 5, 2015.

What type of test are these?

They are qualitative tests—you find out if a particular drug may be in the urine, but not how much is present.

When should you do these tests?

You should use these tests when you think someone might be abusing prescription or illegal drugs. If you are worried about a specific drug, make sure to check the label to confirm that this test is designed to detect the drug you are looking for.

How accurate are these tests?

The at-home testing part of this test is fairly sensitive to the presence of drugs in the urine. This means that if drugs are present, you will usually get a preliminary (or presumptive) positive test result. If you get a preliminary positive result, you should send the urine sample to the laboratory for a second test.

It is very important to send the urine sample to the laboratory to confirm a positive at-home result because certain foods, food supplements, beverages, or medicines can affect the results of at-home tests. Laboratory tests are the most reliable way to confirm drugs of abuse.

Many things can affect the accuracy of these tests, including (but not limited to):

- the way you did the test
- the way you stored the test or urine
- what the person ate or drank before taking the test
- any other prescription or over-the-counter drugs the person may have taken before the test

Note that a result showing the presence of an amphetamine should be considered carefully, even when this result is confirmed in the laboratory testing. Some over-the-counter medications will produce the same test results as illegally-abused amphetamines.

Does a positive test mean that you found drugs of abuse?

No. Take no serious actions until you get the laboratory's result. Remember that many factors may cause a false positive result in the home test.

Remember that a positive test for a **prescription** drug does not mean that a person is abusing the drug, because there is no way for the test to indicate acceptable levels compared to abusive levels of prescribed drugs.

If the test results are negative, can you be sure that the person you tested did not abuse drugs?

No. No drug test of this type is 100% accurate. There are several factors that can make the test results negative even though the person is abusing drugs. First, you may have tested for the wrong drugs. Or, you may not have tested the urine when it contained drugs. It takes time for drugs to appear in the urine after a person takes them, and they do not stay in the urine indefinitely; you may have collected the urine too late or too soon. It is also possible that the chemicals in the test went bad because they were stored incorrectly or they passed their expiration date.

If you get a negative test result, but still suspect that someone is abusing drugs, you can test again at a later time. Talk to your doctor if you need more help deciding what steps to take next.

How soon after a person takes drugs, will they show up in a drug test? And how long after a person takes drugs, will they continue to show up in a drug test?

The drug clearance rate tells how soon a person may have a positive test after taking a particular drug. It also tells how long the person may continue to test positive after the last time he or she took the drug. Clearance rates for common drugs of abuse are given below. These are only guidelines, however, and the times can vary significantly from these estimates based on how long the person has been taking the drug, the amount of drug they use, or the person's metabolism.

How do you do a drugs of abuse test?

These tests usually contain a sample collection cup, the drug test (it may be test strips, a test card, a test cassette, or other method for testing the urine), and an instruction leaflet or booklet. It is very important that the person doing the test reads and understands the instructions first, before even collecting the sample. This is important because with most test kits, the result must be visually read within a certain number of minutes after the test is started.

You collect urine in the sample collection cup and test it according to the instructions. If the test indicates the preliminary presence of one or more drugs, the sample should be sent to a laboratory where a more specific chemical test will be used order to obtain a final result. Some home-use kits have a shipping container and pre-addressed mailer in them. If you have questions about using these tests, or the results that you are getting, you should contact your healthcare provider.

Table 52.1. Clearance rates for common drugs of abuse

Drug	How soon after taking drug will there be a positive drug test?	How long after taking drug will there continue to be a positive drug test?
Marijuana/Pot	1–3 hours	1–7 days
Crack (Cocaine)	2–6 hours	2–3 days
Heroin (Opiates)	2–6 hours	1–3 days
Speed/Uppers (Amphetamine, methamphetamine)	4–6 hours	2–3 days
Angel Dust/PCP	4–6 hours	7–14 days
Ecstacy	2–7 hours	2–4 days
Benzodiazepine	2–7 hours	1–4 days
Barbiturates	2–4 hours	1–3 weeks
Methadone	3–8 hours	1–3 days
Tricyclic Antidepressants	8–12 hours	2–7 days
Oxycodone	1–3 hours	1–2 days

Chapter 53

Direct-to-Consumer Genetic Testing

Traditionally, genetic tests have been available only through health-care providers such as physicians, nurse practitioners, and genetic counselors. Healthcare providers order the appropriate test from a laboratory, collect and send the samples, and interpret the test results. Direct-to-consumer genetic testing refers to genetic tests that are marketed directly to consumers via television, print advertisements, or the Internet. This form of testing, which is also known as at-home genetic testing, provides access to a person's genetic information without necessarily involving a doctor or insurance company in the process.

If a consumer chooses to purchase a genetic test directly, the test kit is mailed to the consumer instead of being ordered through a doctor's office. The test typically involves collecting a DNA sample at home, often by swabbing the inside of the cheek, and mailing the sample back to the laboratory. In some cases, the person must visit a health clinic to have blood drawn. Consumers are notified of their results by mail or over the telephone, or the results are posted online. In some cases, a genetic counselor or other healthcare provider is available to explain the results and answer questions. The price for this type of at-home genetic testing ranges from several hundred dollars to more than a thousand dollars.

Text in this chapter is excerpted from "What is Direct-to-Consumer Genetic Testing?" Genetics Home Reference (GHR), September 14, 2015.

The growing market for direct-to-consumer genetic testing may promote awareness of genetic diseases, allow consumers to take a more proactive role in their health care, and offer a means for people to learn about their ancestral origins. At-home genetic tests, however, have significant risks and limitations. Consumers are vulnerable to being misled by the results of unproven or invalid tests. Without guidance from a healthcare provider, they may make important decisions about treatment or prevention based on inaccurate, incomplete, or misunderstood information about their health. Consumers may also experience an invasion of genetic privacy if testing companies use their genetic information in an unauthorized way.

Genetic testing provides only one piece of information about a person's health—other genetic and environmental factors, lifestyle choices, and family medical history also affect a person's risk of developing many disorders. These factors are discussed during a consultation with a doctor or genetic counselor, but in many cases are not addressed by at-home genetic tests. More research is needed to fully understand the benefits and limitations of direct-to-consumer genetic testing.

How can consumers be sure a genetic test is valid and useful?

Before undergoing genetic testing, it is important to be sure that the test is valid and useful. A genetic test is valid if it provides an accurate result. Two main measures of accuracy apply to genetic tests: analytical validity and clinical validity. Another measure of the quality of a genetic test is its usefulness, or clinical utility.

- Analytical validity refers to how well the test predicts the presence or absence of a particular gene or genetic change. In other words, can the test accurately detect whether a specific genetic variant is present or absent?

- Clinical validity refers to how well the genetic variant being analyzed is related to the presence, absence, or risk of a specific disease.

- Clinical utility refers to whether the test can provide information about diagnosis, treatment, management, or prevention of a disease that will be helpful to a consumer.

All laboratories that perform health-related testing, including genetic testing, are subject to federal regulatory standards called the

Clinical Laboratory Improvement Amendments (CLIA) or even stricter state requirements. CLIA standards cover how tests are performed, the qualifications of laboratory personnel, and quality control and testing procedures for each laboratory. By controlling the quality of laboratory practices, CLIA standards are designed to ensure the analytical validity of genetic tests.

CLIA standards do not address the clinical validity or clinical utility of genetic tests. The Food and Drug Administration (FDA) requires information about clinical validity for some genetic tests. Additionally, the state of New York requires information on clinical validity for all laboratory tests performed for people living in that state. Consumers, health providers, and health insurance companies are often the ones who determine the clinical utility of a genetic test.

It can be difficult to determine the quality of a genetic test sold directly to the public. Some providers of direct-to-consumer genetic tests are not CLIA-certified, so it can be difficult to tell whether their tests are valid. If providers of direct-to-consumer genetic tests offer easy-to-understand information about the scientific basis of their tests, it can help consumers make more informed decisions. It may also be helpful to discuss any concerns with a health professional before ordering a direct-to-consumer genetic test.

Chapter 54

Hepatitis C Home Test

What does this test do?

This is a home-use collection kit to determine if you may have a hepatitis C infection now or had one in the past. You collect a blood sample and send it to a testing laboratory for analysis.

What is hepatitis C infection?

Hepatitis C infection is caused by the hepatitis C virus (HCV). Untreated, hepatitis C can cause liver disease.

What type of test is this?

This is a qualitative test—you find out whether or not you may have this infection, not how advanced your disease is.

Why should you do this test?

You should do this test if you think you may have been infected with HCV. If you are infected with HCV, you should take steps to avoid spreading the disease to others. At least 8 out of 10 people with acute hepatitis C develop chronic liver infection, and 2 to 3 out of 10 develop cirrhosis. A small number of people may also develop liver cancer. Hepatitis C infection is the number 1 cause for liver transplantation in the US.

Text in this chapter is excerpted from "Hepatitis C," U.S. Food and Drug Administration (FDA), June 5, 2014.

When should you do this test?

The Centers for Disease Control (CDC) recommend that you do this test if you:

- have ever injected illegal drugs

- received clotting factor concentrates produced before 1987

- were ever on long-term dialysis

- received a blood transfusion before July 1992

- received an organ transplant before July 1992 or

- are a health care, emergency medicine, or public safety worker who contacted HCV-positive blood through needlesticks, sharps, or mucosal exposure

How accurate is this test?

This test is about as accurate as the test your doctor uses, but you must carefully follow the directions about getting the sample and sending it the testing laboratory. Proper sample collection is important for obtaining accurate results. Researchers found that about 90 of 100 home users were able to obtain acceptable samples to send to the laboratory. After the laboratory got these 90 samples, it could get results for about 81 of them. Of these 81 samples, the laboratory got correct results in 77 and incorrect results in 4.

Does a positive test mean you have HCV?

If you have a positive test, you either are infected with HCV now or you have been infected with HCV in the past. You need to see your doctor to find out if you have an active infection and what therapy you should have. Some people who become infected with HCV develop antibodies and then are no longer infected.

If your test results are negative, can you be sure that you do not have HCV infection?

A negative test does not guarantee that you don't have HCV infection since it takes some time for you to develop antibodies after you are infected with this virus. If you think you were exposed to the virus and might be infected, you should see your doctor for a more accurate laboratory test.

How do you do this test?

The test kit comes with a small piece of filter paper, a lancet, and instructions for obtaining a blood sample and placing it on the filter paper. You first prick your finger with the lancet to get a drop of blood. Then, you put your drop of blood on a piece of filter paper and send it in a special container to the testing laboratory. You get the results of your test by phone from the laboratory. The laboratory does a preliminary (screening) test that separates the samples into three groups

- Samples that are clearly positive,

- Samples that *might* be positive, and

- Samples that are negative.

All samples that "**might** be positive" receive a more specific (confirmatory) test to find those that are truly positive. All the "clearly positives" from the preliminary test and the "truly positives" from the more specific test are reported to you as positive.

You should note that a positive result does not mean that you are infected with HCV. If you receive a positive result from this test, you should see your doctor for further testing and information.

Chapter 55

HIV Home Test

What does this test do?

This is a home-use collection kit to detect whether or not you have antibodies to HIV (human immunodeficiency virus).

What is HIV?

HIV is the virus that causes AIDS (acquired immunodeficiency syndrome).

What type of test is this?

This is a qualitative test—you find out whether or not you have this infection, not how advanced your disease is.

Why should you do this test?

You should do this test to find out if you have an HIV infection. If you know that you have an HIV infection,

- you can obtain medical treatment that helps slow the course of the disease, and

- you can take precautions to keep from infecting others.

Text in this chapter is excerpted from "Human Immunodeficiency Virus (HIV)," U.S. Food and Drug Administration (FDA), June 5, 2014.

Untreated, HIV destroys your immune system. The most advanced stage of HIV infection is AIDS, an often-fatal disease.

When should you do this test?

You should do this test if you believe there is a chance you may have an HIV infection. You are at greatest risk for HIV if you:

- have ever shared injection drug needles and syringes or "works"
- have ever had sex without a condom with someone who had HIV
- have ever had a sexually transmitted disease, like chlamydia or gonorrhea
- received a blood transfusion or a blood-clotting factor between 1978 and 1985 or
- have ever had sex with someone who has done any of the above-said things

If you use this test, no one but you will know you were tested for HIV or what the results showed.

How accurate is this test?

This test is similar to the test your doctor would use. Researchers have found that about 90 of 100 home users were able to obtain acceptable samples for sending to the laboratory. After the laboratory got these 90 samples, they could get results for about 81 of 100 of them. Of these 81 samples, the laboratory almost always shows whether or not the person tested had HIV infection.

Does a positive test mean you have HIV?

If you test positive in this test, you are infected with the HIV virus. You should take precautions so you do not spread this infection to your sexual partners or others who might be at risk. You should not donate blood because this infection could spread to others. Having HIV infection does not necessarily mean you have AIDS. You should see your doctor so you can learn the status of your disease and decide what therapy, if any, you need.

If your results are negative, can you be sure that you do not have HIV infection?

If you test negative for HIV, it means you did not have antibodies to HIV at the time of the test. However, if you are newly infected, it will take time for you to make antibodies. It is uncertain how long it may take you to develop antibodies--it may take more than 3 months. So, although you may be infected, the results of your testing will not verify that you are infected for several months. If you think you were exposed to the virus and might be infected, you should test yourself again in a few months.

How do you do this test?

The test comes with sterile lancets, an alcohol pad, gauze pads, a blood specimen collection card, a bandage, a lancet disposal container, a shipping pouch, and instructions. To do the test, you

- call a specified telephone number,
- register a code number that is included with the specimen collection kit,
- prick your finger with a lancet to get a drop of blood,
- place drops of blood on the card,
- send the shipping pouch by express courier service to the central testing laboratory,
- receive results by phone after 3-7 business days later, and
- if you test positive for HIV, you get counseling on what to do about your infection.

Chapter 56

Menopause Home Test

What Is Menopause?

Menopause is a normal part of life, just like puberty. It is the time of your last menstrual period. You may notice changes in your body before and after menopause. The transition usually has three parts: *perimenopause*, *menopause*, and *postmenopause*.

Changes usually begin with *perimenopause*. This can begin several years before your last menstrual period. Changing levels of estrogen and progesterone, which are two female hormones made in your ovaries, might lead to symptoms. *Menopause* comes next, the end of your menstrual periods. After a full year without a period, you can say you have been "through menopause," and perimenopause is over. *Postmenopause* follows perimenopause and lasts the rest of your life.

The average age of a woman having her last period, menopause, is 51. But, some women have their last period in their forties, and some have it later in their fifties.

Smoking can lead to early menopause. So can some types of operations. For example, surgery to remove your uterus (called a hysterectomy) will make your periods stop, and that's menopause. But you might not have menopause symptoms like hot flashes right then because if your ovaries are untouched, they still make hormones. In

This chapter includes excerpts from "Menopause," National Institute on Aging (NIA), December 2013; and text from "Menopause," U.S. Food and Drug Administration (FDA), June 5, 2014.

time, when your ovaries start to make less estrogen, menopause symptoms could start. But, sometimes both ovaries are removed (called an oophorectomy), usually along with your uterus. In this case, menopause symptoms can start right away, no matter what age you are, because your body has lost its main supply of estrogen.

What Are the Signs of Menopause?

Women may have different signs or symptoms at menopause. That's because estrogen is used by many parts of your body. As you have less estrogen, you could have various symptoms. Here are the most common changes you might notice at midlife. Some may be part of aging rather than directly related to menopause.

Change in your period. This might be what you notice first. Your periods may no longer be regular. They may be shorter or last longer. You might bleed less than usual or more. These are all normal changes, but to make sure there isn't a problem, see your doctor if:

- Your periods come very close together
- You have heavy bleeding
- You have spotting
- Your periods last more than a week
- Your periods resume after no bleeding for more than a year

Hot flashes. Many women have hot flashes, which can last a few years after menopause. They may be related to changing estrogen levels. A *hot flash* is a sudden feeling of heat in the upper part or all of your body. Your face and neck become flushed. Red blotches may appear on your chest, back, and arms. Heavy sweating and cold shivering can follow. Flashes can be very mild or strong enough to wake you from your sleep (called *night sweats*). Most hot flashes last between 30 seconds and 10 minutes.

Vaginal health and bladder control. Your vagina may get drier. This could make sexual intercourse uncomfortable. Or, you could have other health problems, such as vaginal or bladder infections. Some women also find it hard to hold their urine long enough to get to the bathroom. This loss of bladder control is called incontinence. You may have a sudden urge to urinate, or urine may leak during exercise, sneezing, or laughing.

Sleep. Around midlife, some women start having trouble getting a good night's sleep. Maybe you can't fall asleep easily, or you wake too early. Night sweats might wake you up. You might have trouble falling back to sleep if you wake up during the night.

Sex. You may find that your feelings about sex are changing. You could be less interested. Or, you could feel freer and sexier after menopause. After 1 full year without a period, you can no longer become pregnant. But remember, you could still be at risk for sexually transmitted diseases (STDs), such as gonorrhea or even HIV/AIDS. You increase your risk for an STD if you are having sex with more than one person or with someone who is having sex with others. If so, make sure your partner uses a condom each time you have sex.

Mood changes. You might find yourself more moody or irritable around the time of menopause. Scientists don't know why this happens. It's possible that stress, family changes such as growing children or aging parents, a history of depression, or feeling tired could be causing these mood changes.

Your body seems different. Your waist could get larger. You could lose muscle and gain fat. Your skin could get thinner. You might have memory problems, and your joints and muscles could feel stiff and achy. Are these a result of having less estrogen or just related to growing older? Experts don't know the answer.

What About My Heart and Bones?

Two common health problems can start to happen at menopause, and you might not even notice.

Osteoporosis. Day in and day out, your body is busy breaking down old bone and replacing it with new healthy bone. Estrogen helps control bone loss, and losing estrogen around the time of menopause causes women to lose more bone than is replaced. In time, bones can become weak and break easily. This condition is called osteoporosis. Talk to your doctor to see if you should have a bone density test to find out if you are at risk. Your doctor can also suggest ways to prevent or treat osteoporosis.

Heart disease. After menopause, women are more likely to have heart disease. Changes in estrogen levels may be part of the cause. But, so is getting older. As you age, you may gain weight and develop other problems, like high blood pressure. These could put you at greater risk for heart disease. Be sure to have your blood pressure and levels of triglycerides, fasting blood glucose, and cholesterol, including LDL and HDL, checked regularly. Talk to your healthcare provider to find out what you should do to protect your heart.

How Can I Stay Healthy after Menopause?

Staying healthy after menopause may mean making some changes in the way you live.

- Don't smoke. If you do use any type of tobacco, stop—it's never too late to benefit from quitting smoking.

- Eat a healthy diet, low in fat, high in fiber, with plenty of fruits, vegetables, and whole-grain foods, as well as all the important vitamins and minerals.

- Make sure you get enough calcium and vitamin D—in your diet or with vitamin/mineral supplements if recommended by your doctor.

- Learn what your healthy weight is, and try to stay there.

- Do weight-bearing exercise, such as walking, jogging, or dancing, at least 3 days each week for healthy bones. But try to be physically active in other ways for your general health.

Other things to remember:

- Take medicine if your doctor prescribes it for you, especially if it is for health problems you cannot see or feel—for example, high blood pressure, high cholesterol, or osteoporosis.

- Use a water-based vaginal lubricant (not petroleum jelly) or a vaginal estrogen cream or tablet to help with vaginal discomfort.

- Get regular pelvic and breast exams, Pap tests, and mammograms. You should also be checked for colon and rectal cancer and for skin cancer. Contact your doctor right away if you notice a lump in your breast or a mole that has changed.

Menopause is not a disease that has to be treated. But you might need help if symptoms like hot flashes bother you. Here are some ideas that have helped some women:

- Try to keep track of when hot flashes happen—a diary can help. You might be able to use this information to find out what triggers your flashes and then avoid those triggers.

- When a hot flash starts, try to go somewhere cool.

- If night sweats wake you, sleep in a cool room or with a fan on.

- Dress in layers that you can take off if you get too warm.

- Use sheets and clothing that let your skin "breathe."

- Have a cold drink (water or juice) when a flash is starting.

You could also talk to your doctor about whether there are any medicines to manage hot flashes. A few drugs that are approved for other uses (for example, certain antidepressants) seem to be helpful to some women.

What about Those Lost Hormones?

These days you hear a lot about whether or not you should use hormones to help relieve some menopause symptoms. It's hard to know what to do, although there is some information to help you.

During perimenopause, some doctors suggest birth control pills to help with very heavy, frequent, or unpredictable menstrual periods. These pills might also help with symptoms like hot flashes, as well as prevent pregnancy.

If you are bothered by symptoms like hot flashes, night sweats, or vaginal dryness, your doctor might suggest taking estrogen (as well as progesterone, if you still have a uterus). This is known as *menopausal hormone therapy (MHT)* . Some people still call it hormone replacement therapy or HRT. Taking these hormones will probably help with menopause symptoms. It also can prevent the bone loss that can happen at menopause.

Menopausal hormone therapy has risks. That is why the U.S. Food and Drug Administration suggests that women who want to try MHT to manage their hot flashes or vaginal dryness use the lowest dose that works for the shortest time it's needed.

Home-Use Tests

What does this test do?

This is a home-use test kit to measure follicle stimulating hormone (FSH) in your urine. This may help indicate if you are in menopause or perimenopause.

What is menopause?

Menopause is the stage in your life when menstruation stops for at least 12 months. The time before this is called perimenopause and could last for several years. You may reach menopause in your early 40's or as late as your 60's.

What is FSH?

Follicle stimulating hormone (FSH) is a hormone produced by your pituitary gland. FSH levels increase temporarily each month to stimulate your ovaries to produce eggs. When you enter menopause and your ovaries stop working, your FSH levels also increase.

What type of test is this?

This is a qualitative test—you find out whether or not you have elevated FSH levels, not if you definitely are in menopause or perimenopause.

Why should you do this test?

You should use this test if you want to know if your symptoms, such as irregular periods, hot flashes, vaginal dryness, or sleep problems are part of menopause. While many women may have little or no trouble when going through the stages of menopause, others may have moderate to severe discomfort and may want treatment to alleviate their symptoms. This test may help you be better informed about your current condition when you see your doctor.

How accurate is this test?

These tests will accurately detect FSH about 9 out of 10 times. This test does not detect menopause or perimenopause. As you grow older, your FSH levels may rise and fall during your menstrual cycle. While your hormone levels are changing, your ovaries continue to release eggs and you can still become pregnant.

Your test will depend on whether you

- used your first morning urine,

- drank large amounts of water before the test,

- use, or recently stopped using, oral or patch contraceptives, hormone replacement therapy, or estrogen supplements.

How do you do this test?

In this test, you put a few drops of your urine on a test device, put the end of the testing device in your urine stream, or dip the test device into a cup of urine. Chemicals in the test device react with FSH and produce a color. Read the instructions with the test you buy to learn exactly what to look for in this test.

Are the home menopause tests similar to the ones my doctor uses?

Some home menopause tests are identical to the one your doctor uses. However, doctors would not use this test by itself. Your doctor would use your medical history, physical exam, and other laboratory tests to get a more thorough assessment of your condition.

Does a positive test mean you are in menopause?

A positive test indicates that you may be in a stage of menopause. If you have a positive test, or if you have any symptoms of menopause, you should see your doctor. Do not stop taking contraceptives based on the results of these tests because they are not foolproof and you could become pregnant.

Do negative test results indicate that you are not in menopause?

If you have a negative test result, but you have symptoms of menopause, you may be in perimenopause or menopause. You should not assume that a negative test means you have not reached menopause, there could be other reasons for the negative result. You should always discuss your symptoms and your test results with your doctor. Do not use these tests to determine if you are fertile or can become pregnant. These tests will not give you a reliable answer on your ability to become pregnant.

Chapter 57

Fecal Occult Blood Test

What does this test do?

This is a home-use test kit to measure the presence of hidden (occult) blood in your stool (feces).

What is fecal occult blood?

Fecal occult blood is blood in your feces that you cannot see in your stool or on your toilet paper after you use the toilet.

What type of test is this?

This is a qualitative test—you find out whether or not you have occult blood in your feces, not how much is present.

Why should you do this test?

You should do this test, because blood in your feces may be an early sign of a digestive condition, for example abnormal growths (polyps) or cancer in your colon.

How often should you test for fecal occult blood?

The American Cancer Society recommends that you test for fecal occult blood every year after you turn 50. Some doctors suggest that

---

Text in this chapter is excerpted from "Fecal Occult Blood," U.S. Food and Drug Administration (FDA), June 5, 2014.

you start testing at age 40, if your family is thought to be at increased risk. Follow your doctor's recommendations about how often you test for fecal occult blood.

How accurate is this test?

This test is about as accurate as the test your doctor uses, but you must follow the directions carefully. For accurate results, you must prepare properly for the test and get a good stool sample.

Does a positive test mean you have hidden blood in your stool?

A positive result means that the test has detected blood. This does not mean you have tested positive for cancer or any other illness. False positive results may be caused by diet or medications. Further testing and examinations should be performed by the physician to determine the exact cause and source of the occult blood in the stool.

If the test results are negative, can you be sure that you do not have a bowel condition?

No. You could still have bowel condition that you should know about. You should use this test again in a year.

How do you do this test?

There are several different methods for detecting hidden blood in the stool.

In one method, you collect stool samples and smear them onto paper cards in a holder. You then either send these cards to a laboratory for testing or test them at home. If you test them at home, you add a special solution from your test kit to the paper cards to see if they change color. If the paper cards change color, it means there was blood in the stool.

In another method, you put special paper in the toilet after a bowel movement. If the special paper changes color, it indicates there was blood in the toilet.

You will need to test your feces from three separate bowel movements. These bowel movements should be three in a row, closely spaced in time to minimize the time you need to be on the special diet. This is necessary because if you have polyps, they may not bleed all the time.

You improve your chances of catching any bleeding if you sample three different bowel movements.

- Unless you use the method where you put a test solution into the toilet, it is best to catch your feces before it enters the toilet. You can do this by holding a piece of toilet paper in your hand. After you catch it, cut it apart in two places with the little wooden stick you get in the kit. Take a little bit of the feces from each place where you cut it apart and put these bits on one place in the cardboard in the kit. You use the second and third spots on the cardboard for other bowel movements.

What interferes with this test?

To get good results with this test, you have to follow the instructions. You may find it difficult because you need to things you do not ordinarily do.

Because the test is for blood, any source of blood will give a positive test. Blood from another source, like bleeding hemorrhoids or your menstrual period will interfere with the test, so you won't be able to tell what made the test positive.

Pay attention to your diet before the test:

- Eat a high fiber diet, such as one that has cereals and breads with bran.

- Cook your fruits and vegetables *well*.

- Don't eat *raw* turnips, radishes, broccoli, or horseradish. These foods can make it look like you have hidden blood when you don't.

- Don't eat *red* meat. (You may eat poultry or fish). Red meat in your diet can make it look like you have hidden blood when you don't.

Avoid the following drugs for the 7 days before the test—they can make it look like you have hidden blood when you don't:

- Aspirin

- Anti-inflammatory drugs, such as Motrin

Don't take Vitamin C supplements for the 7 days before the test. Then can prevent the test from detecting your hidden blood.

Chapter 58

Gynecological Concerns Home Tests

Ovulation (Urine Test)

What does this test do?

This is a home-use test kit to measure luteinizing hormone (LH) in your urine. This helps detect the LH surge that happens in the middle of your menstrual cycle, about 1–1½ days before ovulation. Some tests also measure another hormone—estrone-3-glucuronide (E3G).

What is LH?

Luteinizing hormone (LH) is a hormone produced by your pituitary gland. Your body always makes a small amount of LH, but just before you ovulate, you make much more LH. This test can detect this LH surge, which usually happens 1–1½ days before you ovulate.

What is E3G?

E3G is produced when estrogen breaks down in your body. It accumulates in your urine around the time of ovulation and causes your cervical mucus to become thin and slippery. Sperm may swim

---

Text in this chapter is excerpted from "Home Use Tests," U.S. Food and Drug Administration (FDA), June 5, 2014.

more easily in your thin and slippery cervical mucus, increasing your chances of getting pregnant.

What type of test is this?

This is a qualitative test—you find out whether or not you have elevated LH or E3G levels, not if you will definitely become pregnant.

Why should you do this test?

You should do this test if you want to know when you expect to ovulate and be in the most fertile part of your menstrual cycle. This test can be used to help you plan to become pregnant. You should not use this test to help prevent pregnancy, because it is not reliable for that purpose.

How accurate is this test?

How well this test will predict your fertile period depends on how well you follow the instructions. These tests can detect LH and E3G reliably about 9 times out of 10, but you must do the test carefully.

How do you do this test?

You add a few drops of your urine to the test, hold the tip of the test in your urine stream, or dip the test in a cup of your urine. You either read the test by looking for colored lines on the test or you put the test device into a monitor. You can get results in about 5 minutes. The details of what the color looks like, or how to use the monitor varies among the different brands.

Most kits come with multiple tests to allow you to take measurements over several days. This can help you find your most fertile period, the time during your cycle when you can expect to ovulate based on your hormone levels. Follow the instructions carefully to get good results. You will need to start your testing at the proper time during your cycle, otherwise the test will be unreliable, and you will not find your hormonal surges or your fertile period.

Is this test similar to the one my doctor uses?

The fertility tests your doctor uses are automated, and they may give more consistent results. Your doctor may use other tests that are not yet available for home use (i.e., blood and urine laboratory tests) and information about your history to get a better view of your fertility status.

Pregnancy

What does this test do?

This is a home-use test kit to measure human chorionic gonadotropin (hCG) in your urine. You produce this hormone only when you are pregnant.

What is hCG?

hCG is a hormone produced by your placenta when you are pregnant. It appears shortly after the embryo attaches to the wall of the uterus. If you are pregnant, this hormone increases very rapidly. If you have a 28 day menstrual cycle, you can detect hCG in your urine 12-15 days after ovulation.

What type of test is this?

This is a qualitative test—you find out whether or not you have elevated hCG levels indicating that you are pregnant.

Why should you do this test?

You should use this test to find out if you are pregnant.

How accurate is this test?

The accuracy of this test depends on how well you follow the instructions and interpret the results. If you mishandle or misunderstand the test kit, you may get poor results.

Most pregnancy tests have about the same ability to detect hCG, but their ability to show whether or not you are pregnant depends on how much hCG you are producing. If you test too early in your cycle or too close to the time you became pregnant, your placenta may **not** have had enough time to produce hCG. This would mean that you are pregnant but you got a **negative** test result.

Because many women have irregular periods, and women may miscalculate when their period is due, 10 to 20 pregnant women out of every 100 will not detect their pregnancy on the first day of their missed period.

How do you do this test?

For most home pregnancy tests, you either hold a test strip in your urine stream or you collect your urine in a cup and dip your test strip into the cup. If you are pregnant, most test strips produce a colored line, but this will depend on the brand you purchased. Read the instructions for the test you bought and follow them carefully. Make sure you know how to get good results. The test usually takes only about 5 minutes.

The different tests for sale vary in their abilities to detect low levels of hCG. For the most reliable results, test 1-2 weeks after you miss your period. There are some tests for sale that are sensitive enough to show you are pregnant before you miss your period.

You can improve your chances for an accurate result by using your first morning urine for the test. If you are pregnant, it will have more hCG in it than later urines. If you think you are pregnant, but your first test was negative, you can take the test again after several days. Since the amount of hCG increases rapidly when you are pregnant, you may get a positive test on later days. Some test kits come with more than one test in them to allow you to repeat the test.

Is this test similar to the one my doctor uses?

The home pregnancy test and the test your doctor uses are similar in their abilities to detect hCG, however your doctor is probably more experienced in running the test. If you produce only a small amount of hCG, your doctor may not be able to detect it any better than you could. Your doctor may also use a blood test to see if you are pregnant. Finally, your doctor may have more information about you from your history, physical exam, and other tests that may give a more reliable result.

Does a positive test mean you are pregnant?

Usually, yes, but you must be sure to read and interpret the results correctly.

Do negative test results mean that you are not pregnant?

No, there are several reasons why you could receive false negative test results. If you tested too early in your cycle, your placenta may not have had time to produce enough hCG for the test to detect. Or, you may not have waited long enough before you took this test.

If you have a negative result, you would be wise to consider this a tentative finding. You should not use medications and should consider avoiding potentially harmful behaviors, such as smoking or drinking alcohol, until you have greater certainty that you are not pregnant.

You will probably recognize incorrect results with the passage of time. You may detect false negatives by the unexpected onset of menses (regular vaginal bleeding associated with "periods".) Repeat testing and/or other investigations such as ultrasound may provide corrected results.

Vaginal pH

What does this test do?

This is a home-use test kit to measure the pH of your vaginal secretions.

What is pH?

pH is a way to describe how acidic a substance is. It is given by a number on a scale of 1-14. The lower the number, the more acidic the substance.

What type of test is this?

This is a quantitative test—you find out how acidic your vaginal secretions are.

Why should you do this test?

You should do this test to help evaluate if your vaginal symptoms (i.e., itching, burning, unpleasant odor, or unusual discharge) are likely caused by an infection that needs medical treatment. The test is not intended for HIV, chlamydia, herpes, gonorrhea, syphilis, or group B streptococcus.

How accurate is this test?

Home vaginal pH tests showed good agreement with a doctor's diagnosis. However, just because you find changes in your vaginal pH, doesn't always mean that you have a vaginal infection. pH changes also do not help or differentiate one type of infection from another. Your doctor diagnoses a vaginal infection by using a combination of: pH, microscopic examination of the vaginal discharge, amine odor, culture, wet preparation, and Gram stain.

Does a positive test mean you have a vaginal infection?

No, a positive test (elevated pH) could occur for other reasons. If you detect elevated pH, you should see your doctor for further testing and treatment. There are no over-the-counter medications for treatment of an elevated vaginal pH.

If test results are negative, can you be sure that you do not have a vaginal infection? No, you may have an infection that does not show up in these tests. If you have no symptoms, your negative test could suggest the possibility of chemical, allergic, or other noninfectious irritation of the vagina. Or, a negative test could indicate the possibility of a yeast infection. You should see your doctor if you find changes in your vaginal pH or if you continue to have symptoms.

How do you do this test?

You hold a piece of pH paper against the wall of your vagina for a few seconds, then compare the color of the pH paper to the color on the chart provided with the test kit. The number on the chart for the color that best matches the color on the pH paper is the vaginal pH number.

Is the home test similar to your doctor's test?

Yes. The home vaginal pH tests are practically identical to the ones sold to doctors. But your doctor can provide a more thorough assessment of your vaginal status through your history, physical exam, and other laboratory tests than you can using a single pH test in your home.

Part Eight

Additional Help and Information

Chapter 59

Glossary of Terms Related to Medical Tests

angiography: A procedure to X-ray blood vessels. The blood vessels can be seen because of an injection of a dye that shows up in the X-ray.

assessment: In health care, a process used to learn about a patient's condition. This may include a complete medical history, medical tests, a physical exam, a test of learning skills, tests to find out if the patient is able to carry out the tasks of daily living, a mental health evaluation, and a review of social support and community resources available to the patient.

barium swallow: The process of getting X-ray pictures of the esophagus or the upper gastrointestinal (GI) tract (esophagus, stomach, and duodenum). The X-ray pictures are taken after the patient drinks a liquid that contains barium sulfate (a form of the silver-white metallic element barium). The barium sulfate coats and outlines the inner walls of the esophagus and the upper GI tract so that they can be seen on the X-ray pictures.

biopsy: The removal of cells or tissues for examination by a pathologist. The pathologist may study the tissue under a microscope or perform other tests on the cells or tissue. There are many different types of biopsy procedures. The most common types include: (1) incisional

---

This glossary contains terms excerpted from documents produced by several sources deemed reliable.

biopsy, in which only a sample of tissue is removed; (2) excisional biopsy, in which an entire lump or suspicious area is removed; and (3) needle biopsy, in which a sample of tissue or fluid is removed with a needle. When a wide needle is used, the procedure is called a core biopsy. When a thin needle is used, the procedure is called a fine-needle aspiration biopsy.

body mass index (BMI): A measure that relates body weight to height. BMI is sometimes used to measure total body fat and whether a person is a healthy weight. Excess body fat is linked to an increased risk of some diseases including heart disease and some cancers.

bone mineral density scan: see DEXA scan.

bronchoscopy: A procedure that uses a bronchoscope to examine the inside of the trachea, bronchi (air passages that lead to the lungs), and lungs. A bronchoscope is a thin, tube-like instrument with a light and a lens for viewing. It may also have a tool to remove tissue to be checked under a microscope for signs of disease.

cardiovascular: Having to do with the heart and blood vessels.

complete blood count (CBC): A test to check the number of red blood cells, white blood cells, and platelets in a sample of blood.

colonoscopy: Examination of the inside of the colon using a colonoscope, inserted into the rectum. A colonoscope is a thin, tube-like instrument with a light and a lens for viewing. It may also have a tool to remove tissue to be checked under a microscope for signs of disease.

computed tomography scan (CT): A series of detailed pictures of areas inside the body taken from different angles. The pictures are created by a computer linked to an X-ray machine. Also called computerized axial tomography (CAT) scan.

contrast material: A dye or other substance that helps show abnormal areas inside the body. It is given by injection into a vein, by enema, or by mouth. Contrast material may be used with X-rays, CT scans, magnetic resonance imaging (MRI), or other imaging tests.

cystoscopy: Examination of the bladder and urethra using a cystoscope, inserted into the urethra. A cystoscope is a thin, tube-like instrument with a light and a lens for viewing. It may also have a tool to remove tissue to be checked under a microscope for signs of disease.

deoxyribonucleic acid (DNA): The molecules inside cells that carry genetic information and pass it from one generation to the next.

DEXA scan: An imaging test that measures bone density (the amount of bone mineral contained in a certain volume of bone) by passing X-rays with two different energy levels through the bone. It is used to diagnose osteoporosis (decrease in bone mass and density). Also, called BMD scan, bone mineral density scan, DEXA, dual energy X-ray absorptiometric scan, dual X-ray absorptiometry, and DXA.

electrocardiogram (EKG): A line graph that shows changes in the electrical activity of the heart over time. It is made by an instrument called an electrocardiograph. The graph can show that there are ab-normal conditions, such as blocked arteries, changes in electrolytes (particles with electrical charges), and changes in the way electrical currents pass through the heart tissue.

electronic medical record: A collection of a patient's medical information in a digital (electronic) form that can be viewed on a computer and easily shared by people taking care of the patient.

endoscopic retrograde cholangiopancreatography (ERCP): A procedure that uses an endoscope to examine and X-ray the pancreatic duct, hepatic duct, common bile duct, duodenal papilla, and gallbladder. An endoscope is a thin, tube-like instrument with a light and a lens for viewing.

endoscopy: A procedure that uses an endoscope to examine the inside of the body. An endoscope is a thin, tube-like instrument with a light and a lens for viewing. It may also have a tool to remove tissue to be checked under a microscope for signs of disease.

false-positive test result: A test result that indicates that a person has a specific disease or condition when the person actually does not have the disease or condition.

fine-needle aspiration (FNA) biopsy: The removal of tissue or fluid with a thin needle for examination under a microscope.

fluoroscopy: An X-ray procedure that makes it possible to see internal organs in motion.

genetic counseling: A communication process between a specially trained health professional and a person concerned about the genetic risk of disease. The person's family and personal medical history may be discussed, and counseling may lead to genetic testing.

genetic testing: Analyzing DNA to look for a genetic alteration that may indicate an increased risk for developing a specific disease or disorder.

imaging: In medicine, a process that makes pictures of areas inside the body. Imaging uses methods such as X-rays (high-energy radiation), ultrasound (high-energy sound waves), and radio waves.

intravenous pyelogram: An X-ray image of the kidneys, ureters, and bladder. It is made after a substance that shows up on X-rays is injected into a blood vessel. The substance outlines the kidneys, ureters, and bladder as it flows through the system and collects in the urine. An intravenous pyelogram is usually made to look for a block in the flow of urine.

kidney function test: A test in which blood or urine samples are checked for the amounts of certain substances released by the kidneys. A higher- or lower-than-normal amount of a substance can be a sign that the kidneys are not working the way they should. Also, called renal function test.

laboratory test: A medical procedure that involves testing a sample of blood, urine, or other substance from the body. Tests can help determine a diagnosis, plan treatment, check to see if treatment is working, or monitor the disease over time.

lower gastrointestinal (GI) series: X-rays of the colon and rectum that are taken after a person is given a barium enema. lumbar puncture: A procedure in which a thin needle called a spinal needle is put into the lower part of the spinal column to collect cerebrospinal fluid or to give drugs. Also, called spinal tap.

lung function test: See pulmonary function test. magnetic resonance imaging: A procedure in which radio waves and a powerful magnet linked to a computer are used to create detailed pictures of areas inside the body. These pictures can show the difference between normal and diseased tissue. Magnetic resonance imaging makes better images of organs and soft tissue than other scanning techniques, such as computed tomography (CT) or X-ray. Magnetic resonance imaging is especially useful for imaging the brain, the spine, the soft tissue of joints, and the inside of bones. Also, called MRI, NMRI, and nuclear magnetic resonance imaging.

monitor: In medicine, to regularly watch and check a person or condition to see if there is any change. Also refers to a device that records and or displays patient data, such as for an electrocardiogram (EKG).

myelogram: An X-ray of the spinal cord after an injection of dye into the space between the lining of the spinal cord and brain.

nuclear magnetic resonance imaging: A procedure in which radio waves and a powerful magnet linked to a computer are used to create detailed pictures of areas inside the body. These pictures can show the difference between normal and diseased tissue. Nuclear magnetic resonance imaging is especially useful for imaging the brain, the spine, the soft tissue of joints, and the inside of bones.

optical coherence tomography: A procedure that uses infrared light waves to give three-dimensional (3-D) pictures of structures inside tissues and organs. The pictures are made by a computer linked to the light source.

Pap test: A procedure in which cells are scraped from the cervix for examination under a microscope. It is used to detect cancer and changes that may lead to cancer. Also, called Pap smear and Papanicolaou test.

pelvic exam: A physical examination in which the healthcare professional will feel for lumps or changes in the shape of the vagina, cervix, uterus, fallopian tubes, ovaries, and rectum. The healthcare professional will also use a speculum to open the vagina to look at the cervix and take samples for a Pap test. Also, called internal examination.

positron emission tomography (PET) scan: A procedure in which a small amount of radioactive glucose (sugar) is injected into a vein, and a scanner is used to make detailed, computerized pictures of areas inside the body where the glucose is used. Because cancer cells often use more glucose than normal cells, the pictures can be used to find cancer cells in the body.

positive test result: A test result that reveals the presence of a specific disease or condition for which the test is being done.

radiology: The use of radiation (such as X-rays) or other imaging technologies (such as ultrasound and magnetic resonance imaging) to diagnose or treat disease.

reference range: In medicine, a set of values that a doctor uses to interpret a patient's test results. The reference range for a given test is based on test results for 95% of the healthy population. The reference range for a test may be different for different groups of people (for example, men and women). Also, called normal range, reference interval, and reference values.

sigmoidoscopy: Examination of the lower colon using a sigmoidoscope, inserted into the rectum. A sigmoidoscope is a thin, tube-like instrument with a light and a lens for viewing. It may also have a tool to remove tissue to be checked under a microscope for signs of disease.

screening: Checking for disease when there are no symptoms. Since screening may find diseases at an early stage, there may be a better chance of curing the disease. Examples of cancer screening tests are the mammogram (breast), colonoscopy (colon), Pap smear (cervix), and PSA blood level and digital rectal exam (prostate). Screening can also include checking for a person's risk of developing an inherited disease by doing a genetic test.

sentinel lymph node biopsy: Removal and examination of the sentinel node(s) (the first lymph node(s) to which cancer cells are likely to spread from a primary tumor).

single photon emission computed tomography (SPECT): A special type of computed tomography (CT) scan in which a small amount of a radioactive drug is injected into a vein and a scanner is used to make detailed images of areas inside the body where the radioactive material is taken up by the cells. Single-photon emission computed tomography can give information about blood flow to tissues and chemical reactions (metabolism) in the body.

skin test: A test for an immune response to a compound by placing it on or under the skin. slit-lamp eye exam: An eye exam using an instrument that combines a low-power microscope with a light source that makes a narrow beam of light. The instrument may be used to examine the retina, optic nerve, and other parts of the eye. Also, called slit-lamp biomicroscopy.

sonogram: See ultrasound.

spiral CT scan: detailed picture of areas inside the body. The pictures are created by a computer linked to an X-ray machine that scans the body in a spiral path. Also, called helical computed tomography.

symptom: An indication that a person has a condition or disease. Some examples of symptoms are headache, fever, fatigue, nausea, vomiting, and pain.

ultrasound: A procedure in which high-energy sound waves are bounced off internal tissues or organs and make echoes. The echo patterns are shown on the screen of an ultrasound machine, forming a picture of body tissues called a sonogram. Also, called ultrasonography.

upper endoscopy: Examination of the inside of the stomach using an endoscope, passed through the mouth and esophagus. An endoscope is a thin, tube-like instrument with a light and a lens for viewing. It may also have a tool to remove tissue to be checked under a microscope for signs of disease. Also, called gastroscopy.

upper gastrointestinal (GI) series: A series of X-ray pictures of the esophagus, stomach, and duodenum (the first part of the small intestine). The X-ray pictures are taken after the patient drinks a liquid containing barium sulfate (a form of the silver-white metallic element barium). The barium sulfate coats and outlines the inner walls of the upper gastrointestinal tract so that they can be seen on the X-ray pictures.

ureteroscopy: Examination of the inside of the kidney and ureter, using a ureteroscope. A ureteroscope is a thin, tube-like instrument with a light and a lens for viewing. It may also have a tool to remove tissue to be checked under a microscope for signs of disease. The ureteroscope is passed through the urethra into the bladder, ureter, and renal pelvis (part of the kidney that collects, holds, and drains urine).

urinalysis: A test that determines the content of the urine.

venous sampling: A procedure in which a sample of blood is taken from a certain vein and checked for specific substances released by nearby organs and tissues.

virtual colonoscopy: A method to examine the inside of the colon by taking a series of X-rays. A computer is used to make 2-dimensional (2-D) and 3-D pictures of the colon from these X-rays. The pictures can be saved, changed to give better viewing angles, and reviewed after the procedure, even years later. Also, called computed tomographic colonography, computed tomography colonography, CT colonography, and CTC.

X-ray: A type of high-energy radiation. In low doses, X-rays are used to diagnose diseases by making pictures of the inside of the body. In high doses, X-rays are used to treat cancer.

Chapter 60

Online Health Screening Tools

Alcoholism, Drug Dependence, and Addictions

About My Drinking and Other Drug Use
Hazelden
Website: http://www.aboutmydrinking.org

Drug Abuse Screening Test (DAST)
Project Cork Online
Website: http://www.projectcork.org/clinical_tools/html/DAST.html

Food Addiction
Addicted.com
Website: http://addicted.com/self-tests/food-addiction/

Tobacco Dependence
Addicted.com
Website: http://addicted.com/self-tests/tobacco-addiction/

Resources in this chapter were compiled from several sources deemed reliable; all contact information was verified and updated in September 2015. Inclusion does not imply endorsement. This list is not comprehensive, it is intended as a starting point for gathering of information. Discuss findings and questions with your health care provider.

Auditory

*Hearing Test, Environmental Sounds, and Simulated
Hearing Loss*
Freehearingtest.com
Website: http://www.freehearingtest.com/test.shtml

Sensitivity, equal loudness contours and audiometry
University New South Wales
Website: http://www.freehearingtest.com/test.shtml

Autism

Quick Test
Iautistic
Website: http://iautistic.com/free-autism-tests.php

Milestone Checklist
Centers for Disease Control and Prevention
Website: http://www.cdc.gov/ncbddd/actearly/milestones

AQ Test (Adult Autism)
Autism Research Centre
Website: http://www.wired.com/wired/archive/9.12/aqtest.html

Bone and Joint Risk Assessments

Osteoporosis Risk Questionnaire
Washington University School of Medicine: Your Disease Risk
Website: http://www.yourdiseaserisk.wustl.edu/hccpquiz.
pl?lang=english&func=home&quiz=osteoporosis

Joint Disorders Risk Assessment
Trinity Iowa Health System
Website: https://ha.healthawareservices.com/ra/survey/730

Spine and Back Risk Assessment
Trinity Iowa Health System
Website: https://ha.healthawareservices.com/ra/survey/733

Cancer Risk Assessments

Risk for Developing Bladder Cancer
Washington University School of Medicine: Your Disease Risk
Website: http://www.yourdiseaserisk.wustl.edu/hccpquiz.
pl?lang=english&func=home&quiz=bladder

Risk Assessment for Developing Breast Cancer
Washington University School of Medicine: Your Disease Risk
Website: http://www.yourdiseaserisk.wustl.edu/hccpquiz.
pl?lang=english&func=home&quiz=breast

Breast Cancer Risk Assessment Tool
National Cancer Institute
Website: http://www.cancer.gov/bcrisktool/Default.aspx

Risk Assessment for Developing Cervical Cancer
Washington University School of Medicine: Your Disease Risk
Website: http://www.yourdiseaserisk.wustl.edu/hccpquiz.
pl?lang=english&func=home&quiz=cervical

Risk Assessment for Developing Colon Cancer
Washington University School of Medicine: Your Disease Risk
Website: http://www.yourdiseaserisk.wustl.edu/hccpquiz.
pl?lang=english&func=home&quiz=colon

Risk Assessment for Developing Kidney Cancer
Washington University School of Medicine: Your Disease Risk
Website: http://www.yourdiseaserisk.wustl.edu/hccpquiz.
pl?lang=english&func=home&quiz=kidney

Risk Assessment for Developing Lung Cancer
Washington University School of Medicine: Your Disease Risk
Website: http://www.yourdiseaserisk.wustl.edu/hccpquiz.
pl?lang=english&func=home&quiz=lung

Lung Cancer Prediction Tool for Long-Term Smokers
Memorial Sloan-Kettering Cancer Center
Website: http://www.mskcc.org/mskcc/html/12463.cfm

Risk Assessment for Developing Melanoma Cancer
Washington University School of Medicine: Your Disease Risk
Website: http://www.yourdiseaserisk.wustl.edu/hccpquiz.
pl?lang=english&func=home&quiz=melanoma

Risk Assessment for Developing Ovarian Cancer
Washington University School of Medicine: Your Disease Risk
Website: http://www.yourdiseaserisk.wustl.edu/hccpquiz.
pl?lang=english&func=home&quiz=ovarian

Risk Assessment for Developing Pancreatic Cancer
Washington University School of Medicine: Your Disease Risk
Website: http://www.yourdiseaserisk.wustl.edu/hccpquiz.
pl?lang=english&func=home&quiz=pancreatic

Prostate Cancer Prevention Trial Prostate Cancer Risk Calculator (PCPTRC)
UT Health Science Center–San Antonio
Website: http://deb.uthscsa.edu/URORiskCalc/Pages/uroriskcalc.jsp

Risk Assessment for Developing Stomach Cancer
Washington University School of Medicine: Your Disease Risk
Website: http://www.yourdiseaserisk.wustl.edu/hccpquiz.
pl?lang=english&func=home&quiz=stomach

Risk Assessment for Developing Uterine Cancer
Washington University School of Medicine: Your Disease Risk
Website: http://www.yourdiseaserisk.wustl.edu/hccpquiz.
pl?lang=english&func=home&quiz=uterine

Diabetes and Kidney Disease Risk

Risk Assessment for Developing Diabetes
Washington University School of Medicine: Your Disease Risk
Website: http://www.yourdiseaserisk.wustl.edu/hccpquiz.
pl?lang=english&func=home&quiz=diabetes

Diabetes Risk Test
American Diabetes Association
Website: http://www.diabetes.org/diabetes-basics/prevention/
diabetes-risk-test

Diabetes Risk Score
Diabetes UK
Website: http://www.diabetes.org.uk/riskscore

GFR Calculators for Adults and Children
National Kidney Disease Educational Program
Website: http://www.nkdep.nih.gov/professionals/gfr_calculators

Heart Attack Risk, Heart Disease Risk, and Arterial Age Risk

Heart Disease Risk Calculator
American College of Cardiology
Website: http://www.cardiosmart.org/CardioSmart/Default.
aspx?id=298

Heart Attack Risk Assessment
American Heart Association
Website: http://www.heart.org/HEARTORG/Conditions/
HeartAttack/HeartAttackToolsResources/Heart-Attack-Risk-
Assessment_UCM_303944_Article.jsp

My Life Check: State of Your Heart
American Heart Association
Website: http://mylifecheck.heart.org/PledgePage.
aspx?NavID=5&CultureCode=en-US

Coronary Artery Calcium (CAC) Score Reference Values
University of Washington
Website: http://www.mesa-nhlbi.org/CACReference.aspx

Infectious Disease Risk Assessment

Assess Your Risk for HIV and Other Similarly Transmitted Diseases
Body Health Resources Foundation
Website: http://www.thebody.com/surveys/sexsurvey.html

Malaria Risk Assessment
Centers for Disease Control and Prevention (CDC)
Website: http://www.cdc.gov/malaria/travelers/risk_assessment.html

Mental Health Risk Assessments

Adult Self-Report Scale-V1.1 (ASRS-V1.1) Screener for ADHD
World Health Organization (WHO)
Website: http://webdoc.nyumc.org/nyumc/files/psych/attachments/
psych_adhd_screener.pdf

Adult ADHD Self-Report Scale (ASRS-v1.1)
New York University Medical Center
Website: http://webdoc.nyumc.org/nyumc/files/psych/attachments/
psych_adhd_checklist.pdf

Anxiety Screening Test
New York University (NYU) Langone Medical Center
Website: http://www.med.nyu.edu/psych/patient-care/
screening-tests/anxiety-screening-test

Goldburg Bipolar Screening Quiz
Psych Central
Website: http://psychcentral.com/quizzes/bipolarquiz.htm

Stress Screener
Mental Health America
Website: http://www.mentalhealthamerica.net/llw/stressquiz.html

Pregnancy

Online Pregnancy Test
Live Pregnancy Test
Website: http://www.livepregnancytest.com/pregnancytest

Online Pregnancy Due Date Calculator
Live Pregnancy Test
Website: http://www.livepregnancytest.com/duedate

Ovulation Calendar
Live Pregnancy Test
Website: http://www.livepregnancytest.com/ovulation

Radiation Exposure Risk

RADAR Medical Procedure Radiation Dose Calculator
doseinfo-radar
Website: http://www.doseinfo-radar.com/RADARDoseRiskCalc.html

Sexual Health

Sexual Disorders Screening Test for Men
New York University (NYU) Langone Medical Center
Website: http://www.med.nyu.edu/psych/patient-care/
screening-tests/sexual-disorders-screening-test-men

Sexual Disorders Screening Test for Women
New York University (NYU) Langone Medical Center
Website: http://www.med.nyu.edu/psych/patient-care/
screening-tests/sexual-disorders-screening-test-women

Sleep

Sleep Risk Assessment
Trinity Iowa Health System
Website: https://ha.healthawareservices.com/ra/survey/1138

Stroke

Stroke Risk Questionnaire
Washington University School of Medicine: Your Disease Risk
Website: http://www.yourdiseaserisk.wustl.edu/hccpquiz.
pl?lang=english&func=home&quiz=stroke

Visual Tests

Color Vision Tests
Sight and Hearing Association
Website: http://www.freevisiontest.com/colortest.php

Near Vision Test for Adults
Prevent Blindness America
Website: http://www.preventblindness.org/eye_tests/near_vision_
test.html

Distance Vision Test for Adults
Prevent Blindness America
Website: http://www.preventblindness.org/eye_tests/Adult_distance_
test.html

Self Vision Screening Tests
Sight and Hearing Association
Website: http://www.freevisiontest.com/selfvision.php

Weight Risk

Weight Assessment
Trinity Iowa Health System
Website: https://ha.healthawareservices.com/ra/survey/484

Body Mass Index Calculator
National, Heart, Lung, and Blood Institute (NHLBI)
Website: http://www.nhlbi.nih.gov/health/educational/lose_wt/BMI/bmicalc.htm

Chapter 61

Directory of Breast and Cervical Cancer Early Detection Programs

Alabama
Breast and Cervical Cancer Early Detection Program, Bureau of Family Health Services, AL Dept. of Public Health
P.O. Box 303017
Montgomery, AL 36130
Toll-Free: 877-252-3324
Phone: 334-206-5851
Fax: 334-206-2950
Website: http://www.adph.org/earlydetection

Alaska
Breast and Cervical Health Check Division of Public Health Section of Women's, Children's and Family Health
3601 C St.
Ste. 322
Anchorage, AK 99503
Toll-Free: 800-410-6266
Phone: 907-269-3476
Fax: 907-269-3414
Website:http://dhss.alaska.gov/dph/wcfh/Pages/bchc/default.aspx

Resources in this chapter were excerpted from: "National Breast and Cervical Cancer Early Detection Program: State, U.S. Territory and Organization Program Contacts," Centers for Disease Control and Prevention (CDC). All contact information was verified and updated in September 2015.

American Samoa
Breast and Cervical Cancer
Early Detection Program
Department of Health American
Samoa Government Territory of
American Samoa
Pago Pago, AS 96799
Phone: 684-633-2135
Fax: 684-633-2136

Arizona
Well Woman Healthcheck
Program Bureau of Chronic
Disease Prevention and Control
Arizona Department of Health
Services
1740 W Adams
No. 205
Phoenix, AZ 85007
Toll-Free: 888-257-8502
Fax: 602-542-7520
http://azdhs.gov/hsd/
healthcheck/wellwoman

Arkansas
BreastCare, AR Dept. of Health
4815 W. Markham St.
Slot 11
Little Rock, AR 72205
Toll-Free: 877-670-2273
Website: http://www.healthy
.arkansas.gov/programsServices/
chronicDisease/ArBreastCare

California
Cancer Detection Programs:
Every Woman Counts Cancer
Detection and Treatment Branch
California Department of Health
Services, MS-4600
P.O. Box 997417
Sacramento
Toll-Free: 800-511-2300
Phone: 916-449-5300
Fax: 916-440-5310
www.dhcs.ca.gov/services/
Cancer/ewc/Pages/default.aspx

Colorado
Women's Wellness Connection
Colorado Department of Public
Health and Environment
4300 Cherry Creek Dr S
Denver, CO 80246
Toll-Free: 866-951-9355
Phone: 303-692-2511
Fax: 303-758-3268
https://www.colorado.gov/cdphe/
womens-wellness-connection

*Commonwealth of Northern
Mariana Islands*
Department of Public Health
Breast and Cervical Cancer
Screening Program
P.O. Box 500409
Saipan, MP 96950
Phone: 670-236-8703
Fax: 670-236-8700

Connecticut

Breast and Cervical Cancer
Program, CT Dept. of Public
Health
410 Capitol Ave.
MS Ste. 11CCS
Hartford, CT 06106
Phone: 860-509-7804; or
860-509-8000
Website: http://www.ct.gov/dph/
cwp/view.asp?a=3124&q=388824
&dphPNavCtr=l 47735 l#47737

Delaware

Screening for Life, Div. of Public
Health, DE Dept. of Health and
Social Services
417 Federal St., Jesse Cooper
Bldg.
Dover, DE 19901
Toll-Free: 800-464-4357
Phone: 302-744-4700
Fax: 302-739-6659
Website: http://www.dhss
.delaware.gov/dph/dpc/sfl.html

District of Columbia

Breast and Cervical Cancer
Early Detection Program
District of Columbia Department
of Health
899 N Capitol St, N.E.
Washington, DC 20002
Phone: 202-442-5900
Fax: 202-442-4825
http://doh.dc.gov/node/114122

Florida

Breast and Cervical Cancer
Early Detection Program Bureau
of Chronic Disease Prevention
Florida Department of Health
4052 Bald Cypress Way
Bin Ste. A-18
Tallahassee, FL 32399
Toll-Free: 800-227-2345
Phone: 850-245-4444
Fax: 850-414-6625
http://www.floridahealth.gov/
diseases-and-conditions/cancer/
breast-cancer/bccedp.html

Georgia

Breast and Cervical Cancer
Program (BCCP) Office of
Cancer Prevention, Screening,
and Treatment Health
Promotion and Disease
Prevention Program Georgia
Department of Public Health
2 Peachtree St. N.W., Rm 16-304
Atlanta, GA 30303
Phone: 404-657-7735
http://dph.georgia.gov/BCCP

Guam

Breast and Cervical Cancer
Early Detection Program
Division of Public Health
Department of Public Health
and Social Services
123 Chalan Kareta, Route 10
Mangilao, GU 96913
Phone: 671-735-0671
Fax: 671-734-7626
http://www.dphss.guam.gov/
content/breast-and-cervical-
cancer-early-detection-program

Hawaii

Hawaii Breast and Cervical
Cancer Program Breast and
Cervical Cancer Control
Program Hawaii State
Department of Health
601 Kamokila Blvd., Ste. 344
Kapolei, HI 96707
Phone: 808-692-7460
Fax: 808-692-7478
http://health.hawaii.gov

Idaho

Women's Health Check, Division
of Health, ID Dept. of Health
and Welfare
450 W. State St., 4th Fl.
P.O. Box 83720
Boise, ID 83720
Toll-Free in ID: 800-926-2588
ID Care Line: 211
ID Care Line: 211
Phone: 208-332-7311
Fax: 208-334-0657
Website: http://
healthandwelfare.idaho.gov/
Health/DiseasesConditions/
Cancer/WomensHealthCheck/
tabid/255/Default.aspx

Illinois

Illinois Breast and Cervical
Cancer Program Office of
Women's Health Services Illinois
Department of Public Health
535 W Jefferson St. 1st Fl.
Springfield, IL 62761
Toll-Free: 888-522-1282
Phone: 217-785-1050
Fax: 217-557-3326
http://dph.illinois.gov/topics-
services/life-stages-populations/
womens-health-services/ibccp

Indiana

Breast and Cervical Cancer
Early Detection Program, IN
State Dept. of Health
2 N. Meridian St.
Mailstop 6B-F4
Indianapolis, IN 46204
Toll-Free: 800-433-0746
Phone: 317-233-7405
Fax: 317-234-2275
Website: http://www.in.gov/
isdh/24967.htm

Iowa

Care for Yourself, Iowa Breast
and Cervical Cancer Early
Detection Program, IA Dept. of
Public Health
321 E. 12th St.
Des Moines, IA 50319
Toll-Free: 800-369-2229
Toll-Free TTY: 800-735-2942
Phone: 515-281-7689
Website: http://www.idph.state
.ia.us/careforyourself

Kansas

Early Detection Works, KS Dept.
of Health and Environment,
State Office Bldg.
1000 S.W. Jackson
Ste. 230
Topeka, KS 66612
Toll-Free: 877-277-1368
Phone: 785-296-1207
Fax: 785-368-7287
Website: http://www.kdheks.gov/
edw

Kentucky

Women's Cancer Screening
Program
275 E. Main St.
HS1WF
Frankfort, KY 40621
Toll-Free: 800-422-6237
Phone: 502-564-3236
Fax: 502-564-1552
Website: http://chfs.ky.gov/dph/
info/dwh/cancerscreening.htm

Louisiana

Louisiana Breast and Cervical
Health Program Louisiana State
University Health Sciences
Center School of Public Health
1615 Poydras St.
Ste. 1400
New Orleans, LA 70112
Toll-Free: 888-599-1073
Fax: 504-568-5838

Maine

Breast and Cervical Health
Program Maine Center for
Disease Control and Prevention/
DHHS
286 Water St. Key Bank Plaza,
4th Fl.
11 State House Station
Augusta, ME 04333
Toll-Free: 800-350-5180
Phone: 207-287-8068
Fax: 207-287-4100
http://www.maine.gov/dhhs/
mecdc/population-health/bcp/
index.htm

Maryland

Breast and Cervical Cancer
Screening Program Center for
Cancer Surveillance and Control
Maryland Department of Health
and Mental Hygiene
201 W Preston St. 3rd Fl.
Baltimore, MD 21201
Toll-Free: 800477-9774
Fax: 410-333-7279
http://phpa.dhmh.maryland.gov/
cancer/SitePages/bccp_home.
aspx

Massachusetts

Women's Health Network
Massachusetts Department of
Health
250 Washington St., 4th Fl.
Boston, MA 02108
Toll-Free: 877-414-4447
Phone: 617-624-5441
Fax: 617-624-5055
http://www.mass.gov/eohhs/gov/
departments/dph

Michigan

Breast and Cervical Cancer
Control Program, MI Dept. of
Community Health, Capitol
View Bldg.
201 Townsend St.
Lansing, MI 48913
Toll-Free: 800-922-6266
Toll-Free TTY: 800-649-3777
Phone: 517-373-3740
Website: http://www.michigan
.gov/mdch/1,1607,7-132-
2940_2955-13487--,00.html

Minnesota
SAGE Screening Program, MN
Dept. of Health
85 E. 7th Pl.
P.O. Box 64882
St. Paul, MN 55164
Toll-Free: 888-643-2584
TTY: 651-201-5797
Phone: 651-201-5000
Website: http://www.health.state.
mn.us/divs/hpcd/ccs/screening/
sage

Mississippi
Breast and Cervical Cancer
Early Detection Program, MS
State Dept. of Health
570 E. Woodrow Wilson
P.O. Box 1700
Jackson, MS 39215
Toll-Free: 800-721-7222
Phone: 601-576-7466
Website: http://msdh.ms.gov/
msdhsite/_static/41,0,103.html

Missouri
Show Me Healthy Women
Program, MO Dept. of Health
and Senior Services
P.O. Box 570
Jefferson City, MO 65102
Phone: 573-522-2845
Fax: 573-522-2899
Website: http://health.mo.gov/
living/healthcondiseases/chronic/
showmehealthywomen
E-mail: info@health.mo.gov

Montana
Breast and Cervical Health
Program Montana Department
of Public Health and Human
Services Cogswell Building
1400 Broadway, C-317
P.O. Box 202951
Helena, MT 59620
Toll-Free: 888-803-9343
Phone: 406-444-0063
Fax: 406-444-7465
http://dphhs.mt.gov/
publichealth/cancer

Nebraska
Every Woman Matters Program
Office of Women's Health
Nebraska Health and Human
Services
301 Centennial Mall S 3rd Fl.
P.O. Box 94817
Lincoln, NE 68509
Toll-Free: 800-532-2227
Phone: 402-471-0314
Fax: 402-471-0913
http://dhhs.ne.gov/publichealth/
Pages/womenshealth_ewm.aspx

Nevada
Women's Health Connection
Access to Healthcare Network
4001 S Virginia St
Ste. F
Reno, NV 89502
Toll-Free: 877-385-2345
Phone: 775-284-8989
Fax: 775-284-8991

New Hampshire

Breast and Cervical Cancer
Program, NH Dept. of Health
and Human Services
129 Pleasant St.
Concord, NH 03301
Toll-Free in NH: 800-852-3345
ext. 4931
Phone: 603-271-4886
Fax: 603-271-0539
Website: http://www.dhhs.nh.gov/
dphs/cdpc/bccp

New Jersey

Cancer Education and Early
Detection Program, NJ Dept. of
Health and Senior Services
50 E. State St.
6th Fl., P.O. Box 364
Trenton, NJ 08625
Toll-Free: 800-328-3838
Phone: 609-292-8540
Fax: 609-588-3638
Website: http://www.state.nj.us/
health/cancer/njceed

New Mexico

Breast and Cervical Cancer
Early Detection Program New
Mexico Department of Health
5301 Central Ave N.E.
Ste. 800
Albuquerque, NM 87108
Toll-Free: 877-852-2585
Phone: 505-841-5860
Fax: 505-222-8602
http://nmhealth.org/about/phd/
cdb/bcc/

New York

Cancer Services Program,
Bureau of Chronic Disease
Services, NY State Dept. of
Health
Riverview Ctr.
Ste. 350
Albany, NY 12204
Toll-Free: 866-442-2262
Phone: 518-474-1222
Fax: 518-473-0642
Website: http://www.state.nj.us/
health/cancer/njceed
E-mail: canserv@health.state
.ny.us

North Carolina

Breast and Cervical Cancer
Control Program
1922 Mail Service Ctr.
Raleigh, NC 27699
Phone: 919-707-5300
Fax: 919-870-4812
Website: http://www.bcccp
.ncdhhs.gov

North Dakota

Women's Way, Div. of Cancer
Prevention and Control, ND
Dept. of Health
600 E. Blvd. Ave.
Dept. 301
Bismarck, ND 58505
Toll-Free in ND: 800-449-6636
Phone: 701-328-2333
Website: http://www.ndhealth
.gov/womensway
E-mail: womensway@nd.gov

Ohio

Breast and Cervical Cancer
Project, OH Dept. of Health
246 N. High St.
Columbus, OH 43215
Phone: 614-728-2177
Fax: 614-564-2409
Website: http://www.odh.ohio
.gov/odhPrograms/hprr/bc_canc/
bcanc1.aspx
E-mail: BHPRR@odh.ohio.gov

Oklahoma

Breast and Cervical Cancer
Early Detection Program
Oklahoma State Department of
Health
1000 N.E. 10th St.
Oklahoma City, OK 73117
Toll-Free: 888-669-5934
Phone: 405-271-4072
Fax: 405-271-6315
http://www.ok.gov/health/
Disease,_Prevention,_
Preparedness/Chronic_
Disease_Service/
Cancer_Prevention_Programs_/
Take_Charge,_Oklahoma%27s_
Breast_and_Cervical_Cancer_
Early_Detection_Program/

Oregon

Breast and Cervical Cancer
Program Office of Family Health
Oregon Department of Human
Services
800 N.E. Oregon St.
Ste. 370
Portland, OR 97232
Toll-Free: 877-255-7070
Phone: 971-673-0581
Fax: 971-673-0997
http://public.health.oregon.
gov/HealthyPeopleFamilies/
Women/HealthScreening/
BreastCervicalCancerScreening/
Pages/index.aspx

Pennsylvania

Healthy Woman Program
Pennsylvania Department of
Health
Rm 1011 Health and Welfare
Bldg.
Harrisburg, PA 17120
Toll-Free: 800-215-7494
Fax: 717-772-0608
http://www.portal.state.pa.us/
portal/server.pt/community/
healthy_women/14172/
healthywoman_program_
home/557855

Puerto Rico

Breast and Cervical Cancer
Early Detection Program
University of Puerto Rico
Comprehensive Cancer Center
Medical Sciences Campus
P.O. Box 70344 PMB 371
San Juan, PR 00936
Phone: 787-772-8300
Fax: 787-767-8008

Republic of Palau

Breast and Cervical Cancer
Early Detection Program
Republic of Palau Ministry of
Health
P.O. Box 6027
Koror, PW 96940
Phone: 680-488-4612
Fax: 680-488-1211

Rhode Island

Women's Cancer Screening
Program, RI Cancer Control
Program, RI Dept. of Health
3 Capitol Hill
Providence, RI 02908
Health Information Line:
401-222-4324
Health Information Line:
401-222-4324
Website: http://www.
health.ri.gov/programs/
womenscancerscreening

South Carolina

Best Chance Network Division of
Cancer Prevention and Control
Bureau of Chronic Disease
Prevention, DHEC
1800 St. Julian Pl.
Columbia, SC 29204
Toll-Free: 800-227-2345
Phone: 803-898-1602
Fax: 803-545-4445

South Dakota

All Women Count! South Dakota
Department of Health
615 E 4th St.
Pierre, SD 57501
Toll-Free: 800-738-2301
605-773-5728
Fax: 605-773-8104

Tennessee

Breast and Cervical Cancer
Early Detection Program
Tennessee Department of Health
Cordell Hull Bldg., 6th Fl. 425
5th Ave N
Nashville, TN 37247
Toll-Free: 877-969-6636
Fax: 615-741-3806
http://tn.gov/health

Texas

Breast and Cervical Cancer
Services, TX Dept. of State
Health Services, Preventive and
Primary Care Unit
1100 W. 49th St.
MC 1923, P.O. Box 149347
Austin, TX 78714
Phone: 512-458-7796
Fax: 512-458-7203
Website: http://www.dshs.state
.tx.us/bcccs
E-mail: BCCSprogram@dshs.
state.tx.us

Utah

Utah Cancer Control Program,
Bureau of Health Promotion, UT
Dept. of Health
288 N. 1460 W.
P.O. Box 141010
Salt Lake City, UT 84114
Toll-Free: 800-717-1811
Website: http://www.cancerutah.
org

Vermont

Ladies First, VT Dept. of Health
108 Cherry St.
P.O. Box 70, Drawer 38 (LF)
Burlington, VT 05402
Toll-Free: 800-508-2222
Toll-Free TDD: 800-319-3141
Phone: 802-863-7330
Website: http://healthvermont
.gov/prevent/ladies_first.aspx

Virginia

Every Woman's Life Virginia
Department of Health
109 Governor St., 8th Fl.
Richmond, VA 23219
Toll-Free: 866-395-4968
Phone: 804-864-8204
Fax: 804-864-7763
http://www.vdh.virginia.gov/ofhs/
prevention/ewl/

Washington

Breast, Cervical and Colon
Health Program Washington
State Department of Health
111 Israel Rd., Town Center 2,
3rd Fl.
Tumwater, WA 98501
Toll-Free: 888-438-2247
Phone: 360-236-3672
Fax: 360-664-2619
http://www.doh.wa.gov/
YouandYourFamily/
IllnessandDisease/Cancer/
BreastCervicalandColonHealth

West Virginia

Breast and Cervical Cancer
Screening Program, WV Dept. of
Health and Human Resources
350 Capital St.
Rm. 427
Charleston, WV 25301
Toll-Free in WV: 800-642-8522
Phone: 304-558-5388
Fax: 304-558-7164
Website: http://www.wvdhhr.org/
bccsp

Wisconsin

Well Woman Program, Div.
of Public Health, WI Dept. of
Health Services
1 W. Wilson St.
Rm. 218, P.O. Box 2659
Madison, WI 53701
TTY: 888-701-1251
Phone: 608-261-6872
Website: http://www.dhs.
wisconsin.gov/womenshealth/
wwwp

Wyoming

Breast and Cervical Cancer
Early Detection Program,
Preventive Health and Safety
Div., WY Dept. of Health
6101 Yellowstone Rd.
Ste. 510
Cheyenne, WY 82002
Toll-Free: 800-264-1296
Phone: 307-777-7172
Fax: 307-777-5402
Website: http://www.health.wyo.
gov/PHSD/bccedp

Chapter 62

Organizations with Resources for People Undergoing Medical Tests

Government Organizations

Agency for Healthcare Research and Quality (AHRQ)
540 Gaither Rd.
Rockville, MD 20850
Toll-Free: 800-358-9295
Phone: 301-427-1364
Website: http://www.ahrq.gov

Center for Biologics Evaluation and Research (CBER)
Consumer Affairs Branch
(CBER)
1401 Rockville Pike
Ste. 200N/HFM-47
Rockville, MD 20852
Toll-Free: 800-835-4709
Phone: 301-827-1800
Website: http://www.fda.gov/
BiologicsBloodVaccines/default
.htm

Resources in this chapter were compiled from several sources deemed reliable; all contact information was verified and updated in September 2015.

Centers for Disease Control and Prevention (CDC)
1600 Clifton Rd.
Atlanta, GA 30333
Toll-Free: 800-CDC-INFO (232-4636)
Toll-Free TTY: 888-232-6348
Website: http://www.cdc.gov
E-mail: cdcinfo@cdc.gov

Centers for Medicare and Medicaid Services
7500 Security Blvd.
Baltimore, MD 21244
Toll-Free: 800-633-4227
Toll-Free TTY: 877-486-2048
Website: http://www.cms.hhs.gov

FDA Center for Devices and Radiological Health (CDRH)
Website: http://www.fda.gov/ MedicalDevices/default.htm

FDA MedWatch
Toll-Free: 800-FDA-1088
Website: http://www.fda.gov/ Safety/MedWatch

Federal Trade Commission (FTC)
Consumer Response Center
600 Pennsylvania Ave., N.W.
Washington, DC 20850
Toll-Free: 877-FTC-HELP (382-4357)
Toll-Free TTY: 866-653-4261
Phone: 202-326-2222
Website: http://www.ftc.gov

National Breast and Cervical Cancer Early Detection Program
Toll-Free: 800-232-4636
Toll-Free TTY: 888-232-6348
Website: http://www.cdc.gov/ cancer/nbccedp

National Cancer Institute (NCI)
NCI Public Inquiries Office
6116 Executive Blvd.
Rm. 3036A
Bethesda, MD 20892
Toll-Free: 800-4-CANCER (800-422-6237)
Website: http://www.cancer.gov

National Diabetes Education Program
1 Diabetes Way
Bethesda, MD 20814
Toll-Free: 888-693-NDEP (6337)
Toll-Free TTY: 866-569-1162
Fax: 703-738-4929
Website: http://www.ndep.nih .gov
E-mail: ndep@mail.nih.gov

National Eye Institute
31 Center Dr.
MSC 2510
Bethesda, MD 20892
Phone: 301-496-5248
Website: http://www.nei.nih.gov/ index.asp
E-mail: 2020@nei.nih.gov

National Institute of Diabetes and Digestive and Kidney Diseases (NIDDK)
Bldg. 31, Rm. 9A06, 31 Center Dr.
MSC 2560
Bethesda, MD 20892
Phone: 301-496-3583
Website: http://www2.niddk.nih
.gov

National Institute of Mental Health (NIMH)
6001 Executive Blvd.
Rm. 8184, MSC 9663
Bethesda, MD 20892
Toll-Free: 866-615-6464
Toll-Free TTY: 866-415-8051
TTY: 301-443-8431
Phone: 301-443-4513
Fax: 301-443-4279
Website: http://www.nimh.nih .gov
E-mail: nimhinfo@nih.gov

National Institute of Neurological Disorders and Stroke (NINDS)
P.O. Box 5801
Bethesda, MD 20894
Toll-Free: 800-352-9424
TTY: 301-468-5981
Phone: 301-496-5751
Website: http://www.ninds.nih .gov

National Institute on Aging (NIA)
Bldg. 31, Rm. 5C27, 31 Center Dr.
MSC 2292
Bethesda, MD 20892
Toll-Free: 800-222-2225
Toll-Free TTY: 800-222-4225
Phone: 301-496-1752
Fax: 301-496-1072
Website: http://www.nia.nih.gov

National Institute on Deafness and Other Communication Disorders (NIDCD)
Information Clearinghouse
1 Communication Ave.
Bethesda, MD 20892
Toll-Free: 800-241-1044
Toll-Free TTY: 800-241-1055
Fax: 301-770-8977
Website: http://www.nidcd.nih
.gov
E-mail: nidcdinfo@nidcd.nih.gov

National Library of Medicine (NLM)
8600 Rockville Pike
Bethesda, MD 20894
Toll-Free: 888-346-3656
Phone: 301-594-5983
Fax: 301-402-1384
Website: http://www.nlm.nih.gov

Substance Abuse and Mental Health Services Administration (SAMHSA)
P.O. Box 2345
Rockville, MD 20847
Toll-Free: 877-SAMHSA-7
(877-726-4727)
Toll-Free TTY: 800-487-4889
Fax: 240-221-4292
Website: http://www.samhsa.gov
E-mail: SAMHSAinfo@samhsa
.hhs.gov

U.S. Department of Health and Human Services
200 Independence Ave., S.W.
Washington, DC 20201
Toll-Free: 877-696-6775
Website: http://www.hhs.gov

U.S. Food and Drug Administration (FDA)
10903 New Hampshire Ave.
Silver Spring, MD 20993
Toll-Free: 888-INFO-FDA
(463-6332)
Website: http://www.fda.gov

U.S. Preventive Services Task Force (USPSTF)
540 Gaither Rd.
Rockville, MD 20850
Website: http://www.
uspreventiveservicestaskforce
.org

Private Organizations

American Academy of Allergy, Asthma, and Immunology
555 E. Wells St.
Ste. 1100
Milwaukee, WI 53202
Phone: 414-272-6071
Website: http://www.aaaai.org
E-mail: info@aaaai.org

American Academy of Family Physicians
11400 Tomahawk Crk. Pkwy.
Leawood, KS 66211
Toll-Free: 800-274-2237
Phone: 913-906-6000
Fax: 913-906-6075
Website: http://www.aafp.org
E-mail: contactcenter@aafp.org

American Academy of Pediatrics
141 N.W. Point Blvd.
Elk Grove Village, IL 60007
Phone: 847-434-4000
Fax: 847-434-8000
Website: http://www.aap.org
E-mail: kidsdocs@aap.org

American College of Physicians
American Society of Internal Medicine
190 N. Independence Mall W.
Philadelphia, PA 19106
Toll-Free: 800-523-1546
Phone: 215-351-2600
Website: http://www.acponline.org

American Association of Neurological Surgeons
5550 Meadowbrook Dr.
Rolling Meadows, IL 60008
Toll-Free: 888-566-AANS (2267)
Phone: 847-378-0500
Fax: 847-378-0600
Website: http://www.aans.org
E-mail: info@aans.org

American Cancer Society
Toll-Free: 800-227-2345
Toll-Free TTY: 866-228-4327
Website: http://www.cancer.org

American College of Radiology
1891 Preston White Dr.
Reston, VA 20191
Toll-Free: 800-227-5463
Phone: 703-648-8900
Website: http://www.acr.org
E-mail: info@acr.org

American Diabetes Association
1701 N. Beauregard St.
Alexandria, VA 22311
Toll-Free: 800-DIABETES
(342-2383)
Website: http://www.diabetes.org
E-mail: AskADA@diabetes.org

American Gastroenterological Association
4930 Del Ray Ave.
Bethesda, MD 20814
Phone: 301-654-2055
Fax: 301-654-5920
Website: http://www.gastro.org
E-mail: member@gastro.org

American Heart Association
7272 Greenville Ave.
Dallas, TX 75231
Toll-Free: 800-242-8721
Website: http://www.heart.org

American Kidney Fund
6110 Executive Blvd.
Ste. 1010
Rockville, MD 20852
Toll-Free: 800-638-8299
Website: http://www.kidneyfund.org
E-mail: helpline@kidneyfund.org

American Society of Echocardiography
2100 Gateway Centre Blvd.
Ste. 310
Morrisville, NC 27560
Phone: 919-861-5574
Fax: 919-882-9900
Website: http://www.asecho.org

American Society of Radiologic Technologists
15000 Central Ave. SE
Albuquerque, NM 87123
Toll-Free: 800-444-2778
Phone: 505-298-4500
Fax: 505-298-5063
Website: http://www.asrt.org
E-mail: memberservices@asrt.org

American Speech-Language-Hearing Association
2200 Research Blvd.
Rockville, MD 20850
Toll-Free: 800-638-8255
TTY: 301-296-5650
Phone: 301-296-5700
Fax: 301-296-8580
Website: http://www.asha.org
E-mail: actioncenter@asha.org

American Stroke Association
7272 Greenville Ave.
Dallas, TX 75231
Toll-Free: 888-478-7653
Website: http://www.strokeassociation.org

Glaucoma Research Foundation
251 Post St.
Ste. 600
San Francisco, CA 94108
Toll-Free: 800-826-6693
Phone: 415-986-3162
Fax: 415-986-3763
Website: http://www.glaucoma.org
E-mail: grf@glaucoma.org

725

Health Physics Society
1313 Dolley Madison Blvd.
Ste. 402
McLean, VA 22101
Phone: 703-790-1745
Fax: 703-790-2672
Website: http://www.hps.org
E-mail: HPS@BurkInc.com

Healthline
Healthline Networks, Inc.
660 Third St.
San Francisco, CA 94107
Phone: 415-281-3100
Website: http://www.healthline
.com

International Foundation for Functional Gastrointestinal Disorders
P.O. Box 170864
Milwaukee, WI 53217
Toll-Free: 888-964-2001
Phone: 414-964-1799
Fax: 414-964-7176
Website: http://www.iffgd.org
E-mail: iffgd@iffgd.org

The Joint Commission
One Renaissance Blvd.
Oakbrook Terrace, IL 60181
Phone: 630-792-5000
Fax: 630-792-5000
Website: http://www.
jointcommission.org

Juvenile Diabetes Research Foundation International
26 Broadway
14th Fl.
New York, NY 10004
Toll-Free: 800-533-CURE (2873)
Fax: 212-785-9595
Website: http://www.jdrf.org
E-mail: info@jdrf.org

March of Dimes
1275 Mamaroneck Ave.
White Plains, NY 10605
Phone: 914-997-4488
Website: http://www.
marchofdimes.com
E-mail: askus@marchofdimes.
com

MedicineNet.com
Website: http://www.
medicinenet.com

Mental Health America
2000 N. Beauregard St.
6th Fl.
Alexandria, VA 22311
Toll-Free: 800-969-6642
Phone: 703-684-7722
Fax: 703-684-5968
Website: http://www.
mentalhealthamerica.net

National Kidney Foundation
30 East 33rd St.
New York, NY 10016
Toll-Free: 800-622-9010
Phone: 212-889-2210
Website: http://www.kidney.org

National Newborn Screening and Genetics Resource Center
1912 W. Anderson Ln., Ste. 210
Austin, TX 78757
Phone: 512-454-6419
Fax: 512-454-6509
Website: http://genes-r-us
.uthscsa.edu

National Sleep Foundation
1010 N. Glebe Rd., Ste. 310
Arlington, VA 22201
Phone: 703-243-1697
Website: http://www.
sleepfoundation.org
E-mail: nsf@sleepfoundation.org

National Stroke Association
9707 E. Easter Ln., Ste. B
Centennial, CO 80112
Toll-Free: 800-STROKES
(787-6537)
Fax: 303-649-1328
Website: http://www.stroke.org
E-mail: info@stroke.org

Nemours Foundation
1600 Rockland Rd.
Wilmington, DE 19803
Phone: 302-651-4000
Website: http://www.kidshealth .org
E-mail: info@kidshealth.org

Radiological Society of North America (RSNA)
820 Jorie Blvd.
Oak Brook, IL 60523
Toll-Free: 800-381-6660
Phone: 630-571-2670
Fax: 630-571-7837
Website: http://www.rsna.org
E-mail: webmaster@rsna.org

RESOLVE
The National Infertility
Association
1760 Old Meadow Rd., Ste. 500
McLean, VA 22102
Phone: 703-556-7172
Fax: 703-506-3266
Website: http://www.resolve.org
E-mail: info@resolve.org

Society of American Gastrointestinal Endoscopic Surgeons (SAGES)
11300 W. Olympic Blvd., Ste. 600
Los Angeles, CA 90064
Phone: 310-437-0544
Fax: 310-437-0585
Website: http://www.sages.org
E-mail: sagesweb@sages.org

Susan G. Komen for the Cure
5005 LBJ Fwy.
Ste. 250
Dallas, TX 75244
Toll-Free: 877-465-6636
Website: http://www.komen.org

University of Maryland Medical Center
22 S. Greene St.
Baltimore, MD 21201
Toll-Free: 800-492-5538
Toll-Free TDD: 800-735-2258
Physician Referral:
800-373-4111
Physician Referral:
800-373-4111
Phone: 410-328-8667
Website: http://www.umm.edu

WebMD
Website: http://www.webmd.com

Index

Index

Page numbers followed by 'n' indicate a footnote. Page numbers in italics indicate a table or illustration.

A

AAFP *see* American Academy of Family Physicians
abnormal lipid levels, electrocardiography 109
abdominal aortic aneurysm, screening 162
abdominal ultrasound, ultrasound imaging 292
actigraphy, described 607
acanthosis nigricans, insulin resistance 552
addictions, online screening tools 703
adenocarcinoma
 defined 469
 esophageal cancer 477
adolescents
 cholesterol 656
 obesity 73
 sleep apnea 85
adrenal glands, neuroblastoma 505
Agatston score, coronary calcium scan 342

Agency for Healthcare Research and Quality (AHRQ)
 contact 721
 publications
  hepatitis test 580n
  medical tests 23n
  questions about medical tests 31n
  recommended screening 116n
AHRQ *see* Agency for Healthcare Research and Quality
Alabama, breast and cervical cancer early detection program 711
Alaska, breast and cervical cancer early detection program 711
alcoholism, dietary guidelines 25
alpha-fetoprotein, tumor markers 483
alpha-1 antitrypsin deficiency, chronic obstructive pulmonary disease 103
Alzheimer's disease, preventive care 167
amblyopia, children 88
amebiasis, antigen detection 243
American Academy of Allergy, Asthma and Immunology, contact 724
American Academy of Family Physicians (AAFP), contact 724
American Academy of Pediatrics, contact 724
American Association of Neurological Surgeons, contact 724